Hospital Medicine and Clinical Education

Editors

NANCY D. SPECTOR
AMY J. STARMER

PEDIATRIC CLINICS OF NORTH AMERICA

www.pediatric.theclinics.com

Consulting Editor
BONITA F. STANTON

August 2019 • Volume 66 • Number 4

ELSEVIER

1600 John F. Kennedy Boulevard • Suite 1800 • Philadelphia, Pennsylvania, 19103-2899

http://www.theclinics.com

THE PEDIATRIC CLINICS OF NORTH AMERICA Volume 66, Number 4
August 2019 ISSN 0031-3955, ISBN-13: 978-0-323-68233-6

Editor: Kerry Holland
Developmental Editor: Casey Potter

The Pediatric Clinics of North America (ISSN 0031-3955) is published bimonthly by Elsevier Inc., 360 Park Avenue South, New York, NY 10010-1710. Months of issue are February, April, June, August, October, and December. Periodicals postage paid at New York, NY and additional mailing offices. Subscription prices are $229.00 per year (US individuals), $653.00 per year (US institutions), $315.00 per year (Canadian individuals), $868.00 per year (Canadian institutions), $345.00 per year (international individuals), $868.00 per year (international institutions), $100.00 per year (US students and residents), and $165.00 per year (international and Canadian residents and students). To receive students/resident rare, orders must be accompanied by name of affiliated institution, date of term, and the signature of program/residency coordinator on institution letterhead. Orders will be billed at individual rate until proof of status is received. Foreign air speed delivery is included in all *Clinics* subscription prices. All prices are subject to change without notice. **POSTMASTER:** Send address changes to *The Pediatric Clinics of North America*, Elsevier Health Sciences Division, Subscription Customer Service, 3251 Riverport Lane, Maryland Heights, MO 63043. **Customer Service: 1-800-654-2452 (US and Canada). From outside of the US and Canada: 1-314-447-8871. Fax: 1-314-447-8029. For print support, E-mail: JournalsCustomerService-usa@elsevier.com**. **For online support, E-mail: JournalsOnlineSupport-usa@elsevier.com**.

Reprints. For copies of 100 or more, of articles in this publication, please contact the Commercial Reprints Department, Elsevier Inc., 360 Park Avenue South, New York, NY 10010-1710. Tel.: 212-633-3874; Fax: 212-633-3820; E-mail: reprints@elsevier.com.

The Pediatric Clinics of North America is also published in Spanish by McGraw-Hill Inter-americana Editores S.A., Mexico City, Mexico; in Portuguese by Riechmann and Affonso Editores, Rua Comandante Coelho 1085, CEP 21250, Rio de Janeiro, Brazil; and in Greek by Althayia SA, Athens, Greece.

The Pediatric Clinics of North America is covered in *MEDLINE/PubMed (Index Medicus), Excerpta Medica, Current Contents, Current Contents/Clinical Medicine, Science Citation Index, ASCA, ISI/BIOMED*, and *BIOSIS*.

Printed in the United States of America.

PROGRAM OBJECTIVE

The goal of the *Pediatric Clinics of North America* is to keep practicing physicians and residents up to date with current clinical practice in pediatrics by providing timely articles reviewing the state-of-the-art in patient care.

TARGET AUDIENCE

All practicing pediatricians, physicians and healthcare professionals who provide patient care to pediatric patients.

LEARNING OBJECTIVES

Upon completion of this activity, participants will be able to:

1. Review patient- and family-centered care strategies for promoting coproduction in pediatric hospital medicine.
2. Discuss the selection, development, and use of process and outcome measures for pediatric hospital medicine quality improvement initiatives.
3. Recognize current challenges and growth opportunities of interprofessional practice in pediatric hospital medicine.

ACCREDITATIONS

Physician Credit

The Elsevier Office of Continuing Medical Education (EOCME) is accredited by the Accreditation Council for Continuing Medical Education (ACCME) to provide continuing medical education for physicians.

The EOCME designates this journal-based activity for a maximum of 14 *AMA PRA Category 1 Credit*(s)™. Physicians should claim only the credit commensurate with the extent of their participation in the activity.

All other healthcare professionals requesting continuing education credit for this this journal-based activity will be issued a certificate of participation.

ABP Maintenance of Certification Credit

Successful completion of this CME activity, which includes participation in the activity and individual assessment of and feedback to the learner, enables the learner to earn up to 14 MOC points in the American Board of Pediatrics' (ABP) Maintenance of Certification (MOC) program. It is the CME activity provider's responsibility to submit learner completion information to ACCME for the purpose of granting ABP MOC credit.

DISCLOSURE OF CONFLICTS OF INTEREST

The EOCME assesses conflict of interest with its instructors, faculty, planners, and other individuals who are in a position to control the content of CME activities. All relevant conflicts of interest that are identified are thoroughly vetted by EOCME for fair balance, scientific objectivity, and patient care recommendations. EOCME is committed to providing its learners with CME activities that promote improvements or quality in healthcare and not a specific proprietary business or a commercial interest.

The planning committee, staff, authors and editors listed below have identified no financial relationships or relationships to products or devices they or their spouse/life partner have with commercial interest related to the content of this CME activity:

Wilma Alvarado-Little, MA, MSW; Michele Ashland, BA; Jennifer Baird, PhD, MPH, MSW, RN; Rebecca Blankenburg, MD, MPH; Cindy Brach, MPP; Sharon Calaman, MD; Arti D. Desai, MD, MSPH; Lauren A. Destino, MD; Benard P. Dreyer, MD; Jennifer L. Everhart, MD; Alexander F. Glick, MD, MS; Brian Good, MB BCh, BAO; Helen Haskell, MA; Duncan Henry, MD; Jennifer H. Hepps, MD; Kerry Holland; Alison Kemp; Hans B. Kersten, MD; Alisa Khan, MD, MPH; Irene Kocolas, MD, MS; Nicholas Kuzma, MD; Christopher P. Landrigan, MD, MPH; Christy J.W. Ledford, PhD; Kheyandra D. Lewis, MD; Joseph O. Lopreiato, MD, MPH, FAAP, CHSE; Rajkumar Mayakrishnan; Jennifer K. O'Toole, MD, MEd; Shilpa J. Patel, MD; Aarti Patel, MD, MEd; Matthew W. Ramotar, BA; Glenn Rosenbluth, MD; Theodore C. Sectish, MD; Samir S. Shah, MD, MSCE; Nancy D. Spector, MD; Raj Srivastava, MD, MPH; Bonita F. Stanton, MD; Amy J. Starmer, MD, MPH; Anupama Subramony, MD, MBA; Eric Douglas Thompson, MD, MMM; Daniel C. West, MD; Hsiang Shonna Yin, MD, MS; Clifton E. Yu, MD.

The planning committee, staff, authors and editors listed below have identified financial relationships or relationships to products or devices they or their spouse/life partner have with commercial interest related to the content of this CME activity:

Thuy L. Ngo, DO, MEd: is a consultant/advisor for Welch Allyn.

UNAPPROVED/OFF-LABEL USE DISCLOSURE

The EOCME requires CME faculty to disclose to the participants:

1. When products or procedures being discussed are off-label, unlabelled, experimental, and/or investigational (not US Food and Drug Administration [FDA] approved); and
2. Any limitations on the information presented, such as data that are preliminary or that represent ongoing research, interim analyses, and/or unsupported opinions. Faculty may discuss information about pharmaceutical agents that is outside of FDA-approved labelling. This information is intended solely for CME and is not intended to promote off-label use of these medications. If you have any questions, contact the medical affairs department of the manufacturer for the most recent prescribing information.

TO ENROLL

To enroll in the *Pediatric Clinics of North America* Continuing Medical Education program, call customer service at 1-800-654-2452 or sign up online at http://www.theclinics.com/home/cme. The CME program is available to subscribers for an additional annual fee of USD 301.60.

METHOD OF PARTICIPATION

In order to claim credit, participants must complete the following:

1. Complete enrolment as indicated above.
2. Read the activity.
3. Complete the CME Test and Evaluation. Participants must achieve a score of 70% on the test. All CME Tests and Evaluations must be completed online.

In order to claim MOC points, participants must complete the following:

1. Complete steps listed above for claiming CME credit.
2. Provide ABP specialty board ID#, birth date (MM/DD), and attestation.
3. Online MOC submission is only available for the American Board of pediatrics' (ABP) Maintenance of Certification (MOC) program. Find ABP ID# on the ABP website at https://www.abp.org/content/verification-certification.

CME INQUIRIES/SPECIAL NEEDS

For all CME inquiries or special needs, please contact elsevierCME@elsevier.com

Contributors

CONSULTING EDITOR

BONITA F. STANTON, MD
Founding Dean, Hackensack Meridian School of Medicine at Seton Hall University, President, Academic Enterprise, Hackensack Meridian Health Robert C. and Laura C. Garrett Endowed Chair for the School of Medicine, Professor of Pediatrics, Nutley, New Jersey

EDITORS

NANCY D. SPECTOR, MD
Professor of Pediatrics, Executive Director, Executive Leadership in Academic Medicine, Associate Dean of Faculty Development, Drexel University College of Medicine, Philadelphia, Pennsylvania

AMY J. STARMER, MD, MPH
Assistant Professor of Pediatrics, Associate Medical Director of Quality, Department of Pediatrics, Boston Children's Hospital, Harvard Medical School, Boston, Massachusetts

AUTHORS

WILMA ALVARADO-LITTLE, MA, MSW
Associate Commissioner, New York State Department of Health, Director, Office of Minority Health and Health Disparities Prevention, Albany, New York

MICHELE ASHLAND, BA
Family Advisor, Lucile Packard Children's Hospital Stanford, Palo Alto, California

JENNIFER BAIRD, PhD, MPH, MSW, RN
Director, Institute for Nursing and Interprofessional Research, Children's Hospital Los Angeles, Los Angeles, California

REBECCA BLANKENBURG, MD, MPH
Clinical Associate Professor, Pediatric Hospital Medicine, Associate Chair of Education, Stanford School of Medicine, Palo Alto, California

CINDY BRACH, MPP
Center for Evidence and Practice Improvement, Agency for Healthcare Research and Quality, Rockville, Maryland

SHARON CALAMAN, MD
Pediatric Residency Program Director, Simulation Center Director, St. Christopher's Hospital for Children, Professor of Pediatrics, Drexel University College of Medicine, Philadelphia, Pennsylvania

ARTI D. DESAI, MD, MSPH
Assistant Professor of Pediatrics, University of Washington, Seattle Children's Research Institute, Seattle, Washington

LAUREN A. DESTINO, MD
Clinical Associate Professor, Stanford University, Lucile Packard Children's Hospital Stanford, Palo Alto, California

BENARD P. DREYER, MD
Professor of Pediatrics, NYU School of Medicine, NYU Langone Health, Bellevue Hospital Center, New York, New York

JENNIFER L. EVERHART, MD
Clinical Associate Professor, Department of Pediatrics, Division of Pediatric Hospital Medicine, Stanford University School of Medicine, Pediatric Hospitalist, Lucile Packard Children's Hospital Stanford, Stanford, California

ALEXANDER F. GLICK, MD, MS
Assistant Professor, Department of Pediatrics, NYU School of Medicine, NYU Langone Health, Bellevue Hospital Center, New York, New York

BRIAN GOOD, MB BCh, BAO
Associate Professor, University of Utah, Primary Children's Hospital, Salt Lake City, Utah

HELEN HASKELL, MA
President, Mothers Against Medical Error, Columbia, South Carolina

DUNCAN HENRY, MD
Assistant Professor, Department of Pediatrics, University of California, San Francisco, San Francisco, California

JENNIFER H. HEPPS, MD
Transitional Internship Program Director, Associate Professor, Department of Pediatrics, Walter Reed National Military Medical Center, Uniformed Services University of the Health Sciences, Bethesda, Maryland

HANS B. KERSTEN, MD
Professor, Department of Pediatrics, Drexel University College of Medicine, St. Christopher's Hospital for Children, Philadelphia, Pennsylvania

ALISA KHAN, MD, MPH
Instructor, Department of Pediatrics, Harvard Medical School, Staff Physician, Division of General Pediatrics, Boston Children's Hospital, Boston, Massachusetts

IRENE KOCOLAS, MD, MS
Assistant Professor, Division of Inpatient Medicine, Department of Pediatrics, University of Utah School of Medicine/Primary Children's Hospital, Intermountain Healthcare, Salt Lake City, Utah

NICHOLAS KUZMA, MD
Assistant Professor, Department of Pediatrics, Drexel University College of Medicine, St. Christopher's Hospital for Children, Philadelphia, Pennsylvania

CHRISTOPHER P. LANDRIGAN, MD, MPH
Professor of Pediatrics, Boston Children's Hospital, Brigham & Women's Hospital, Harvard Medical School, Boston, Massachusetts

CHRISTY J.W. LEDFORD, PhD
Associate Professor, Department of Family Medicine, Uniformed Services University, Bethesda, Maryland

KHEYANDRA D. LEWIS, MD
Assistant Professor of Pediatrics, Section of Hospital Medicine, St. Christopher's Hospital for Children, Drexel University College of Medicine, Philadelphia, Pennsylvania

JOSEPH O. LOPREIATO, MD, MPH, FAAP, CHSE
Professor of Pediatrics, Medicine and Nursing, Uniformed Services University of the Health Sciences, Bethesda, Maryland

THUY L. NGO, DO, MEd
Assistant Professor, Pediatric Emergency Medicine, Associate Program Director, Pediatric Emergency Medicine Fellowship, Johns Hopkins School of Medicine, Baltimore, Maryland

JENNIFER K. O'TOOLE, MD, MEd
Associate Professor of Pediatrics and Internal Medicine, Pediatrics, Program Director of the Internal Medicine-Pediatrics Residency Program, Departments of Pediatrics and Internal Medicine, Cincinnati Children's Hospital Medical Center, University of Cincinnati College of Medicine, Cincinnati, Ohio

AARTI PATEL, MD, MEd
Assistant Clinical Professor of Pediatrics, Division of Pediatric Hospital Medicine, Rady Children's Hospital, University of California, San Diego, San Diego, California

SHILPA J. PATEL, MD
Associate Professor of Pediatrics, John A. Burns School of Medicine, Pediatric Hospitalist, Kapi'olani Medical Center for Women & Children, Physician Liaison for Quality & Safety, Hawaii Pacific Health, Honolulu, Hawaii

MATTHEW W. RAMOTAR, BA
Research Specialist, I-PASS Study Group, Division of General Pediatrics, Department of Medicine, Boston Children's Hospital, Boston, Massachusetts

GLENN ROSENBLUTH, MD
Clinical Professor of Pediatrics, Director of Quality and Safety Programs, Office of Graduate Medical Education, Associate Director, Pediatrics Residency Training Program, Department of Pediatrics, University of California, San Francisco, San Francisco, California

THEODORE C. SECTISH, MD
Vice Chair for Education, Program Director, Boston Combined Residency Program, Division of General Pediatrics, Department of Medicine, Boston Children's Hospital, Professor of Pediatrics, Harvard Medical School, Boston, Massachusetts

SAMIR S. SHAH, MD, MSCE
Professor, Cincinnati Children's Hospital Medical Center, University of Cincinnati College of Medicine, Cincinnati, Ohio

RAJ SRIVASTAVA, MD, MPH
Professor, Division of Inpatient Medicine, Department of Pediatrics, University of Utah School of Medicine/Primary Children's Hospital, Assistant Vice-President, Healthcare Delivery Institute, Intermountain Healthcare, Murray, Utah

AMY J. STARMER, MD, MPH
Assistant Professor of Pediatrics, Associate Medical Director of Quality, Department of Pediatrics, Boston Children's Hospital, Harvard Medical School, Boston, Massachusetts

ANUPAMA SUBRAMONY, MD, MBA
Assistant Professor, Department of Pediatrics, Cohen Children's Medical Center, Donald and Barbara Zucker School of Medicine at Hofstra/Northwell, New Hyde Park, New York

ERIC DOUGLAS THOMPSON, MD, MMM
Associate Professor, Department of Pediatrics, Drexel University College of Medicine, St. Christopher's Hospital for Children, Philadelphia, Pennsylvania

DANIEL C. WEST, MD
Professor, Department of Pediatrics, University of California, San Francisco, San Francisco, California

HSIANG SHONNA YIN, MD, MS
Associate Professor of Pediatrics, NYU School of Medicine, NYU Langone Health, Bellevue Hospital Center, New York, New York

CLIFTON E. YU, MD
Deputy Director for Education, Training, and Research, Professor, Department of Pediatrics, Walter Reed National Military Medical Center, Uniformed Services University of the Health Sciences, Bethesda, Maryland

Contents

Foreword: How Did We Ever Do Without Them? xv

Bonita F. Stanton

Preface: An Evolving Clinical Setting for Education: Pediatric Hospital Medicine xix

Nancy D. Spector, Matthew W. Ramotar, and Amy J. Starmer

Section 1: Hospital-Based Practice

Pediatric Hospitalists Improving Patient Care Through Quality Improvement 697

Anupama Subramony, Irene Kocolas, and Raj Srivastava

This article reviews the industrial underpinnings of the quality improvement (QI) movement and describes how QI became integrated within the larger health care landscape, including hospital medicine. QI methodologies and a framework for using them are described. Key components that make up a successful QI clinical project are outlined, with a focus on the essential role of pediatric hospitalists and practical professional tips to be successful. QI training opportunities are reviewed with opportunities for hospitalists to get involved in QI on a national level. National QI networks are showcased, with multiple examples of advanced improvement projects that have significantly improved patient outcomes highlighted.

Evidence-Based Medicine in the Clinical Learning Environment of Pediatric Hospital Medicine 713

Nicholas Kuzma, Hans B. Kersten, and Eric Douglas Thompson

The article begins with an overview of evidence-based medicine (EBM), including its history and core principles. Next, the article discusses how the current clinical learning environment has shaped EBM, including the accessibility and portability of technology; the access to electronic search engines and libraries; and the movement toward applying the best evidence through order sets, clinical guidelines, and pathways to work toward standardizing care. The article ends with a focus on how educators can influence a trainee's knowledge, skills, attitudes, and behaviors regarding EBM.

Process Metrics and Outcomes to Inform Quality Improvement in Pediatric Hospital Medicine 725

Arti D. Desai and Amy J. Starmer

This article provides an overview of the selection, development, and use of process and outcome measures for pediatric hospital medicine quality improvement initiatives. It reviews commonly used categories of process and outcome measures and provides a list of common sources and repositories of previously validated measures. It also provides a blueprint for the development of novel measures. The relative merits of various data collection methods are discussed (eg, medical record abstraction, administrative,

surveys), along with guiding principles for disseminating the results of quality improvement evaluations on a local and national level.

Interprofessional Teams: Current Trends and Future Directions 739

Jennifer Baird, Michele Ashland, and Glenn Rosenbluth

This article addresses the current and desired future state of interprofessional practice in pediatric hospital medicine. It focuses on identifying optimal team composition and work patterns, describing the value of parent involvement on both the patient's care team and on operational teams, describing the need for interprofessional education, and identifying outcomes associated with interprofessional teamwork. The article also identifies challenges and opportunities for growth as interprofessional teamwork increasingly becomes a standard practice within healthcare settings.

Communication at Transitions of Care 751

Shilpa J. Patel and Christopher P. Landrigan

Communication errors during transitions of care are a leading source of adverse events for hospitalized patients. This article provides an overview of the role of communication errors in adverse events, describes the complexities of communication for hospitalized patients, and provides evidence regarding the positive effects of applying high-reliability principles to transitions of care and culture of safety. Elements of effective handoffs and a detailed approach for successful implementation of a handoff program are provided. The role of handoff communication in medical education at all levels, as well as for the interprofessional team, is discussed.

Section 2: Patient Centered Care

Patient- and Family-Centered Care: Leveraging Best Practices to Improve the Care of Hospitalized Children 775

Jennifer L. Everhart, Helen Haskell, and Alisa Khan

This article aims to broaden pediatric hospital medicine providers' understanding of patient- and family-centered care (PFCC) and equip them to both implement and advance PFCC. The article discusses the origins and history of PFCC and reviews selected relevant literature. The article shares an overview of several existing frameworks for patient-centeredness, emphasizing an emerging concept called coproduction. The article reviews several attitudes, skills, and infrastructure components that are considered essential prerequisites for effective coproduction. The article then highlights several strategies for promoting coproduction in Hospital Medicine, organized around 4 key tenets of coproduction (cocommissioning, codesign, codelivery, and coassessment).

Communication with Diverse Patients: Addressing Culture and Language 791

Jennifer K. O'Toole, Wilma Alvarado-Little, and Christy J.W. Ledford

Effective communication is key when providing quality health care. The dynamics of communication within the health care team and with the patient and family can be challenging. These challenges stem from the sharing of complex information, highly emotional topics, and health literacy barriers.

Linguistic and cultural barriers can further aggravate these challenges. This section provides an overview of linguistic and cultural challenges related to patient-provider communication, strategies for effective communication with patients with limited English Proficiency via the use of interpreter services, and tips for how to teach these skills to health care providers.

Health Literacy in the Inpatient Setting: Implications for Patient Care and Patient Safety **805**

Alexander F. Glick, Cindy Brach, Hsiang Shonna Yin, and Benard P. Dreyer

Health literacy plays a role in the events leading up to children's hospitalizations, during hospital admission, and after discharge. Hospitals and providers should use a universal precautions approach and routinely incorporate health-literacy-informed strategies in communicating with all patients and families to ensure that they can understand health information, follow medical instructions, participate actively in their own/their child's care, and successfully navigate the health care system. Interventions that incorporate health-literacy-informed strategies and that target patients/families and health care systems should be implemented to improve patient outcomes and patient-centered and family-centered care.

Family-Centered Rounds: Past, Present, and Future **827**

Lauren A. Destino, Samir S. Shah, and Brian Good

Bedside rounds have evolved concurrently with hospitalist medicine and patient-centered care. Family-centered rounds are the foundation of effective communication in the in-patient pediatric setting. Participant perspectives (family members, patients, nurses, faculty, and trainees) on family-centered rounds differ and goals may not always align. Further, the practical components of how rounds are conducted varies and have continued opportunities for improvement. This article summarizes the most recent experience with rounds in an attempt to identify unified and effective strategies moving forward.

Section 3: Education in the Inpatient Setting

The Clinical Learning Environment and Workplace-Based Assessment: Frameworks, Strategies, and Implementation **839**

Duncan Henry and Daniel C. West

This article provides an overview of the role played by the clinical learning environment in providing opportunities for assessment of trainee performance and how those assessments can guide learning. It reviews the importance of competency models as frameworks to facilitate the creation of a shared mental model of what is to be learned between learners and supervisors. In addition, it discusses how assessment can be used to drive mastery learning as well as the components necessary for a program of assessment.

Simulation in Medical Education for the Hospitalist: Moving Beyond the Mock Code **855**

Jennifer H. Hepps, Clifton E. Yu, and Sharon Calaman

Simulation in medical education has grown due to an evolution in health care. It uses 4 main modalities to re-create a situation from the clinical

environment to allow experiential learning and improve patient care. Simulation must be considered as an educational strategy within a larger curriculum. Building an exercise requires first developing goals and objectives and then designing the scenario. There are 4 phases of implementation, wherein the final debrief phase is critical for learning. Educators have used simulation for multiple curricular needs: communication skills, interprofessional education, clinical reasoning, procedural training, and patient safety, which apply to the inpatient setting.

A Focus on Feedback: Improving Learner Engagement and Faculty Delivery of Feedback in Hospital Medicine **867**

Kheyandra D. Lewis, Aarti Patel, and Joseph O. Lopreiato

Feedback is an integral part of medical education. However, there is great variation of training and effectiveness of feedback delivery, especially in the inpatient setting. The unique learning environment provided in hospital medicine allows teachers the opportunity to provide feedback on learner performance under several longitudinal observations in areas such as direct patient care, procedural tasks, and interdisciplinary team leadership skills. Most important, feedback should occur on more than one occasion to truly empower change in knowledge, attitude, and skills. This article aims to provide the reader with foundational theories on feedback and strategies to use best practices for delivery.

Teaching at the Bedside: Strategies for Optimizing Education on Patient and Family Centered Rounds **881**

Thuy L. Ngo, Rebecca Blankenburg, and Clifton E. Yu

Resident and attending concern about the potential for decreased teaching has been cited as one of the drawbacks to the adoption of family-centered rounds (FCR). Despite these concerns, FCR can enhance clinical education through direct exposure to multiple patients by all team members, as well as by allowing faculty to teach, model, observe, and assess learners' clinical skills more effectively than in nonbedside settings. This article provides many strategies and approaches to bedside teaching designed to enhance education and communication among care team members as well as patients and their families.

Pediatric Hospital Medicine: Where We Are, Where We Are Headed: State of the Specialty, Looking Forward **891**

Matthew W. Ramotar and Theodore C. Sectish

Although pediatric hospital medicine (PHM) is in its adolescence, it is already having a major impact on patient care, quality, safety, and education. Pediatric hospitalists have been front-and-center in the safety and quality movement, driving change as clinicians, applying evidence-based medicine to standardize practice and promulgate evidence-based guidelines, and playing a central role in optimizing the function of interprofessional teams. Pediatric hospitalists have championed the importance of patient-and family-centeredness of care and the need to incorporate principles of health literacy into all aspects of clinical care and research. Beyond delivering care, pediatric hospitalists have prominent

roles as hospital leaders, educators, and researchers and have played a critical role in promoting improvements in health and health care outcomes. In its continued evolution, clinical care will undoubtedly remain the major focus, though with subspecialty status, the field will be expected to accelerate innovations in systems-based practice, advance clinical learning environments, and drive further improvements in quality of care.

Hospital Medicine and Clinical Education

PEDIATRIC CLINICS OF NORTH AMERICA

FORTHCOMING ISSUES

October 2019
Pediatric Immunology and Allergy
Elizabeth Secord, *Editor*

December 2019
Substance Abuse
David R. Rosenberg and Leslie H. Lundahl, *Editors*

February 2020
Pediatric Orthopedics
Paul T. Haynes, *Editor*

RECENT ISSUES

February 2019
Clinical Disorders of the Kidney
James C. Chan, *Editor*

June 2018
International Migration: Caring for Children and Families
Stephen Ludwig, Andrew P. Steenhoff, and Julie M. Linton, *Editors*

April 2018
Current Advances in Neonatal Care
Beena G. Sood and Dara D. Brodsky, *Editors*

Foreword
How Did We Ever Do Without Them?

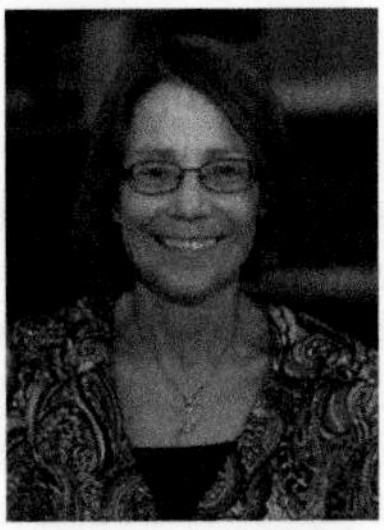

Bonita F. Stanton, MD
Consulting Editor

Now a central component of most departments of pediatrics, the emergence of the unique role of the "hospitalist" dates back less than 40 years. It is difficult to imagine a hospital without hospitalists now given their central role in patient care throughout the nation. Likewise, it is difficult to imagine a department of pediatrics without hospitalists, given their roles in teaching.

A confluence of changes at the end of the twentieth century in the manner in which physicians in the United States were practicing in-hospital care, charging for in-patient care, and teaching in-patient care served as the background for this "new" form of pediatrician. The roles demanded from these changes were not under the purview of any other pediatric subspecialty but required focus and specific skills. The changes reflected a range of issues occurring in the field of medicine, including significant philosophical, organizational, and financial concerns.

Included among these significant changes were important rethinking about residency training and whether it was reflecting the humanism central to our profession and whether it was serving its primary purpose, educating tomorrow's physicians, rather than providing inexpensive labor. Practice realities were also changing as many community-based physicians who admitted their patients into the hospital found it increasingly difficult to meet the growing expectations associated with being the responsible attending. While it is beyond the scope of this preface to discuss all of the changes that were occurring, I will give 2 examples.

Up until the 1980s, resident duty hours were not uniformly restricted; there were great variations by specialty and by residency program. The overall "role" of residents was called into question in the years leading up to 1988 when the Accreditation Council for Graduate Medical Education began to impose restrictions, beginning with the "80-hour work week." Over the next several years, additional recommendations

Pediatr Clin N Am 66 (2019) xv–xvii
https://doi.org/10.1016/j.pcl.2019.05.002

and restrictions were imposed as increasing scrutiny was brought to the topic of resident fatigue and impaired performance by several different professional groups, including the Institute of Medicine.[1] With the restrictions imposed on resident time in the hospital (as well as the establishment of required "rest time" during overnight shifts after a certain number of hours), the resident workforce was not large enough in most hospitals to fully cover patient care. A new workforce for in-hospital care was needed to replace the new loss of time committed to patient care that had existed prior to the institution of "duty hours."

OBSERVATION VERSUS IN-PATIENT ADMISSIONS

Over the last few decades of the twentieth century and the first decade of the current century for both pragmatic reasons and financial reasons, the practice of either discharging a patient from the emergency department or admitting them to the hospital began to be called into question. Emergency departments had been witnessing very long wait periods both to "see a physician" and to reach a clinical disposition plan. This reality resulted from growing volumes of emergency department patients due to a shortage of available beds on the floors, the availability of an increasing array of studies that could be done for an individual patient to inform the decision regarding disposition, legal considerations, concerns regarding the insurance status of the individual and, in some cases, a policy of reserving a certain number of beds for patients with particular diagnoses or needs. In this context, the concept of the "observation bed" or "24-hour admission" arose. At the same time, the financial institutions (Medicare, Medicaid, private insurance) had begun to scrutinize and redefine the criteria for "admissions." These and other realities led to the now widespread practice of "observation status."[2,3] Hospitals vary in their allocation of beds for "observation," with some distributing these patients among "available beds" throughout the hospital, while others use specific "Observation Units." In either case, hospitals are realizing the benefits of placing the care of these patients under physicians with experience in the many demands of an observation patient, including the need for rapid diagnosis and treatment, capacity to simultaneously develop a hospital-treatment plan and a discharge plan, including the necessary medications and outpatients treatments, attend to the billing and insurer needs, and possess and execute the ability to develop an empathetic relationship with the patient and his/her family in a compressed timeframe.

These are but 2 examples of the many "needs" that arose during this time period for which a specific, trained physician group did not exist. For several years, various ad hoc arrangements were made to address the limitations in the workforce with the reduced hours with existing attendings, part-time physicians, and similar, and the observation beds were covered by the general ward attendings or the emergency department staff. Over time it became clear that the physicians filling these roles required special skills and training and that their services would be necessary "around the clock." To meet these and many other needs, several fields, including pediatrics, saw the advent of the hospitalist. Originally an informal category, typically made up of general pediatricians, the Pediatric Hospitalist was approved as a subspecialty in 2015 by the American Board of Pediatrics and in 2016 by the American Board of Medical Specialties.[4]

This now vibrant subspecialty in the field of pediatrics plays a critical role in patient care, clinical administration, and student and resident education. So critical is the cadre of pediatric hospitals to the functioning of our children's hospitals and departments, I can only wonder how we ever "did without them." Under the leadership of

Nancy D. Spector, MD and Amy J. Starmer, MD, MPH, this issue contains contributions from among the finest Pediatric Hospitalists in the United States.

Bonita F. Stanton, MD
Hackensack Meridian School of Medicine at Seton Hall University
Academic Enterprise
340 Kingsland Street, Building 123
Nutley, NJ 07110, USA

E-mail address:
bonita.stanton@shu.edu

REFERENCES

1. ACGME. History of duty hours. Available at: https://www.acgme.org/What-We-Do/Accreditation/Clinical-Experience-and-Education-formerly-Duty-Hours/History-of-Duty-Hours. Accessed May 2, 2019.
2. American Medical Association. Payment and coverage for hospital admissions: inpatient versus observation care. Available at: https://www.ama-assn.org/sites/ama-assn.org/files/corp/media-browser/public/about-ama/councils/Council%20Reports/council-on-medical-service/issue-brief-inpatient-v-observation-care.pdf. Accessed May 2, 2019.
3. Macy ML, Hall M, Shah SS, et al. Pediatric observation status: are we overlooking a growing population in children's hospitals? J Hosp Med 2012;7(7):530–6.
4. American Board of Pediatrics. ABMS approves hospital medicine certification. Available at: https://www.abp.org/news/abms-approves-pediatric-hospital-medicine-certification. Accessed May 2, 2019.

Preface

An Evolving Clinical Setting for Education: Pediatric Hospital Medicine

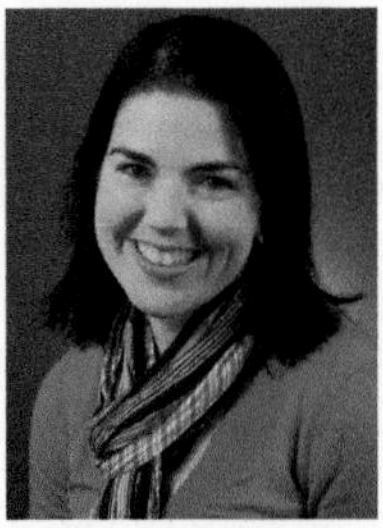

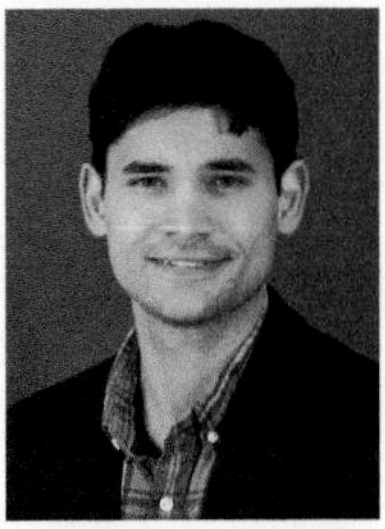

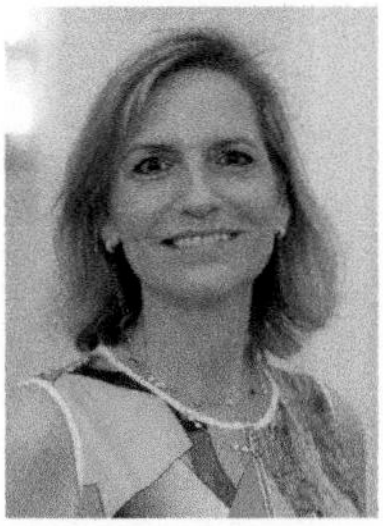

Amy J. Starmer, MD, MPH, *Editor*

Matthew W. Ramotar, BA, *Editorial Assistant*

Nancy D. Spector, MD, *Editor*

This issue of the *Pediatric Clinics of North America* focuses on the rapidly evolving field of Pediatric Hospital Medicine (PHM). Although the articles within this issue broadly address the ways in which pediatric hospitalists and their colleagues have advanced child health in the inpatient setting, each article also specifically focuses on the way in which the role of education and training has also rapidly adapted and progressed within this changing landscape.

Five years have passed since Mary Ottolini and colleagues devoted an issue of *Pediatric Clinics of North America* to the specialty of PHM,[1] and more than a decade has passed since Drs Robert Wachter and Lee Goldman coined the term **hospitalist** in their *New England Journal of Medicine* article in 1996.[2] Hospital Medicine is now the fastest growing medical specialty in the United States due in part to the evolution of inpatient care. As evidence of this growth, while the original meeting of the professional society of PHM in 2003 had just 136 attendees, by 2018 the attendance had increased nearly 10-fold with an attendance just under 1250 individuals.

In 2015, the American Board of Pediatrics and the American Board of Medical Specialties approved PHM as an official subspecialty. It was noted that as a new subspecialty, PHM addresses specialized areas of focus related to (1) quality, cost, and access to pediatric health care; (2) current pediatric residency training; (3) the evolving body of knowledge in pediatrics; and (4) the impact on both primary care generalists and existing subspecialists.[3]

In this issue, we examine the changing nature of inpatient care, including the major movements and trends that have influenced hospital-based practice, patient-centered care, and education in this clinical learning environment. The intended audience for this

Pediatr Clin N Am 66 (2019) xix–xx
https://doi.org/10.1016/j.pcl.2019.05.001

issue is frontline providers who provide care in community hospitals and faculty in academic medical centers.

It was a tremendous pleasure to work with so many talented and diverse colleagues as collaborators and coauthors of this issue addressing such a dynamic and impactful field. We hope that their contributions will be appreciated by a wide variety of readers and that the articles will serve as a valuable resource and context for the specialty of PHM in the years to come. In this regard, we are honored to provide a guidepost by way of this issue as the field continues efforts to provide the highest-quality clinical care for our nation's hospitalized children as well as to train future professionals who will guide PHM on the next phase of this ongoing and exciting journey.

Amy J. Starmer, MD, MPH
Department of Pediatrics
Boston Children's Hospital
Harvard Medical School
300 Longwood Avenue
Boston MA 02115, USA

Matthew W. Ramotar, BA
Boston Children's Hospital
300 Longwood Avenue
Boston, MA 02115, USA

Nancy D. Spector, MD
Drexel University College of Medicine
245 North 15th Street
Mail Stop 400
Philadelphia, PA 19102, USA

E-mail addresses:
amy.starmer@childrens.harvard.edu (A.J. Starmer)
matthew.ramotar@childrens.harvard.edu (M.W. Ramotar)
nds24@drexel.edu (N.D. Spector)

REFERENCES

1. Ottolini MC. Preface. Pediatr Clin 2014;61(4):xix–xx.
2. Wachter RM, Goldman L. The emerging role of "hospitalists" in the American health care system. N Engl J Med 1996;335(7):514–7.
3. Barrett DJ, McGuinness GA, Cunha CA, et al. Pediatric hospital medicine: a proposed new subspecialty. Pediatrics 2017;139(3):e20161823.

Section 1: Hospital-Based Practice

Pediatric Hospitalists Improving Patient Care Through Quality Improvement

Anupama Subramony, MD, MBA[a,*,1], Irene Kocolas, MD, MS[b,1],
Raj Srivastava, MD, MPH[c,2]

KEYWORDS

• Quality improvement • Hospital medicine • Pediatric hospitalists • Children

KEY POINTS

- Quality improvement has been successfully used in pediatric hospital medicine.
- Hospitalists should take advantage of training opportunities, use the methods and tools, work on hospital-based projects, and partner on national projects.

INTRODUCTION

Quality improvement (QI) has become a major lever for health care transformation over the last 20 years; stimulated by a recognition that, whereas research advances have increased, the reliable practice of clinical care within complex health care systems has lagged behind. This article reviews the industrial underpinnings of the QI movement and describes how QI became integrated within the larger health care landscape, as well as within the burgeoning field of hospital medicine. QI methodologies and a framework for using them is described. Key components in a successful QI

Disclosure Statement: Dr R. Srivastava works for Intermountain Healthcare, which holds equity in the I-PASS Patient Safety Institute. Dr R. Srivastava is an Executive Council member of the Pediatric Research in Inpatient Settings (PRIS) network. PRIS has received funding from the Children's Hospital Association and federal grant agencies to conduct multicenter research. Dr R. Srivastava has received monetary awards, honoraria, and travel reimbursements from multiple academic and professional organizations for talks about pediatric hospitalist research networks and quality of care. Dr I. Kocolas and Dr A. Subramony have nothing to disclose.
[a] Department of Pediatrics, Cohen Children's Medical Center, Donald and Barbara Zucker School of Medicine at Hofstra/Northwell, 269-01 76th Avenue, New Hyde Park, NY 11040, USA; [b] Division of Inpatient Medicine, Department of Pediatrics, University of Utah School of Medicine/Primary Children's Hospital, Intermountain Healthcare, 100 Mario Capecchi Drive, Salt Lake City, UT 84113, USA; [c] Division of Inpatient Medicine, Department of Pediatrics, University of Utah School of Medicine/Primary Children's Hospital, Healthcare Delivery Institute, Intermountain Healthcare, 5026 State Street, Murray, UT 84107, USA
[1] Co-first authors.
[2] Senior author.
* Corresponding author.
E-mail address: asubramony@northwell.edu

Pediatr Clin N Am 66 (2019) 697–712
https://doi.org/10.1016/j.pcl.2019.03.009 pediatric.theclinics.com

project are outlined. The role of pediatric hospitalists within QI is introduced, with practical tips for pediatric hospitalists getting started. Next, QI training opportunities are reviewed for hospitalists, trainees, and other providers, with a robust discussion on ways hospitalists can get involved in QI on a national level. Showcasing the advanced level of QI initiatives, national QI networks are described, and examples of how national collaboratives improve patient care are highlighted. This article provides an overview and references subsequent chapters for further discussion.

What is Quality Improvement?

QI is a systematic approach to transform organizations to produce better outcomes.[1] Although many distinct methodologies have been developed, the basic components of QI include: (1) a defined measure regarding what the quality outcome should be, (2) a systematic evaluation of processes and identification of variation within these processes related to this outcome, (3) improvement of the aforementioned processes concordantly while the process is occurring, (4) continuous monitoring of the process, (5) use of indicators to measure performance and to benchmark against expected performance, and finally (6) commitment from leadership to achieve these aims.[2]

QI overlaps with traditional research methodologies in numerous ways. Both entities involve seeking order, discerning patterns, and categorizing information in a systematic way. QI is based on the theory of systems, originating from engineering, and the primary aim differs from that of research.[3] Traditionally, the aim of classical research is to develop new knowledge that is generalizable, whereas QI's aim is much more practical; to improve the use of knowledge in a certain setting, embedding processes into an individual context. These distinctions, however, are increasingly blurred as new forms of evaluation of QI efforts are being reported; in addition, many of the implementation concepts that are used in QI projects can be translated from context to context, suggesting that there are increasingly generalizable principles that can be learned from QI projects.[4,5]

Brief History of Quality Improvement

QI's historical roots go back to the industrial revolution and the birth of scientific management.[6] Industry mavens such as Frederick Taylor first suggested that the scientific method could be applied to the factory to improve efficiency and production. In the late nineteenth century, Taylor first used methodologies to improve individual worker efficiency by developing processes for scheduled work using flowcharts and process maps, computing time frames to measure efficiency of each step. Taylor's work became the basis for the development of the discipline of organizational systems theory. From this point, study in organizational behavior shifted away from front-line processes to understanding the role of management, identifying the need for leadership related to change and improvement.

By the mid-twentieth century, the study of organizational behavior had advanced and implications for use in the health care industry started to emerge. Walter Shewhart, a physicist and statistician who worked initially at Bell laboratories, became interested in applying the scientific method to production of telephones.[7] In his measurement of product data across time, he noted that variation in effective production could be categorized into either common cause variation, meaning variation due to chance, which was measurable and predictable within acceptable limits, or special cause variation, meaning variation because of factors that were unpredictable. Shewhart's work at Bell became the basis of the development of statistical quality control, whereby data plotted at regular and frequent intervals show variation encapsulated by control limits representing 2 SD above and below the mean/median showing both common cause and special cause variation.[8] The innovation that Shewhart brought to this methodology was to emphasize that this type of monitoring should be done in the midst of the process, as opposed to measurement of performance only at the end of the production line; with this, special cause variation (data points outside of the control limits) could be identified and fixed before the end of the production line. To achieve this, he believed that front-line workers should be trained on QI methods to be able to conduct this type of analysis and stop, find, and fix issues as they came up. Pioneers such as W. Edwards Deming and Joseph M. Juran were key in transforming the use of QI methodologies to other settings. Importantly, because of these scholars, the use and adaptation of the statistical control chart evolved from the manufacturing process to a broader audience targeted at organizational transformation.[9–13]

Quality Improvement in Health Care

As organizational behavior and management was evolving, it became apparent that many of these principles could be adopted in the health care industry to address certain inadequacies in health care delivery. By the mid-twentieth century, the Joint Commission on Healthcare Accreditation was first formed, conglomerating entities such as the American Medical Association, the American College of Surgeons, and the American Hospital Association, to develop standards for health care organizations, in parallel to what was occurring in the manufacturing industry.[14] Concurrently, scholars such as Avedis Donabedian began to develop a roadmap to transform QI into the health care setting.[15] By 1999, stimulated by the Institute of Medicine's report on preventable harm, the imperative to decrease rapidly increasing health care costs because of poor quality became abundantly clear.[16] The Institute of Medicine quickly followed up their report on preventable errors with a second report, establishing a framework for improvement in health care settings.[17] In their report, the Institute of Medicine cited multiple key drivers for poor quality care delivery, including growing complexity of research, increasing prevalence of patients with chronic disease, and poorly designed health care delivery systems. The report established 6 aims to guide improvement work in health care settings: care that is safe, effective, patient centered, efficient, timely, and equitable. Concurrently with this seminal work, researchers began to show unnecessary variation in clinical practice patterns for a wide array of clinical conditions, further establishing the need for QI. There is a significant body of research showing variability in practice for several common pediatric diagnoses, including asthma,[18] bronchiolitis,[19] gastroenteritis,[20] community-acquired pneumonia,[21] and diabetic ketoacidosis.[22]

Several QI frameworks have emerged to bridge these gaps in health care settings. Many of these, originally birthed in industrial quality assurance, are derived from common conceptual underpinnings. Three of these common frameworks that have increasingly been used in health care include Lean, Six Sigma, and the Model for Improvement (**Table 1**).

The Lean methodology focuses on eliminating waste and improving flow in a process. It focuses on standardizing work, minimizing wait time and time between steps, and signals between downstream operations and upstream operations to be able to flex to fill a need.[23] In the health care world, there is a plethora of ways waste can occur, whether in inventory, motion, rework, waiting, staff potential, and so forth. Healthcare experts estimate there is ~30% of waste in the US health care spend.[24] Lean uses a tool called value stream mapping to lay out all the steps in a process, with each step designated as either value added or nonvalue added. This then allows a visual representation of time spent and opportunities to reduce nonvalue added time. Lean has been used in pediatric settings in numerous ways, including improving

Table 1
Common QI framework

	Model for Improvement	Lean	Six Sigma
Aim	What are we trying to accomplish?	Decrease the gap between current state and standard performance/ideal state	Define the problem as it relates to the consumer
Measures	How will we know a change is an improvement?	Identify value	Measure and validate the outcome metric
Change concepts	What small tests of change can we make that will result in improvement?	Understand value stream to eliminate waste, establish flow, enable pull through value stream mapping	Analyze to identify and prioritize root causes
Change cycles	Plan-Do-Study-Act cycles to increase confidence that the change can improve performance on the aim	Reduction of nonvalue added steps	Improve process performance by addressing and eliminating the root causes to decrease defects
Sustain			Control to achieve sustainability

Adapted from The Improvement Guide: A Practical Approach to Enhancing Organizational Performance, 2nd Edition. Langley, Moen, Nolan, Nolan, Normal, and Provost. Jossey-Bass; with permission.

efficiency of rounding in the intensive care unit[25] and decreasing time of transfer from the operating room to the pediatric intensive care unit.[26]

Six Sigma focuses on using iterative change cycles to measure and reduce variability to decrease "defects." The Six Sigma improvement methodology uses DMAIC (define, measure, analyze, improve, and control) as a structure to define the root causes of a problem, measure current process, analyze the process to understand opportunities for improvement, conduct change cycles, then control to process by developing systems that will lead to process sustainability.[27] Six Sigma has been used to improve multiple areas of pediatric care including: reducing unplanned extubations in the neonatal intensive care unit (NICU),[28] reducing breast milk administration errors in the NICU,[29] and reducing unnecessary head computed tomography orders in children with hydrocephalus.[30]

The Model for Improvement is likely the most used improvement methodology in health care.[31] The methodology uses the following framework for improvement: (1) What are we trying to accomplish? (2) How will we know that a change is an improvement? (3) What change can we make that will result in improvement? After developing a team, setting a SMART (specific, measurable, actionable, relevant, and time bound) aim, in serial Plan-Do-Study-Act cycles, small tests of change are adopted, adapted, or abandoned until they are ramped up to scale to meet the a priori set aim.[31] Specific tools that are part of the Model for Improvement methodology include the key driver diagram (**Table 2**). The Model for Improvement has been used to improve a variety of pediatric care in both single-institutions including: increasing the number of patients with asthma discharged with asthma controller medication,[32] increasing use of nasogastric hydration among hospitalized patients with bronchiolitis,[33] and use of

Table 2
Specific QI tools in model of improvement methodology

Specific QI Tools	
Fishbone	• Understand causes that led to a poor outcome
Key driver diagram	• Describes entities that contribute to an aim
Run chart	• A way to describe data monthly to show progress to an aim
Control chart	• Statistical process control chart showing performance that is within control • Displays special cause and common cause variation
Process maps and swim lanes	• Describes a process from start to finish • Swim lanes describe a process where multiple players do overlapping activities
Value stream mapping	• Process map that identifies steps that are value added or nonvalue added
SIPOC tool	• Tool to identify stakeholders to create a multidisciplinary team • Uses a high-level process map to assure accurate participation

appropriate hand hygiene in pediatric inpatient settings[34] as well as in multicenter collaboratives.[35,36]

Whatever the specific methodology, for improvement projects to be successful, there are a few key elements necessary (**Table 3**). A first key step is to build a comprehensive team with key stakeholders; a good improvement team is multidisciplinary, and membership should reflect disciplines that will be affected by the change. Creating a charter that clearly delineates the problem that needs to be addressed and outlines the anticipated resources necessary to conduct the QI project is helpful in assuring that the project has a defined scope that is agreed on by all stakeholders. Leadership engagement and executive sponsorship for the improvement project, also delineated in the charter, allows for removal of barriers that may emerge or assignment of resources necessary for the improvement project and process change. In addition, leadership engagement helps to align projects with strategic goals of the institution and provide the framework for sustainability. Developing a clear and concise global aim and aim statement summarizes the project by specifically defining the primary outcome measure for the project and laying out a time frame to see the project carried through. Lastly, tests of change should initially be small, and ramped up with iterative cycles in which changes are adapted, adopted, or abandoned based on process measures identified during each test of change. It is imperative that these tests be sequential, and that data are collected at each step to assure that the change in fact will lead to an improvement in the outcome measure. In practice, cycles of change are not uniformly positive; that is, failed cycles of change are often encountered and lessons learned in these failed cycles are as valuable as cycles that produce a positive outcome.[37] Finally, a plan for sustainability is imperative to assure that the project results remain viable.

Quality Improvement and the Pediatric Hospitalist

The pediatric hospitalist cares for patients with a wide range of disease processes, severity of illness, and complexity of comorbidities.[4] From a clinical perspective, pediatric hospitalists are in a unique position within the inpatient world as a consistent presence on pediatric floors. Traditional evidence is often lacking to guide care plans and leads to a struggle in providing highest-quality care, even for some common

Table 3
Key elements to a successful QI project

Key Element	Components and Purpose
Build a team	• Identify and engage key stakeholders in the local context • Assure multidisciplinary and front-line representation (eg, hospitalists, nurses, residents, fellows, pharmacists, allied staff) • Solicit support of an executive sponsor or key influencer who can facilitate removal of barriers
Develop a charter	• Defining the problem that the quality improvement project will be addressing in a concise manner • Listing key members of the team and assigning roles to assure accountability • Outlining anticipated resources necessary to complete the project • Determine project scope
Develop an aim	• Define a global aim as well as a SMART (specific, measurable, achievable, relevant, and time bound) primary metric • Collect baseline data and understand current state through quantitative and qualitative methods • Use structured brainstorming methodologies to organize project with concept maps for improvement (eg, key driver diagrams, fishbone diagrams, value stream mapping) • Engage data analysts if available to collect data efficiently
Conduct change cycles	• Plan small tests of change affecting the process • Collect process data associated with tests • Adopt, adapt, or abandon change based on data • Ramp up cycles of change to widen to desired scope
Plan for sustainability	• Understand and mitigate risks to sustainability • Develop plans for routine monitoring and reporting of outcome data • Create a process to address failures to sustain the new process

inpatient pediatric diagnosis. Within this challenge, the role for QI emerges as a catalyst for more rapid understanding of systems and processes, leading to change and dissemination of best practice.

For the pediatric hospitalist engaged in QI there are practical tips using the key elements described in the previous section that can improve the likelihood of success. For the pediatric hospitalist developing a multidisciplinary team, key stakeholders could include front-line nurses, unit managers, unit receptionists, residents, and other allied staff including respiratory therapists or physical therapists depending on the project. Developing a charter that clearly defines an aim that is within control of the team is imperative; this could be measuring a process that occurs on a specific hospitalist unit. Leadership and executive sponsorship of the project could vary depending on the scope of the project; it may entail including the medical and nursing director of the unit, it may also necessitate including other leaders in the organization, including residency directors, Chief Medical and Nursing Officers, as well as Chief Quality Officers. Pulling the multidisciplinary team together for structured brainstorming allows for the pediatric hospitalist to include alternate views of the process or understand a new process in more detail. Developing a concept map using an improvement tool (eg, fishbone, key driver diagram or value stream map) helps assure that all team members have a consistent understanding of the underlying problem to be solved. Pursing change cycles should initially start small—for example, testing a change in process for 1 pediatric hospitalist on 1 day, and then slowly ramping it up. Data collection can be done concurrently with the tests; although designing reports from the electronic medical records may seem the best approach, manual data collection, especially in the beginning, may result in a new understanding of the process in question. Finally, connecting the work to strategic goals of the organization may facilitate sustainability plans to assure that there is little drift once the project is completed and the aim is initially achieved.

By networking and collaborating as outlined above, pediatric hospitalists use skills developed by leading QI projects to further professional advancement. In working on health care-acquired condition reduction teams and national collaboratives, pediatric hospitalists use these experiences to partner with hospital leadership and provide a key clinical understanding in the realm of hospital administration. In doing so, career trajectories of pediatric hospitalists have expanded beyond traditional academic positions. Hospitalists have used these capabilities largely in conjunction with advanced degrees to become hospital leaders including Chief Medical Officers, Chief Quality Officers, Chief Patient Safety Officers, Chief Patient Experience Officers, and Chief Executive Officers. Using these skills on the academic side, there is opportunity for leadership as division chiefs, department chairs, and deans.

Training in Quality Improvement

To participate in, and then subsequently lead, a successful QI project as mapped out above, pediatric hospitalists and trainees need to be educated in the basics of QI. The tools below are useful to all clinicians caring for patients, including advanced practice nurses, physician assistants, charge and bedside nurses, respiratory therapists, and physical therapists. There are local and national resources available in learning how to incorporate QI techniques into clinical practice. Pediatric health care providers should be aware of these resources because many organizations use pediatric providers to lead hospital-wide tactical QI and safety teams, necessitating an understanding of basic QI and leadership techniques for professional development; in addition, hospitalists and clinicians may more effectively mentor housestaff and trainees on their own QI projects.

Pediatric hospitalists and providers

There are opportunities for QI training on local and national levels. Clinicians are encouraged to meet with a senior leader such as the Chief Quality Officer or Chief Medical Officer of the hospital and identify local resources, understand hospital team structures and the current QI projects underway. Clinicians should consider joining one of the hospital QI projects with the goal of establishing a mentor and learning how the process works. There also may be ongoing interactive QI workgroup sessions offered within the hospital/institution. In addition, often hospital-wide lectures such as grand rounds or invited speakers discuss QI projects and opportunities for participation.

There are several training opportunities for self-training available. Below, we offer a basic introduction to QI as well as in-depth pediatric hospital initiatives aimed at improving pediatric inpatient care. The Institute for Healthcare Improvement (IHI) offers free resources, including tools, change ideas, measures, guidelines, and literature sources. IHI resources may serve as a foundation for QI for any level of learner. Webinars and in-person training sessions are also available to build on the basics (**Table 4**).[38] The American Board of Pediatrics Maintenance of Certification part IV is currently being used as a way to assure ongoing QI as part of recertification for pediatricians. A variety of Web-based tools are available from the American Board of Pediatrics, including the ability to participate in collaborative QI projects, and other

Table 4
Local, online, and national QI training opportunities

		Examples
Local	Continuous improvement meetings	"Research/QI in Progress" workgroups
	Educational lectures	Grand rounds, visiting lecturers
	Continuous Medical Education (CME)	Local American Board of Pediatrics (ABP) Maintenance of Certification (MOC) part IV collaboratives, hospital-sponsored CME QI activities
Online	ABP	MOC part IV
	American Academy of Pediatrics (AAP)	Education in Quality Improvement for Pediatric Practices (EQIPP) (EQIPP.aap.org). Modules: asthma, bronchiolitis
	Institute of Healthcare Improvement (IHI)	Leadership training, webinars • Courses: "Leading Quality Improvement" QI 105 "Why Engage Trainees in Quality and Safety" course GME 201 (http://www.ihi.org/education/IHIOpenSchool/Chapters/Groups/Faculty/Pages/Courses.aspx#gme1) • Hospitalist specific: IHI White Paper "Using Care Bundles to Improve Health Care Quality" (http://www.ihi.org/resources/Pages/IHIWhitePapers/UsingCareBundles.aspx)
National	Collaborative meetings	Pediatric Hospital Medicine (PHM), Society Hospital Medicine (SHM), Pediatric Academic Society (PAS), AAP National Conference Exhibition, IHI
	Leadership courses	Intermountain Healthcare Advance Training Program, Cincinnati Children's Hospital Medical Center Intermediate Improvement Science Series (I^2S^2), Nationwide Children's Clinical Fellowship in Quality and Safety Leadership

Web-based improvement activities.[39] Training modules geared to "teach systematic measurement and improvement to improve child health" are also available. The American Academy of Pediatrics (AAP) also houses Education in Quality Improvement for Pediatric Practices, an online learning program that uses QI methods to improve children's health outcomes. Courses are available for individuals and groups, including residents.[40]

Nationally recognized sponsoring organizations and hospitals provide advanced QI training programs relevant to pediatric hospitalists. For example, Intermountain Healthcare in Utah offers the Advanced Training Program.[41] This program is aimed at health care leaders and clinicians on how to use QI to investigate and implement solutions in their home organizations and use outcome measurements and management of clinical and nonclinical processes. Cincinnati Children's Hospital offers the Intermediate Improvement Science Series (I^2S^2), an accredited course aimed at QI leadership development in transforming health care.[42] Nationwide Children's Hospital offers a Clinical Fellowship in Quality and Safety Leadership. The focus of the fellowship is to prepare trainees to lead quality and safety programs in hospital systems and offers an advanced degree.[43] The Geisinger Administrative Fellowship is a leadership training program in health care administration, offering opportunity to apply principles in an integrated health care delivery system.[44] Participation in these advanced training opportunities may add skills to a pediatric hospitalist's armamentarium and improve the value to an organization seeking to further develop a robust QI program.

Hospital medicine fellows

Pediatric hospital medicine (PHM) fellowship programs are growing in number. Fellowship completion will soon be required for pediatricians to qualify for PHM subspecialty board certification. Despite our expanding field, there is no standardized curriculum for QI training within hospital medicine fellowships. A national group of PHM fellowship directors have published a curricular framework focused on 3 sections comprised of clinical care, systems and scholarships, and individualized curriculum.[45] The curricular framework describes that a required portion of fellow education is dedicated to QI, leadership, business administration, medical education, and advocacy. Most fellowship education consists of an individualized curriculum, whereby a trainee may choose to focus on QI. Examples of career tracks and suggestions on how to allocate educational time are described. This individualized curriculum offers flexibility for a wide scope of clinical practice. For example, a fellow interested in community practice may choose to focus on QI in leadership within the community, whereas a fellow with a research focus may choose to focus on QI in safety/advocacy. Both fellows may then participate in pertinent QI projects for each career trajectory.[45] Stucky and colleagues[46] have also published the *Pediatric Hospital Medicine Core Competencies*, which define the standards for the knowledge, skills, attitudes, and focus on systems improvements that are expected of all pediatric hospitalists, regardless of practice setting or location. The section on continuous QI provides essential knowledge, skills, and attitudes that pediatric hospitalists should know. Lastly, many PHM fellowship programs offer advanced degrees that may have an emphasis in QI. Although this is not an official requirement, advanced training in QI methodologies, data analysis, and statistical methods would be beneficial.

Housestaff

For many pediatric hospitalists in academic and community practices, resident education is woven into daily responsibilities. Hospitalists have the opportunity to partner with residents in hospital QI projects. The Accreditation Council for Graduate Medical Education (ACGME) has recently required targeted education in QI within pediatric residency training.[47] Under the auspices of the ACGME, the Clinical Learning Environment Review (CLER) was created to provide specific and more frequent feedback to ACGME-accredited institutions and programs. Areas of focus include patient safety and health care quality. The goal of CLER feedback is to enhance engagement of resident and fellow physicians to provide safe, high-quality patient care. CLER has published "Pathways to Excellence" as an expectation for pediatric residency programs and offers guidelines on QI curriculum.[48] These guidelines are general and allow for flexibility in training programs, ranging from academic centers to community hospitals and rural settings, allowing the opportunity to involve housestaff in hospital quality initiatives and enhance the teamwork of existing projects.

Hospitalists interested in teaching QI to housestaff may find webinars and further resources online.[47] Although the ACGME outlines the framework for QI training, other resources exist to help educators teach QI in effective ways. Multiple curricula have been published in MedEdPORTAL that may be adapted to individual clinical and educational settings to engage trainees in QI; examples include a game-based approach to QI for early learners, and experiential training in QI design.[49] For assessment of these skills in the clinical setting, please see Duncan Henry and Daniel C. West's article, "The Clinical Learning Environment and Workplace-based Assessment: Frameworks, Strategies, and Implementation," in this issue.

Interprofessional team training

In our experience, effective team communication is an important contributor to successful QI projects.[50] IHI offers leadership training for clinicians leading interdisciplinary teams.[51] The Agency for Healthcare Research and Quality also sponsors a widely recognized tool in team training called Team STEPPS (Team Strategies and Tools to Enhance Performance and Patient Safety).[52] Online curriculum is available in addition to training modified to the needs of institutions. Several academic centers offer their own tailored Team STEPPS training. Other avenues for this training include programs such as QIPS (QI and Patient Safety), a simulation created for interdisciplinary teamwork.[53] Please refer to Jennifer Baird and Colleagues' article, "Interprofessional Teams: Current Trends and Future Directions," in this issue.

Pediatric Hospital Medicine and Quality Improvement

National meetings

National meetings are ideal for attending in-person workshops, tutorials, plenary sessions, and networking. QI courses are offered across the continuum, targeting trainees and fellows to seasoned experts in QI. The PHM annual conference is sponsored by the AAP, the Academic Pediatric Association, and the Society of Hospital Medicine (SHM). PHM is geared specifically for pediatric hospitalists and focuses on clinical tracks including QI. The AAP National Conference and Exhibition, SHM, and Pediatric Academic Society annual meetings also offer QI educational sessions and workshops for pediatricians. The IHI National Forum on Quality Improvement in Health Care offers the longest standing QI conference in the United States, exploring how improvement science methodologies can be used to effect real change in patient safety and care.[54]

Impact

Pediatric hospitalists are poised to engage in QI activities at multiple levels. Pediatric hospitalists have been integral in improvement projects locally and also establishing a presence at the national level—by securing large federal grants to study how to improve the quality of care in inpatient settings, publishing in high-tier medical journals, and taking on academic leadership roles in the education and research arenas of academic medicine.

QI projects related to guideline adherence for asthma,[55] bronchiolitis,[35] community-acquired pneumonia,[36] and osteomyelitis[56] have shown improvements both in single-site projects as well as in collaboratives. These not only span traditional general pediatric inpatient services,[57] but also include areas such as newborn nursery.[58] Local improvement outside of traditional pediatric hospitalist medicine topics also provides a way for pediatric hospitalists to become involved; most organizations have teams dedicated to improving quality measures such as reduction of health care-acquired conditions, such as central line-associated bloodstream infections, catheter-associated urinary tract infections, and readmissions. Work done internally in a pediatric hospitalist team can be spread to the rest of the hospital.

Networks

QI efforts in PHM have improved patient outcomes and safety through collaborative efforts.[59] There are several national QI opportunities within PHM. The AAP sponsors the Value in Inpatient Pediatrics (VIP) network. The mission of VIP is to improve the value of care given to inpatient pediatric patients. VIP works by conducting large-scale national collaboratives in QI. The VIP network educates providers to implement clinical guidelines and assess the impact in preventing overuse.[60] By virtue of the projects, VIP allows pediatric hospitalists to network with national colleagues and collaborate on QI projects and best practices. Large-impact VIP-sponsored projects include decreasing unnecessary care in bronchiolitis patients and decreasing patient identification errors.[61]

As described in the first section, often there is a hazy line between QI and QI research. One conduit established to merge QI and QI research is the Pediatric Research Inpatient Setting (PRIS). PRIS is a research network aimed at improving health care delivery to hospitalized children.[62] The PRIS network orchestrates multicenter research studies in the inpatient setting. PRIS work has included working with leadership from over 40 children's hospitals, identifying high-priority clinical conditions that are prevalent, costly, and exhibit high interhospital variation in care, identifying unwarranted variation in clinical services for specific hospital conditions (eg, diabetic ketoacidosis or routine tonsillectomies), and assessing which high-priority conditions would be amenable to QI interventions based on national guidelines.[22,63,64] PRIS also offers hospitalists who are site investigators authorship on published work. There are specific opportunities for fellow and junior faculty involvement in national initiatives with mentorship offered by the PRIS Executive Council.

Another strong national collaborative shown to improve patient safety is the Children's Hospitals' Solutions for Patient Safety (SPS).[65] It is a network of over 130 children's hospitals that has decreased preventable patient harm by sharing bundles, best practices, and tools disseminated through collaboration and learning opportunities.[66] SPS focuses on reducing hospital-acquired conditions including readmissions and serious safety events through rigorous QI and a focus on culture and leadership; importantly, the network fosters sharing between hospitals to help develop best practices to promote patient safety.[67] SPS partners with other safety networks, such as the Child Health Patient Safety Organization sponsored by the Children's Hospital Association.[68] This organization allows for children's hospitals to share adverse events in real time with legal protection, allowing organizations to conduct their own risk assessments and develop prevention measures to mitigate risks before safety events occur.

The Children's Hospital Association owns the Pediatric Health Information System (PHIS). PHIS is a comparative pediatric database that houses information for hospitalized children including over 45 children's hospitals.[69] Opportunities exist to improve local processes by comparing hospital-specific data with other similar hospitals. Leadership within hospitals often use these data for both QI projects, given the comparisons in care that can be made, as well as understanding the sources of inpatient variation in care.[70,71]

Networks such as VIP and PRIS and databases such as PHIS support research studies to improve patient safety and outcomes. PRIS was a sponsor of a large multicenter QI and research study that implemented a resident handoff bundle in several children's hospitals. The resident handoff bundle standardized provider communication specifically at the transition of care and was associated with a reduction in medical errors.[72] Much of the success of that project used QI principles, tools, teams, and outcomes data to drive the improvement in change. I-PASS and other standardized handoff tools are further discussed in Shilpa J. Patel and Christopher P. Landrigan's article,

"Handoffs for Hospital Medicine Physicians: Creating a Shared Mental Model", in this issue.

SUMMARY

QI is a key part of the health care industry; understanding its usefulness and applying its principles is an important part of pediatric hospital practice. Pediatric hospitalists can use QI in many ways; to transform daily clinical care locally and to improve outcomes nationally. In addition, QI can provide a platform for education for trainees, serve as a catalyst for research opportunities and provide a framework for career growth. As PHM comes into its own as a distinct specialty, the field must develop its own QI agenda that integrates with local hospitals as well as partners with national groups. This partnership is a vital component to assuring the success of improving pediatric care both at the individual doctor-patient level and at the system level.

REFERENCES

1. Colton D. Quality improvement in health care, vol. 23. Conceptual and Historical Foundations; 2000. Available at: http://journals.sagepub.com/doi/pdf/10.1177/016327800220344462. Accessed August 7, 2018.
2. Martin L. Total quality management in human service organizations 1993. Available at: https://books.google.com/books?hl=en&lr=&id=qZZrjpFG4RwC&oi=fnd&pg=PR9&dq=%22total+quality+management+in+human+service+organzations%22&ots=QgDChu3Cr0&sig=vj_M7nXIys3AqI2XSDXfvO9NhGs. Accessed September 19, 2018.
3. Baker F. Quality assurance and program evaluation. Eval Health Prof 1983;6(2):149–60.
4. Simon TD, Starmer AJ, Conway PH, et al. Quality improvement research in pediatric hospital medicine and the role of the Pediatric Research in Inpatient Settings (PRIS) network. Acad Pediatr 2013;13(6):S54–60.
5. Ogrinc G, Davies L, Goodman D, et al. SQUIRE 2.0 (*Standards for Quality Improvement Reporting Excellence)*: revised publication guidelines from a detailed consensus process. BMJ Qual Saf 2016;25(12):986–92.
6. Taylor FW. The principles of scientific management. Management 1911;6:144. https://doi.org/10.2307/257617.
7. Best M, Neuhauser D. Walter A Shewhart, 1924, and the Hawthorne factory. Qual Saf Health Care 2006;15(2):142–3.
8. Carey RG. How do you know that your care is improving? Part II: using control charts to learn from your data. J Ambul Care Manage 2002;25(2):78–88. Available at: http://www.ncbi.nlm.nih.gov/pubmed/11995199. Accessed September 19, 2018.
9. Deming WE. Improvement of quality and productivity through action by management. Natl Product Rev 1981;1(1):12–22.
10. Anderson JC, Rungtusanatham M, Schroeder RG. A theory of quality management underlying the Deming management method. Acad Manage Rev 1994; 19(3):472–509.
11. Godfrey AB, Kenett RS, Joseph M. Juran, a perspective on past contributions and future impact. Qual Reliab Eng Int 2007;23(6):653–63.
12. Juran J. Juran on leadership for quality 2003. Available at: https://books.google.com/books?hl=en&lr=&id=_30uNnb6dQIC&oi=fnd&pg=PP7&dq=joseph+m,+juran+the+life+and+contribution&ots=P0p5mM7n2B&sig=D7sWu8LaE8nizGwagIuOAKwBvfQ. Accessed November 6, 2018.

13. Juran J. A history of managing for quality: the evolution, trends, and future directions of managing for quality 1995. Available at: http://book-catdof.com/a-history-of-managing-for-quality-the-evolution-trends-and-future-directions-of-managing-for-qual-ebooks-are-digitized-written-text.pdf. Accessed November 6, 2018.
14. Roberts JS, Coale JG, Redman RR. A history of the joint commission on accreditation of hospitals. JAMA 1987;258(7):936.
15. Donabedian A. Evaluating the quality of medical care. Milbank Q 2005;83(4): 691–729.
16. Institute of Medicine (US) Committee on Quality of Health Care, Kohn LT, Corrigan JM, Donaldson MS. To err is human. Washington (DC): National Academies Press (US); 2000. https://doi.org/10.17226/9728.
17. Institute of Medicine (US) Committee on Quality of Health Care in America. Crossing the quality chasm: a new health system for the 21st century. Washington, DC: National Academies Press (US); 2001. Available at: http://www.ncbi.nlm.nih.gov/books/NBK222274/. Accessed December 22, 2014.
18. Tsai C-L, Sullivan AF, Gordon JA, et al. Quality of care for acute asthma in 63 US emergency departments. J Allergy Clin Immunol 2009;123(2):354–61.
19. Macias CG, Mansbach JM, Fisher ES, et al. Variability in inpatient management of children hospitalized with bronchiolitis. Acad Pediatr 2015;15(1):69–76.
20. Tieder JS, Robertson A, Garrison MM. Pediatric hospital adherence to the standard of care for acute gastroenteritis. Pediatrics 2009;124(6):e1081–7.
21. Brogan TV, Hall M, Williams DJ, et al. Variability in processes of care and outcomes among children hospitalized with community-acquired pneumonia. Pediatr Infect Dis J 2012;31(10):1.
22. Tieder JS, McLeod L, Keren R, et al. Variation in resource use and readmission for diabetic ketoacidosis in children's hospitals. Pediatrics 2013;132(2):229–36.
23. Womack J, Byrne A, Flume O. Going lean in health care. IHI Innovation Series white paper. Cambridge (MA): Institute for Healthcare Improvement; 2005.
24. Berwick DM, Hackbarth AD. Eliminating waste in US health care. JAMA 2012; 307(14):1513–6.
25. Vats A, Goin KH, Villarreal MC, et al. The impact of a lean rounding process in a pediatric intensive care unit. Crit Care Med 2012;40(2):608–17.
26. Gleich SJ, Nemergut ME, Stans AA, et al. Improvement in patient transfer process from the operating room to the PICU using a lean and six sigma-based quality improvement project. Hosp Pediatr 2016;6(8):483–9.
27. Knapp S. Lean Six Sigma implementation and organizational culture. Int J Health Care Qual Assur 2015;28(8):855–63.
28. Powell BM, Gilbert E, Volsko TA. Reducing unplanned extubations in the NICU using lean methodology. Respir Care 2016;61(12):1567–72.
29. Drenckpohl D, Bowers L, Cooper H. Use of the six sigma methodology to reduce incidence of breast milk administration errors in the NICU. Neonatal Netw 2007; 26(3):161–6.
30. Tekes A, Jackson EM, Ogborn J, et al. How to reduce head CT orders in children with hydrocephalus using the lean six sigma methodology: experience at a major quaternary care Academic Children's Center. AJNR Am J Neuroradiol 2016;37(6): 990–6.
31. Langley GJ, Moen R, Nolan KM, et al. The improvement guide: a practical approach to enhancing organizational performance. San Francisco (CA): Jossey-Bass; 2009. Available at: http://books.google.com/books?id=kE4aEnZgBO8C.
32. Hogan AH, Rastogi D, Rinke ML. A quality improvement intervention to improve inpatient pediatric asthma controller accuracy. Hosp Pediatr 2018;8(3):127–34.

33. Srinivasan M, Pruitt C, Casey E, et al. Quality improvement initiative to increase the use of nasogastric hydration in infants with bronchiolitis. Hosp Pediatr 2017;7(8):436–43.
34. McLean HS, Carriker C, Bordley WC. Good to great: quality-improvement initiative increases and sustains pediatric health care worker hand hygiene compliance. Hosp Pediatr 2017;7(4):189–96.
35. Ralston S, Garber M, Narang S, et al. Decreasing unnecessary utilization in acute bronchiolitis care: results from the value in inpatient pediatrics network. J Hosp Med 2013;8(1):25–30.
36. Parikh K, Biondi E, Nazif J, et al. A multicenter collaborative to improve care of community acquired pneumonia in hospitalized children. Pediatrics 2017; 139(3) [pii:e20161411].
37. Ogrinc G, Shojania KG. Building knowledge, asking questions. BMJ Qual Saf 2014;23(4):265–7.
38. Institute for Healthcare Improvement. Available at: http://www.ihi.org/resources/pages/default.aspx. Accessed May 16, 2018.
39. The American Board of Pediatrics | Certifying excellence in pediatrics – for a healthier tomorrow. Available at: https://www.abp.org/. Accessed May 1, 2018.
40. Available at: Home|eqipp.aap.org. https://eqipp.aap.org/?requestedToken=true&nfstatus=401&nftoken=00000000-0000-0000-0000-000000000000&nfstatusdescription=ERROR%3A+No+local+token. Accessed May 15, 2018.
41. Advanced Training Program. Available at: https://intermountainhealthcare.org/about/transforming-healthcare/institute-for-healthcare-delivery-research/courses/advanced-training-program/. Accessed November 2, 2018.
42. Intermediate Improvement Science Series | Anderson Center. Available at: https://www.cincinnatichildrens.org/service/j/anderson-center/education/i2s2. Accessed May 28, 2018.
43. Clinical fellowship in quality and safety leadership. Available at: https://www.nationwidechildrens.org/for-medical-professionals/education-and-training/fellowship-programs/quality-and-safety-leadership-fellowship. Accessed June 2, 2018.
44. Geisinger administrative fellowship. Available at: https://www.geisinger.org/health-professions/health-professions/administrative-fellowship/program-overview. Accessed May 30, 2018.
45. Jerardi K, Fisher E, Rassbach C, et al. Development of a Curricular Framework for Pediatric Hospital Medicine Fellowships. Pediatrics 2017;140(1). Available at: http://pediatrics.aappublications.org/content/140/1/e20170698.abstract. Accessed November 2, 2018 [pii:e20170698].
46. Stucky ER, Maniscalco J, Ottolini MC. The Pediatric Hospital Medicine core competencies supplement. J Hosp Med 2010;5(S2). i–iv.
47. ACGME program requirements for graduate medical education in pediatrics ACGME program requirements for graduate medical education in pediatrics common program requirements are in BOLD. Available at: https://www.acgme.org/Portals/0/PFAssets/ProgramRequirements/320_pediatrics_2017-07-01.pdf. Accessed November 14, 2018.
48. Health care quality. 2017. Available at: http://www.acgme.org/Portals/0/PDFs/CLER/ACGME_CLER_Health_Care_Quality.pdf. Accessed May 24, 2018.
49. Hanson E, Rosenbluth G, McPeak K. QI olympics: a game-based educational activity in quality improvement. MedEdPORTAL 2013;vol. 9. https://doi.org/10.15766/mep_2374-8265.9421.

50. Brock D, Abu-Rish E, Chiu C-R, et al. Interprofessional education in team communication: working together to improve patient safety. BMJ Qual Saf 2013;22(5): 414–23.
51. Institute for Healthcare Improvement: improve clinical care in your organization. Available at: http://www.ihi.org/education/InPersonTraining/clinicians-leading-improvement/Pages/default.aspx. Accessed November 14, 2018.
52. TeamStepps|Agency for Healthcare Research & Quality. TeamSTEPPS: National implementation. Available at: https://www.ahrq.gov/teamstepps/index.html. Accessed April 4, 2019.
53. Tad-y D, Price L, Cumbler E, et al. An experiential quality improvement curriculum for the inpatient setting – part 1: design phase of a QI project. MedEdPORTAL 2014;10. https://doi.org/10.15766/mep_2374-8265.9841.
54. Institute for Healthcare Improvement: 2018 IHI National Forum. Available at: http://www.ihi.org/education/Conferences/National-Forum-2018/Pages/default.aspx. Accessed June 1, 2018.
55. Nkoy F, Fassl B, Stone B, et al. Improving pediatric asthma care and outcomes across multiple hospitals. Pediatrics 2015;136(6):e1602–10.
56. Brady PW, Brinkman WB, Simmons JM, et al. Oral antibiotics at discharge for children with acute osteomyelitis: a rapid cycle improvement project. BMJ Qual Saf 2014;23(6):499–507.
57. Tchou MJ, Tang Girdwood S, Wormser B, et al. Reducing electrolyte testing in hospitalized children by using quality improvement methods. Pediatrics 2018; 141(5) [pii:e20173187].
58. Patrick SW, Schumacher RE, Horbar JD, et al. Improving care for neonatal Abstinence syndrome. Pediatrics 2016;137(5):e20153835.
59. Landrigan CP, Srivastava R. Pediatric hospitalists: coming of age in 2012. Arch Pediatr Adolesc Med 2012;166(8):696–9.
60. Value in inpatient pediatrics (VIP) network. Available at: https://www.aap.org/en-us/professional-resources/quality-improvement/Quality-Improvement-Innovation-Networks/Value-in-Inpatient-Pediatrics-Network/Pages/Value-in-Inpatient-Pediatrics-Network.aspx. Accessed June 1, 2018.
61. Phillips SC, Saysana M, Worley S, et al. Reduction in pediatric identification band errors: a quality collaborative. Pediatrics 2012;129(6):e1587–93.
62. prisnetwork. Available at: https://www.prisnetwork.org/. Accessed May 15, 2018.
63. Mahant S, Keren R, Localio R, et al. Variation in quality of tonsillectomy perioperative care and revisit rates in children's hospitals. Pediatrics 2014;133(2):280–8.
64. Hester G, Nelson K, Mahant S, et al. Methodological quality of national guidelines for pediatric inpatient conditions. J Hosp Med 2014;9(6):384–90.
65. Solutions for patient safety | Children's Hospitals working together to eliminate harm. Available at: https://www.solutionsforpatientsafety.org/. Accessed November 14, 2018.
66. Lyren A, Brilli RJ, Zieker K, et al. Children's Hospitals' solutions for patient safety collaborative impact on hospital-acquired harm. Pediatrics 2017;140(3) [pii: e20163494].
67. Lyren A, Coffey M, Shepherd M, et al, SPS Leadership Group. We will not compete on safety: how children's hospitals have come together to hasten harm reduction. Jt Comm J Qual Patient Saf 2018;44(7):377–88.
68. Child Health Patient Safety Organization (PSO). Available at: https://www.childrenshospitals.org/Programs-and-Services/Quality-Improvement-and-Measurement/Child-Health-Patient-Safety-Organization. Accessed November 14, 2018.

69. PHIS. Available at: https://www.childrenshospitals.org/Programs-and-Services/Data-Analytics-and-Research/Pediatric-Analytic-Solutions/Pediatric-Health-Information-System. Accessed November 14, 2018.
70. McBride S, Thurm C, Gouripeddi R, et al. Comparison of empiric antibiotics for acute osteomyelitis in children. Hosp Pediatr 2018;8(5):280–7.
71. Chaudhari PP, Monuteaux MC, Bachur RG. Management of urinary tract infections in young children: balancing admission with the risk of emergency department revisits. Acad Pediatr 2018. https://doi.org/10.1016/j.acap.2018.05.011.
72. Starmer AJ, Spector ND, Srivastava R, et al. Changes in medical errors after implementation of a handoff program. N Engl J Med 2014;371(19):1803–12.

Evidence-Based Medicine in the Clinical Learning Environment of Pediatric Hospital Medicine

Nicholas Kuzma, MD*, Hans B. Kersten, MD,
Eric Douglas Thompson, MD, MMM

KEYWORDS

- Evidence-based medicine • Medical education • Hospital medicine

KEY POINTS

- The modern construct for evidence-based medicine (EBM) was created in the 1990s.
- The most commonly used process to apply EBM consists of 5 steps: (1) ask, (2) acquire, (3) appraise, (4) apply, and (5) analyze.
- Changes and advances in the clinical learning environment have influenced how pediatric hospitalists practice EBM.
- Developing the knowledge, skills, attitudes, and behaviors relevant to EBM is an important aspect of medical education.

Evidence-based medicine (EBM) was first defined by Guyatt[1] in 1991 as a process that seeks to integrate the best research evidence with clinical expertise and patient values to optimize clinical outcomes for patients.[2] This process has been adapted and shaped by changes in technology and the clinical learning environment in the almost 30 years since the term EBM was coined.

Although the modern version of EBM was developed in the 1990s, physicians have used the literature to shape clinical practice for centuries. An excellent example of this was James Lind in 1747. He was a surgeon in the Royal Navy who conducted a simple randomized controlled trial that demonstrated the addition of citrus to the diet of sailors with scurvy dramatically improved their symptoms compared with other treatments.[3] Although the study results were quite convincing and citrus fruits eventually became a staple of sailors' diets, it took years for the study to be published, then

The authors of this article have no conflicts of interest.
Section of Hospital Medicine, St Christopher's Hospital for Children, 160 East Erie Avenue, Philadelphia, PA 19134, USA
* Corresponding author.
E-mail address: nck24@drexel.edu

Pediatr Clin N Am 66 (2019) 713–724
https://doi.org/10.1016/j.pcl.2019.03.001
pediatric.theclinics.com

recognized, and then become accepted.[3] EBM was developed as a process to help physicians identify the best available evidence to integrate into the care of their patients and maintain pace with the rapidly expanding body of valid information.[4,5]

The use of EBM has become more common over the past 3 decades because pediatric hospitalists and other healthcare professionals have been encouraged to use EBM to integrate new knowledge into their practice to provide a higher quality of care to their patients.[5] The most commonly used process to practice EBM consists of 5 steps: (1) ask, (2) acquire, (3) appraise, (4) apply, and (5) analyze (**Box 1**).[2]

Another useful construct for understanding EBM is the evidence pyramid. This pyramid organizes different types of evidence from lowest to highest quality.[6] Initially proposed by Haynes[7] in 2001, the pyramid has undergone numerous revisions while becoming increasingly complex.[8] A simplified version of the pyramid was created in 2016, consisting of 5 levels that are practical to conceptualize (**Fig. 1**).[6,8] The base of the pyramid has the highest volume of studies with the evidence becoming stronger at every subsequent level. Toward the top of the pyramid, the evidence has been preappraised and translated into tools that allow active clinicians to readily apply the evidence during their busy clinical schedules.

Pediatric hospitalists have generally welcomed EBM but the limitations of EBM are often discussed. Studies reveal that physicians perceive that practicing EBM can be difficult in a busy clinical practice due to a lack of time, knowledge, and/or resources.[9,10] Additionally, an insufficient number of publications include patient-oriented outcomes.[11] Another challenge for practitioners is staying up to date with the increasing quantity of published evidence, which has been increasing exponentially for decades.[12] Keeping up to date on the relevant evidence to support clinical decisions is not an easily accomplished task. Clinical guidelines developed by professional societies and specialty groups combine research evidence with the consensus views of experts. These guidelines are a possible way for pediatric hospitalists to stay up to date on current evidence and reduce the amount of time spent searching the literature. However, guidelines themselves can be controversial. For example, the increasing number of professional guidelines can lead to variability in suggested approaches to clinical management. More than 10 guidelines with differing clinical recommendations have been developed for the management of group A streptococcus pharyngitis in adults and children.[13] Additionally, many guidelines do not adhere to established standards, making it difficult to compare the discrepancies between guidelines.[14] As these examples show, there are many challenges to practicing EBM in clinical practice. Fortunately, there have been many advancements in the clinical learning environment over the past decade that help pediatric hospitalists overcome these barriers by applying EBM techniques to help determine the best and most appropriate use of the evidence and how to incorporate this into practice.

Box 1
The 5 steps to practicing evidence-based medicine

Ask: Generate clinical questions from a patient encounter

Acquire: Search systematically for the best evidence to answer the clinical question

Appraise: Appraise the evidence critically to assess the validity and importance

Apply: Incorporate the results of the appraisal with clinical expertise and patient values into the care of the patient

Analyze: Evaluate the ability of the EBM process to answer the clinical question

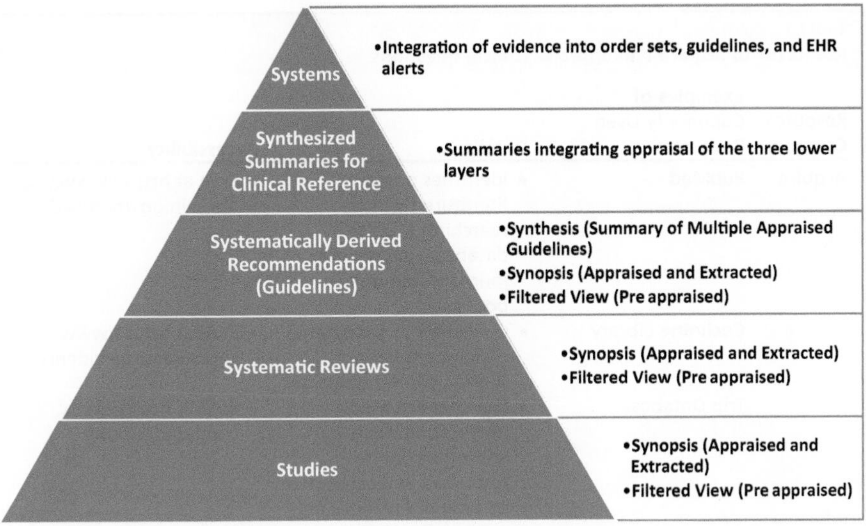

Fig. 1. Evidence-based healthcare pyramid. EHR, electronic health record. (*Adapted from* Alper BS, Haynes RB. EBHC pyramid 5.0 for accessing preappraised evidence and guidance. Evid Based Med. 2016;21(4):123-125; with permission.)

EVIDENCE-BASED MEDICINE IN THE CLINICAL LEARNING ENVIRONMENT

Since the introduction of the term EBM, the clinical learning environment has undergone a tremendous evolution. Advancements in technology, such as laptop computers and cellphones, have transitioned the physical environment, creating the ability to efficiently search the ever-growing medical literature and providing a platform for the integration of evidence into care at the bedside. In addition, external forces, such as regulatory bodies (eg, The Joint Commission, state departments of health) and the multitude of modern payment systems, have further incentivized the use of EBM to obtain the best outcomes for patients at the lowest cost. These factors have all challenged the individual provider to effectively navigate the complexity of medical knowledge and apply this knowledge to clinical care.

Numerous resources are currently available to facilitate the exploration of clinical questions using EBM (**Table 1**). Search engines and databases facilitate the acquisition of information and knowledge in a variety of formats, locations, and costs. Utilization of these resources might depend on the specific scenario. A clinician might turn to the Cochrane Library or the Trip Database to identify systematic reviews or clinical guidelines that can be efficiently applied in a busy clinical setting, whereas a researcher might turn to PubMed and the primary literature to gain an in-depth understanding of the current medical literature. Technology such as desktop and laptop computers and mobile devices, including tablets and cellphones, allows all these resources to be available at the practitioner's fingertips.[15,16] Information gathered through utilization of these resources is often integrated into systems tools that are developed at the hospital level, including disease-specific order sets, clinical guidelines and pathways, and alerts within an electronic medical record. All of these examples encourage providers to apply the highest level of evidence in their care of patients.

Unfortunately, the existence of consensus recommendations and robust clinical literature does not equate to implementation of evidence at the point of care. For example, despite the availability of clinical practice guidelines to support the

Table 1
Resources to acquire and appraise clinical questions

Resource Category	Examples of Commonly Used Resources	Details	Accessibility
Acquire	PubMed	• Identifies primary literature through searching MEDLINE database, life sciences journals, and online books	• Free at https://www.ncbi.nlm.nih.gov/pubmed
	Cochrane Library	• Collection of systematic reviews answering specific clinical questions	• Free at https://www.cochrane.org/evidence
	Trip Database	• Searches PubMed, professional Web sites, and other online resources, and categorizes by type of evidence (eg, primary literature, systematic review, guidelines)	• Free at https://www.tripdatabase.com
	Google Scholar	• Searches scholarly works on the Internet and uses several variables to rank articles based on strength of evidence	• Free at https://scholar.google.com
Appraise	Primary literature (eg, journal articles)	• Requires the reader to be skilled in critical appraisal techniques	• Available electronically or in print through individual or institutional subscription
	—	—	• PubMed Central provides many full text articles free of charge accessible through PubMed citations
	Traditional textbooks	• Useful references for background information but can become outdated quickly as evidence evolves	• Online versions of the paper formats of these textbooks are often available through individual or institutional subscription
	Electronic textbooks (eg, UpToDate, Medscape, or DynaMed Plus)	• Distinguish themselves from traditional textbooks by existing only in electronic format with regular editing to keep current with the medical literature	• Many of these resources require an individual or institutional subscription
	Systematic reviews	• Represent previously appraised material	• Cochrane and traditional journals are the most common sources
	Clinical practice guidelines	• Systematically developed statements about appropriate healthcare decisions for specific clinical circumstances.	• Frequently published through professional organizations and/or in medical journals

management of patients hospitalized with bronchiolitis, Mittal and colleagues[17] demonstrated little impact in the reduction of unnecessary testing and treatment across multiple hospital sites throughout the United States. However, Mittal and colleagues[18] did demonstrate decreased unnecessary resource utilization in patients with bronchiolitis at a single site when applying quality improvement tools to support guideline implementation, such as regular multidisciplinary team meetings, identification of key drivers, implementation of an electronic order set and clinical decision support, clear metrics, and regular feedback of data to clinicians. Similarly, Holmes and colleagues[19] applied quality improvement methodology through a series of plan-do-study-act cycles to implement best practices in the care of newborns with neonatal abstinence syndrome to significantly decrease morphine utilization and length of stay. It is likely that clinical guidelines become more impactful locally when adapted into an institution's cultural practices, which may include tools for implementation, mechanisms for monitoring adherence and patient outcomes, and local expert opinion, as institutional guidelines.

The quality improvement process can serve multiple roles in its relationship to EBM (See Arti D. Desai and Amy J. Starmer's article, "Process Metrics and Outcomes to Inform Quality Improvement in Pediatric Hospital Medicine," in this issue). In the planning phase of a quality improvement project, clinical questions may arise, leading to the acquisition and appraisal of evidence to direct the project. These examples demonstrate how quality improvement can serve as the mechanism to implement the best evidence, as well as to create new knowledge that may be applied by others.

External drivers of the use of EBM in clinical settings include regulatory bodies (eg, The Joint Commission) and insurance companies. In this regard, The Joint Commission requires hospitals caring for pediatric patients to meet certain evidence-based standards related to asthma care as part of their core measures.[20] Insurance companies have used several payment strategies to encourage providers to integrate EBM into their practice in an effort to achieve the best patient outcomes while achieving value.[21–23] Porter[24] outlines the concept of value in healthcare by defining it as patient outcomes per dollar spent. This concept has shaped the discussion regarding current healthcare policy and payment reform. Payment models, such as pay-for-performance, value-based payments, bundled payments, and accountable care organizations, attempt to incentivize practitioners to achieve optimal patient outcomes and cost savings by following best practices and eliminating wasteful and unnecessary care. These models rely on metrics and may provide opportunities to integrate EBM into daily practice. However, care must be taken when designing payment reform to avoid too much focus on the cost portion of the value equation and not enough on patient outcomes. For instance, bundled payments reimbursing providers for episodes of care may encourage the inappropriate underutilization of resources without attention to balancing measures reflecting patient outcomes.[21–23]

EVIDENCE-BASED MEDICINE IN GRADUATE AND UNDERGRADUATE MEDICAL EDUCATION

Advances in the clinical learning environment have strengthened and solidified the role of EBM in pediatric hospital medicine. However, many of the previously discussed challenges to practicing EBM remain. In response, there is now a greater emphasis on teaching the principles of EBM in undergraduate and graduate medical education. Developing the knowledge, skills, attitudes, and behaviors relevant to the 5 steps of practicing EBM has become an important component of medical education and is now mandated in both the graduate and undergraduate settings (**Table 2**).[25,26] In

Table 2
Examples of knowledge, skills, attitudes, and behaviors relevant to each step of the evidence-based medicine process

	Ask	Acquire	Appraise	Apply	Assess
Knowledge	Structure answerable questions	List appropriate databases to search	Select appropriate methods to critically appraise an article or topic	Identify situations in which it is appropriate to apply EBM	Identify successful approaches to translating EBM knowledge
Skills	Generate a focused clinical question based on a patient encounter	Systematically search for the best evidence to answer the clinical question	Complete accurate clinical appraisal of an article or series of articles	Incorporate the results of the critical appraisal to the care of a patient	Reflect on EBM skills and improve them over time
Attitudes	Value designing answerable clinical questions	Value conducting searches to answer clinical questions	Value critical appraisals of topics	Value the use of EBM in clinical practice	Value the evaluation of the EBM process
Behaviors	Ask clinical questions about patients	Perform a search about a relevant clinical situation	Critically appraise evidence related to patient care	Changes clinical behaviors based on EBM	Improve EBM skills based after self-reflection

Adapted from Tilson JK, Kaplan SL, Harris JL, et al. Sicily statement on classification and development of evidence-based practice learning assessment tools. *BMC Med Educ.* 2011;11:78; Figure 2, with permission.

the specific setting of graduate medical education, EBM is addressed in the Medical Knowledge 1 milestone.[27]

In addition to the barriers that all providers struggle with, trainees have unique challenges and obstacles that impede them from learning and practicing EBM. A lack of time due to numerous competing responsibilities is the most frequently cited challenge by resident physicians.[28] Additional barriers trainees may have to practicing EBM include insufficient knowledge, skills, behaviors, and attitudes at each step in the EBM process. Forgetting to look up answers to clinical questions, lack of personal initiative, inadequate searching skills, difficulty recognizing when to stop searching, and insufficient critical appraisal skills are all examples of trainee-level barriers that have been identified in the literature.[28,29] Institutional culture can be another barrier because trainees may not prioritize EBM if they think that faculty are not receptive to changing their practice or have a lack of interest in discussing EBM.[28] Staffing shortages and insufficient information resources are examples of healthcare systems barriers that may affect a trainee's ability to practice EBM.[28]

Numerous strategies and curricula have been designed to teach EBM in both graduate and undergraduate medical education settings and potentially overcome these barriers. Teaching methods reported in the literature include journal clubs, workshops, seminars, didactics, e-learning, problem-based learning, longitudinal EBM curricula, and integration of EBM into other curricula.[30,31] In general, no method of content delivery has been shown to be superior to any other.[30,31] However, studies indicate that the application of EBM in graduate medical education is most effective when it is integrated into clinical practice because improvements in knowledge, skills, attitudes, and behaviors have been shown when this is done.[30,32] Additionally, longitudinal EBM curricula have been shown to be more effective than shorter duration interventions in both undergraduate and graduate medical education.[33–36]

Teaching trainees about the principles of EBM requires time, resources, and expertise. Online learning environments, either used on their own or in a flipped classroom model, are a potential way to overcome these challenges. Studies indicate that online learning is as effective as in-person instruction for teaching EBM knowledge and skills.[30]

No matter the approach to EBM content delivery, it is helpful to design an EBM curriculum in a stepwise approach. One common approach is to use the previously mentioned 5 steps to practicing EBM as a framework. The following sections elaborate the 5 steps and the current best practices for teaching these steps to trainees.

Ask

The patient population, intervention, control, outcome (PICO) format is designed to facilitate the creation of answerable clinical questions from uncertainties that arise during patient encounters (**Fig. 2**). This format improves the clarity of clinical problems,

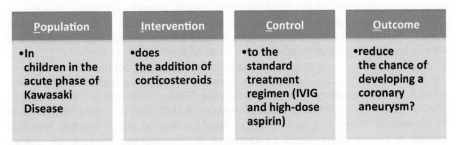

Population	Intervention	Control	Outcome
•In children in the acute phase of Kawasaki Disease	•does the addition of corticosteroids	•to the standard treatment regimen (IVIG and high-dose aspirin)	•reduce the chance of developing a coronary aneurysm?

Fig. 2. Example of a PICO question. IVIG, intravenous immunoglobulin.

allows physicians to perform more complex search strategies, and provides higher quality search results.[37] Teaching trainees to use the PICO structure can lead to improvements in knowledge, skills, and behaviors relevant to the creation of answerable clinical questions.[38,39] Despite some potential challenges in using this format and the existence of several alternative structures, PICO remains a popular strategy for teaching trainees how to ask clinical questions.

Acquire

Electronic databases, including PubMed, have become primary resources for acquiring knowledge that will answer the clinical question. Effectively searching an electronic database requires an understanding of several specific skills. Strategies clinicians can use to narrow electronic searches include using medical subject headings (MeSH); exploding; applying subheadings; using Boolean operators; and applying appropriate limits for publication type, language, or age.[40] Didactic sessions that focus on teaching trainees about search strategies have consistently shown improvements in search skills but there is mixed evidence that these skills are retained over time.[40]

Appraise

Many different teaching strategies have been shown to improve the critical appraisals skills of trainees.[30] Of the many methods by which critical appraisal can be taught, a journal club is both the most frequently used and most studied modality.[41] Journal clubs have consistently been shown to improve both EBM knowledge and skills even though there is no standardized version of what a journal club is.[42] Some best practices for a journal club include the following: establish an overarching long-term goal for the sessions; conduct sessions at regular, predictable intervals; identify a leader for each session and ensure they have a solid grasp of the study's design and analysis; allow participants to review the article before the meeting; and use a standardized approach to critically appraise articles.[42] Essentially, successful journal clubs are multifaceted. They need to role model lifelong learning skills, encourage collaboration and participation, focus on addressing problems relevant to the group of trainees and/or clinicians, and demonstrate how to ingrate theory into clinical practice.[31]

Apply and Assess

Once the clinician has obtained critically appraised evidence, the next step is to apply this evidence to patient care. The practitioner must use their expertise to incorporate the best evidence with the particular clinical scenario and the patient's values. The final step in the EBM process, assess, asks the practitioner to reflect on the effectiveness of the previous 4 steps and apply the lessons learned to future applications of the EBM process. Ideally, trainees will learn how to use EBM to improve patient-centered outcomes and influence their process of care.[41] However, these more difficult to measure steps are not often studied and little is known about the most effective ways to teach them to trainees.[36] Studies that have examined how to teach these steps have varying conclusions. A systematic review found that teaching EBM may lead to changes in physician behavior and clinical decision-making, especially when the EBM coursework is integrated into clinical care.[30] A contrasting Cochrane review found that, despite improvements in knowledge, there is a lack of good quality evidence about whether teaching critical appraisal skills leads to changes in the process of care or patient outcomes.[43]

It is important that educators monitor the impact of EBM curricula on individual and institutional levels. Two tools that evaluate all 5 of the steps of the EBM process have been developed to monitor the impact of EBM curricula on individuals.[44,45] The Berlin Questionnaire is multiple choice and assesses an individual's knowledge about EBM. The Fresno test asks the individual to perform realistic EBM tasks without using multiple choice answers, and assesses both knowledge and skill. A downside is that grading this tool requires more time and expertise.

Many other tools also exist to measure individual steps of the EBM process for trainees. These evaluations tools have variable feasibility, cost, and validity.[33,46,47] Kersten and colleagues[46] developed and validated a tool to evaluate residents' EBM skills in the critical appraisal of research articles. As part of a longitudinal EBM curriculum, Chitkara and colleagues[33] developed a set of evaluation tools to measure resident's knowledge and skills for several important EBM components, including developing PICO questions, performing literature searches, and having the ability to critically appraise articles. Through the Medical Knowledge 1 milestone, all pediatric residency programs are required to evaluate their trainee's knowledge, skills, attitudes, and behaviors regarding EBM.[27]

Few instruments that measure EBM at an institutional level have been published. The Evidence-Based Practice Implementation Scale was created to measure an institution's extent of actual EBM implementation in nursing.[48] Another tool, Evidence-Based Medicine Educational Environment Measure 67, was created to evaluate the perceptions of obstetrics and gynecology residents regarding the environment in which EBM education takes place.[49]

USERS, DOERS, AND REPLICATORS

Whether a pediatric hospitalist or a trainee, there a variety of ways in which one can access and apply clinical evidence in their practice. A model developed by Straus and McAlister[4] describe 3 of these varied approaches using the terms users, doers, and replicators. Most physicians follow the style of a user of evidence because they access resources that have already been acquired and appraised, and use the evidence to inform their clinical practice. The Cochrane Collaboration and Trip Database are examples of resources frequently applied in this manner. Many find the approach practical because it requires less time at the point of care. However, the answers to clinical questions at this level may be limited by the availability of previously appraised topics.

In contrast, doers apply the studies and systematic review levels of the evidence pyramid, and complete all the steps of the EBM process before considering an intervention.[4] Although this can be time-consuming and sometimes impractical at the point of care, this approach is particularly useful in answering important and common clinical questions. To fully understand the body of evidence that drives care, doers ought to have a broad understanding of the EBM process, particularly searching for and critically appraising the evidence. Ideally, trainees have demonstrated their ability to be doers by the end of residency. If not, these skills may be attained through attendance at an EBM course, such as those offered by the Centre for Evidence-Based Medicine, or at several universities around the world.[50] There are also many texts that can be used to learn more about the EBM process.[2]

Replicators follow the recommendations of local opinion experts without reviewing the evidence themselves. This method may work particularly well for patient conditions that are rare, unusual, or unique. Although practical, one may not always know the extent to which an opinion leader is integrating evidence into their clinical care and recommendations. However, a recent Cochrane review concluded that reliance on evidence-based opinion leaders can be very effective in promoting evidence-based practice.[51]

SUMMARY

EBM has become an integral aspect of clinical medicine since its inception 30 years ago. The 5 steps of ask, acquire, appraise, apply, and assess remain a helpful framework for describing the principles of EBM, and can be used for both creating EBM curricula and evaluating individuals and institutions. It is also important to recognize that EBM takes place in a complex learning environment. Clinicians practicing the principles of EBM need to take on many different roles to navigate and apply the multitude of external resources while simultaneously considering the external forces brought about by regulatory bodies and payers.

REFERENCES

1. Guyatt GH. Evidence-based medicine. ACP J Club 1991;114:A16.
2. Straus SE. Evidence-based medicine : how to practice and teach it. 4th edition. Edinburgh (Scotland): Elsevier Churchill Livingstone; 2011.
3. Doherty S. History of evidence-based medicine. Oranges, chloride of lime and leeches: barriers to teaching old dogs new tricks. Emerg Med Australas 2005; 17(4):314–21.
4. Straus SE, McAlister FA. Evidence-based medicine: a commentary on common criticisms. CMAJ 2000;163(7):837–41.
5. Kersten HB, Randis TM, Giardino AP. Evidence-based medicine in pediatric residency programs: where are we now? Ambul Pediatr 2005;5(5):302–5.
6. Alper BS, Haynes RB. EBHC pyramid 5.0 for accessing preappraised evidence and guidance. Evid Based Med 2016;21(4):123–5.
7. Haynes RB. Of studies, syntheses, synopses, and systems: the "4S" evolution of services for finding current best evidence. ACP J Club 2001;134(2):A11–3.
8. Haynes RB. Of studies, syntheses, synopses, summaries, and systems: the "5S" evolution of information services for evidence-based healthcare decisions. Evid Based Med 2006;11(6):162–4.
9. McColl A, Smith H, White P, et al. General practitioner's perceptions of the route to evidence based medicine: a questionnaire survey. BMJ 1998;316(7128):361–5.
10. Tomlin Z, Humphrey C, Rogers S. General practitioners' perceptions of effective health care. BMJ 1999;318(7197):1532–5.
11. Sacristán JA. Patient-centered medicine and patient-oriented research: improving health outcomes for individual patients. BMC Med Inform Decis Mak 2013;13:6.
12. LeFevre M. From authority- to evidence-based medicine: are clinical practice guidelines moving us forward or backward? Ann Fam Med 2017;15(5):410–2.
13. Chiappini E, Regoli M, Bonsignori F, et al. Analysis of different recommendations from international guidelines for the management of acute pharyngitis in adults and children. Clin Ther 2011;33(1):48–58.
14. Kung J, Miller RR, Mackowiak PA. Failure of clinical practice guidelines to meet institute of medicine standards: two more decades of little, if any, progress. Arch Intern Med 2012;172(21):1628–33.
15. Cochrane. Available at: http://www.cochrane.org/. Accessed June 22, 2018.
16. Trip Medical Database. Available at: https://www.tripdatabase.com/. Accessed June 22, 2018.

17. Mittal V, Hall M, Morse R, et al. Impact of inpatient bronchiolitis clinical practice guideline implementation on testing and treatment. J Pediatr 2014;165(3): 570–6.e3.
18. Mittal V, Darnell C, Walsh B, et al. Inpatient bronchiolitis guideline implementation and resource utilization. Pediatrics 2014;133(3):e730–7.
19. Holmes AV, Atwood EC, Whalen B, et al. Rooming-in to treat neonatal abstinence syndrome: improved family-centered care at lower cost. Pediatrics 2016;137(6) [pii:e20152929].
20. Joint Commission. The Joint Commission. Available at: https://www.jointcommission.org/childrens_asthma_care/. Accessed September 27, 2018.
21. Patel KK, Cigarroa JE, Nadel J, et al. Accountable care organizations: ensuring focus on cardiovascular health. Circulation 2015;132(7):603–10.
22. Chee TT, Ryan AM, Wasfy JH, et al. Current state of value-based purchasing programs. Circulation 2016;133(22):2197–205.
23. Shih T, Chen LM, Nallamothu BK. Will bundled payments change health care? examining the evidence thus far in cardiovascular care. Circulation 2015; 131(24):2151–8.
24. Porter ME. What is value in health care? N Engl J Med 2010;363(26):2477–81.
25. Blanco MA, Capello CF, Dorsch JL, et al. A survey study of evidence-based medicine training in US and Canadian medical schools. J Med Libr Assoc 2014; 102(3):160–8.
26. Shaughnessy AF, Torro JR, Frame KA, et al. Evidence-based medicine teaching requirements in the USA: taxonomy and themes. J Evid Based Med 2016;9(2): 53–8.
27. The pediatric milestone project: a joint initiative of the Accreditation Council for Graduate Medical Education and the American Board of Pediatrics. Available at: http://acgme.org/acgmeweb/Portals/0/PDFs/Milestones/PediatricsMilestones.pdf. Accessed June 21, 2018.
28. van Dijk N, Hooft L, Wieringa-de Waard M. What are the barriers to residents' practicing evidence-based medicine? A systematic review. Acad Med 2010; 85(7):1163–70.
29. Green ML, Ruff TR. Why do residents fail to answer their clinical questions? A qualitative study of barriers to practicing evidence-based medicine. Acad Med 2005;80(2):176–82.
30. Coomarasamy A, Khan KS. What is the evidence that postgraduate teaching in evidence based medicine changes anything? A systematic review. BMJ 2004; 329(7473):1017.
31. Ilic D, Maloney S. Methods of teaching medical trainees evidence-based medicine: a systematic review. Med Educ 2014;48(2):124–35.
32. Khan KS, Coomarasamy A. A hierarchy of effective teaching and learning to acquire competence in evidenced-based medicine. BMC Med Educ 2006;6:59.
33. Chitkara MB, Boykan R, Messina CR. A longitudinal practical evidence-based medicine curriculum for pediatric residents. Acad Pediatr 2016;16(3):305–7.
34. Young T, Rohwer A, Volmink J, et al. What are the effects of teaching evidence-based health care (EBHC)? Overview of systematic reviews. PLoS One 2014; 9(1):e86706.
35. Flores-Mateo G, Argimon JM. Evidence based practice in postgraduate healthcare education: a systematic review. BMC Health Serv Res 2007;7:119.
36. Maggio LA, Tannery NH, Chen HC, et al. Evidence-based medicine training in undergraduate medical education: a review and critique of the literature published 2006-2011. Acad Med 2013;88(7):1022–8.

37. Cheng GY. A study of clinical questions posed by hospital clinicians. J Med Libr Assoc 2004;92(4):445–58.
38. Cabell CH, Schardt C, Sanders L, et al. Resident utilization of information technology. J Gen Intern Med 2001;16(12):838–44.
39. Boykan R, Chitkara M, Kenefick C, et al. An integrated practical evidence-based medicine curriculum: two small group sessions to teach PICO question formation and searching strategies. MedEdPORTAL 2013;9:9446.
40. Just M. Is literature search training for medical students and residents effective? a literature review. J Med Libr Assoc 2012;100(4):270–6.
41. Straus SE, Green ML, Bell DS, et al. Evaluating the teaching of evidence based medicine: conceptual framework. BMJ 2004;329(7473):1029–32.
42. Deenadayalan Y, Grimmer-Somers K, Prior M, et al. How to run an effective journal club: a systematic review. J Eval Clin Pract 2008;14(5):898–911.
43. Horsley T, Hyde C, Santesso N, et al. Teaching critical appraisal skills in healthcare settings. Cochrane Database Syst Rev 2011;(11):CD001270.
44. Fritsche L, Greenhalgh T, Falck-Ytter Y, et al. Do short courses in evidence based medicine improve knowledge and skills? Validation of Berlin questionnaire and before and after study of courses in evidence based medicine. BMJ 2002; 325(7376):1338–41.
45. Ramos KD, Schafer S, Tracz SM. Validation of the Fresno test of competence in evidence based medicine. BMJ 2003;326(7384):319–21.
46. Kersten HB, Frohna JG, Giudice EL. Validation of an evidence-based medicine critically appraised topic presentation evaluation tool (EBM C-PET). J Grad Med Educ 2013;5(2):252–6.
47. Boykan R, Jacobson RM. The role of librarians in teaching evidence-based medicine to pediatric residents: a survey of pediatric residency program directors. J Med Libr Assoc 2017;105(4):355–60.
48. Melnyk BM, Fineout-Overholt E, Mays MZ. The evidence-based practice beliefs and implementation scales: psychometric properties of two new instruments. Worldviews Evid Based Nurs 2008;5(4):208–16.
49. Bergh AM, Grimbeek J, May W, et al. Measurement of perceptions of educational environment in evidence-based medicine. Evid Based Med 2014;19(4):123–31.
50. Centre for Evidence-Based Medicine. Available at: https://www.cebm.net/. Accessed June 22, 2018.
51. Flodgren G, Parmelli E, Doumit G, et al. Local opinion leaders: effects on professional practice and health care outcomes. Cochrane Database Syst Rev 2011;(8):CD000125.

Process Metrics and Outcomes to Inform Quality Improvement in Pediatric Hospital Medicine

Arti D. Desai, MD, MSPH[a,*], Amy J. Starmer, MD, MPH[b]

KEYWORDS

• Quality of care • Outcome and process assessment (healthcare) • Hospitals
• Inpatients • Hospitalists • Pediatrics

KEY POINTS

- Evaluating quality improvement interventions typically involves measuring how structures or processes of care affect the health status of patients and populations.
- Selecting appropriate measures requires careful review of the project's goals, stakeholder perspectives, availability of existing measures, validity and feasibility of measures, and measure responsiveness to the quality improvement intervention.
- Developing new measures involves a thorough literature review or conducting a qualitative exploration, drafting measures and specifications, establishing validity and feasibility, and pilot testing the measure in a real-world setting.

INTRODUCTION

One of the core principles of pediatric hospital medicine (PHM) is to improve the quality of care of hospitalized children. (See Anupama Subramony and colleagues' article,

Potential Conflicts of Interest: Dr A.J. Starmer holds equity in and has consulted with the I-PASS Patient Safety Institute. The I-PASS Patient Safety Institute is a company that seeks to train institutions in best handoff practices and aid in their implementation. Dr A.J. Starmer has received monetary awards, honoraria, and travel reimbursement from multiple academic and professional organizations for teaching and consulting on handoffs of care and patient safety, and has served as an expert witness in cases regarding handoffs of care. Dr. Desai's effort is supported by grant number K08HS024299 from the Agency for Healthcare Research and Quality. The content is solely the responsibility of the authors and does not necessarily represent the official views of the Agency for Healthcare Research and Quality. The sponsors had no role in the study design; in the collection, analysis and interpretation of data; in the writing of the report; and in the decision to submit the article for publication.

[a] University of Washington, Seattle Children's Research Institute, 2001 8th Avenue, Suite 400, Seattle, WA 98121, USA; [b] Boston Children's Hospital, Harvard Medical School, 300 Longwood Avenue, Boston, MA 02115, USA

* Corresponding author.

E-mail address: arti.desai@seattlechildrens.org

Pediatr Clin N Am 66 (2019) 725–737
https://doi.org/10.1016/j.pcl.2019.03.002

"Pediatric Hospitalists Improving Patient Care through Quality Improvement," in this issue.) A core component of any quality improvement (QI) initiative is the selection and/or development of quality measures that are directly integrated into the processes and outcomes of daily clinical practice. Efforts to improve quality benefit from measurement to demonstrate whether the improvement initiative has led to a change in the desired direction, to measure unintended results, and to understand whether additional effort will be needed to bring a process back into the desired range.[1]

The identification of meaningful process metrics and outcomes to inform QI within PHM can be challenging due to the diverse nature of the subspecialty.[2] PHM spans multiple clinical settings from general inpatient pediatric care to neonatal care to palliative care.[3] Pediatric hospitalists may be responsible for assisting with perioperative management of surgical patients, providing sedation services, and emergency department consultations. The complexity of hospital systems requires pediatric hospitalists to engage with a multidisciplinary team of providers, administrators, and departments from pharmacy to nutrition services. Furthermore, hospitalized children comprise a diverse population in terms of medical conditions, medical complexity, socioeconomic status, cultural backgrounds, and health plans. The multitude of clinical settings, responsibilities, stakeholders, and diversity of patients provides a wealth of opportunity to engage in QI. However, this poses challenges for QI research; that is, evaluating the effectiveness of QI interventions, to ensure that the chosen process metrics map to key drivers of the project and selected outcomes represent the interests of key stakeholders.

A single QI intervention within PHM may touch on all 6 of the Institute of Medicine's quality dimensions: effectiveness, equity, efficiency, patient-centered, safety, and access.[4] At times, these domains may be at odds with each other as demonstrated by the classic example of length of stay. A shorter length of stay may improve system efficiencies; however, it may also have detrimental effects on patient-centeredness or safety outcomes. Therefore, selecting appropriate measures to evaluate QI interventions and inform future cycles of improvement requires careful consideration of the goals of the improvement project, perspectives of multiple stakeholders, availability of existing measures, the administrative burden of collecting relevant measures, and the ability of the measures to detect meaningful change in response to the QI intervention. This article provides recommendations for selecting appropriate process metrics and outcomes, guidance for the development of new metrics and outcomes, and approaches to applying these metrics and outcomes in PHM practice to fully capture the intended goals of the QI project.

What Is Being Measured?

In 1980, Donabedian[5] provided a useful framework for examining health services and evaluating the quality of healthcare, which encompasses 3 key components: structures, processes, and outcomes. In this model, structures refers to the context in which healthcare is delivered (eg, buildings, staff, equipment). Processes of care refer to the interactions between patients and providers through the delivery of healthcare (eg, did the patient receive X?). Outcomes refer to the effects of healthcare on the health status of patients and populations (eg, morbidity, mortality, quality of life). To understand whether a QI intervention works, the effects of processes of care on health outcomes are often measured. For example, did receipt of patient-tailored discharge instructions (process of care) improve caregiver perceptions of self-efficacy (outcome) after discharge from the hospital? This article focuses on measurement of processes of care (process metrics) as well as health outcomes.

Process metrics within PHM are often categorized as monitoring, treatment, safety, and communication. **Table 1** provides examples of some of the most commonly used

Table 1
Sample process metrics and outcome measures in pediatric hospital medicine

Type of Measure	Measure	Source	Description
Process Metrics			
Monitoring, treatment, communication	Pediatric Respiratory Illness Measurement System (PRIMES)[27]	Medical record	76 evidence-based quality indicators for asthma (n = 36), bronchiolitis (n = 18), community-acquired pneumonia (n = 7), and croup (n = 15) to assess the quality of care in hospital settings
Monitoring, treatment	Choosing Wisely recommendations[28]	Administrative, medical record	5 recommendations to discourage the use of non–evidence-based monitoring and treatment in pediatric inpatients
Safety, communication	I-PASS Handoff assessment tools[29]	Observation	Assessment tools to assess the skills of the giver and receiver of verbal handoffs, as well as to assess the quality of a printed handoff document
Safety, communication	Center of Excellence on Quality of Care Measures for Children with Complex Needs (COE4CCN) care transitions measures[30–32]	Medical record, survey	11 evidence-based metrics related to emergency department-to-home transitions (n = 2), hospital-to-home transitions (n = 8), and intensive care unit-to-floor transitions (n = 1), assessing the quality of discharge education, written discharge instructions, communication between providers, and scheduling follow-up appointments
Outcome Measures			
Health status	Pediatric Quality of Life Inventory (PedsQL) 4.0 Generic Core Scales and PedsQL Infant Scales[33]	Survey	23–45 items (depending on scale and age-group) to assess child health-related quality of life categorized in 4 domains: physical functioning and/or physical symptoms, emotional functioning, social functioning, school or cognitive functioning

(*continued on next page*)

Table 1 (*continued*)			
Type of Measure	**Measure**	**Source**	**Description**
Safety	Medication errors or adverse events[34,35]	—	Various methodologies have leveraged information technology to detect adverse event rates in a systematic way rather than relying on spontaneous reporting, which is known to only detect a minority of errors and adverse events
Patient or family experience	Child Hospital Consumer Assessment of Healthcare Providers and Systems (Child HCAHPS)[36]	Survey	39 items to assess the patient and family experience with inpatient care categorized in 5 domains: communication with parent, communication with child, attention to safety and comfort, hospital environment, and global rating
Psychosocial	Missed school or work	Survey	Typically includes duration of missed school or work while in the hospital and during the recovery phase posthospitalization
Healthcare utilization	Length of stay	Administrative, medical record	Typically measured in hours or days
Healthcare utilization	Readmissions or emergency department return visits	Administrative, medical record, survey	Typically measured as 7-d, 14-d, or 30-d, and categorized as all-cause vs disease-specific or unplanned vs planned readmissions

process metrics that are assessed in the inpatient setting; however, a wide variety of process metrics exist because they depend significantly on the intervention being measured and the context in which the intervention is occurring.[6,7] For the purpose of QI evaluation, process metrics should encompass all aspects of health services delivery using a multidisciplinary approach. For example, for patients hospitalized for an asthma exacerbation, this may include an assessment of (1) obtaining an oxygen saturation measurement in the emergency department (monitoring process metric related to nursing workflow), (2) delivery of a medication within a specific time frame (treatment process metric related to pharmacy workflow or respiratory therapy support), and (3) provision of an asthma action plan (communication process metric related to physician workflow and potentially information technology infrastructure). Using a multidisciplinary approach to QI evaluation ensures that the quality and efficiency of all processes of care that may interface with all relevant stakeholders are being optimized.

One of the challenges of collecting process measures is that it often relies on having reliable, standardized documentation that can be readily abstracted from the electronic medical record. A general rule of thumb for process metrics is that if it is not documented then the interaction did not happen, which may lead to an underestimation of process completion with poor documentation practices or an overestimation of process completion with autopopulated templates that do not accurately reflect the provision of care.

Health outcomes within PHM commonly encompass biomarkers (eg, glycemic control), symptomatology (eg, pain), health status (eg, health-related quality of life), patient safety, patient and/or family experiences with care, psychosocial measures, and healthcare utilization measures, such as length of stay, emergency department (ED) revisits, readmissions, and hospital costs. **Table 1** also reviews some of the more commonly used health outcome measures in PHM. Whenever possible, efforts should be made to elicit the patient and/or family's perspective in QI research because they are the ultimate recipient of care in the hospital setting, and they are likely the best person or persons to evaluate whether the child received high-quality care.[8]

SOURCES OF EXISTING MEASURES IN PEDIATRIC HOSPITAL MEDICINE

Several national repositories of measures have been developed that house validated and previously implemented measures of performance across a variety of clinical domains. A common challenge in the identification of potential existing measures is that a unified repository does not exist; rather, there are numerous national quality measure collections that pertain to pediatric providers. Perhaps the most widely used of these measure databases include the Quality Positioning System (QPS), which is a Web-based tool developed by the National Quality Forum (NQF) to help with the selection and identification of measures.[9] The QPS includes measures that have achieved NQF-endorsement, which is reserved for measures that have been reviewed and recommended through an intensive multistakeholder process. Currently, approximately more than 1000 measures are available through QPS.

The Centers for Medicare and Medicaid Services (CMS) also oversee a quality measure repository, referred to as the CMS Quality Measure Inventory, which compiles measures used by CMS in various quality, reporting, and payment programs.[10] The Inventory lists each measure by program, reporting measure specifications, including but not limited to numerator, denominator, exclusion criteria, Meaningful Measures domain, measure type, and NQF endorsement status.

An additional commonly applied measure set is the Healthcare Effectiveness Data and Information Set (HEDIS), a widely used set of performance measures in the managed care industry that are developed and maintained by the National Committee for Quality Assurance.[11] HEDIS measures span 6 domains of care, including effectiveness of care, access or availability of care, experience of care, utilization and risk-adjusted utilization, health plan descriptive information, and measures collected using electronic clinical data systems. Because HEDIS measures are based primarily on analyses of administrative data sets, their utility is sometimes challenged because different healthcare plans may use different data collection methods and, therefore, lead to inconsistent conclusions about the quality of care delivered by various providers. Additionally, many HEDIS measures focus on aspects of care overseen primarily in ambulatory settings, so there may be less relevance for pediatric hospital inpatient medicine.

The Patient-Reported Outcomes Measurement Information System (PROMIS) is a set of person-centered measures that evaluate and monitor physical, mental, and social outcomes through patient self-reporting mechanisms.[12] More than 25 pediatric-specific measures are available that involve either self-report (ages 8–17 years) or parent proxy (ages 5–17 years). Benefits of PROMIS measures include that they are freely available, they can be administered in multiple ways, and translated versions are available in Spanish and many additional languages in addition to English.

In addition to those previously described, several additional measure repositories are frequently cited and used as a resource for PHM QI leaders. The Joint Commission maintains a set of core measures, many of which are relevant to pediatric providers.[13] In addition, the Agency for Healthcare Research and Quality has developed a set of Pediatric Quality Indicators, which is a set of measures that can be used with hospital inpatient discharge data to screen for potentially preventable complications and iatrogenic events for pediatric patients treated in hospitals, as well as preventable hospital admissions.[14] Given the abundance of available measures and measure repositories, there is an increasing need to streamline existing measures to ensure consistency when possible, as well as to carefully analyze the relative value of existing quality measures to better understand their potential impact on healthcare.[6]

SELECTING APPROPRIATE MEASURES

When designing a QI intervention, thoughtful consideration of process metrics and health outcomes that will be used to evaluate the effectiveness of the intervention should be determined from the outset. Do not just measure for measurement's sake. This section provides guidance on how to select appropriate process metrics and health outcomes in QI evaluation that recognize the unique contexts in which the intervention will take place.

The first step of selecting appropriate measures is to have a clear understanding of the ultimate goal of the intervention.[15] This requires defining the outcomes the intervention was intended to change. The categories described in **Table 1** may provide a useful guide for specifying these outcomes. Assessing more than 1 of these categories of outcomes may prove to be beneficial because a single intervention may have a significant impact on 1 aspect of quality and not on others. However, defining which outcome is the primary outcome of interest versus secondary outcomes should be determined up front to ensure the evaluation is adequately powered to detect a change in the desired outcome.[16] For example, 30-day readmissions continues to be a challenging outcome measure in pediatrics because the ability to detect reductions in readmissions is problematic given the limited number of these events in this population.[17] Furthermore, collecting baseline data on the outcome of interest is invaluable to determine whether there is room for improvement or whether there is sufficient variation to detect changes in response to the intervention. For example, if patient satisfaction scores are 98% with little variation, this should raise questions about whether this is the appropriate outcome of interest to measure or whether the intervention is even necessary.

Unfortunately, some health outcomes are not possible to obtain due to time and logistical constraints. In these cases, process metrics may provide a more proximal assessment of the effectiveness of an intervention if there is strong conceptual rationale linking the process metric to the intended outcomes.[15] Process metrics tend to be more difficult to select because they are highly context and intervention dependent, though key driver diagrams can be useful tools to identify processes of care that affect an intended outcome.[18] (See Anupama Subramony and colleagues' article, "Pediatric Hospitalists Improving Patient Care through Quality Improvement," in this issue.) Therefore, process metrics can be selected (or developed) for each of these key drivers. For example, if the goal of a hospital is to improve communication between providers and families with limited English proficiency, the hospital may choose to implement a QI intervention focused on the use of professional interpreters. If the hospital is unable to obtain outcome measures of communication quality directly from patients and/or family caregivers, a process metric such as the number of times professional interpretation was used in encounters with the family may serve as a proximal measure of the effectiveness of this intervention.[19]

Once process metrics and outcomes are specified, conducting a thorough search of the published literature on the intervention and measures of interest is a useful strategy to identify existing process metrics and outcomes that may be applicable to one's own QI evaluation. A comprehensive literature search may reveal measures that have established validity and reliability for use in a specific context. Whenever possible, these validated measures should be selected over de novo measures to optimize the credibility of the QI evaluation. However, if an existing measure is to be used in a population or manner in which it was not originally validated, further validation in the context of interest should be conducted to enhance measurement accuracy. For example, a survey measure is no longer considered to be validated if one picks and chooses survey items from a measure that was intended to be used and validated in its entirety.[20]

Finally, selecting appropriate measures requires careful consideration of the available resources to collect the data. Survey-based measures are more resource-intensive and costly to administer; however, they may also provide a more accurate patient-centered perspective. In contrast, administrative data are often easier to obtain (especially with the advent of large pediatric hospital databases such as the Pediatric Health Information System); however, measures within this dataset may not be relevant to the specified process metrics or outcomes of interest, which may produce inconsequential findings.

DEVELOPING NEW MEASURES

On occasion, existing validated patient-centered process metrics or outcomes that are relevant to the intervention or evaluation of interest are not available, and clinicians, researchers, or administrators may need to develop de novo measures to evaluate the effectiveness of their QI initiatives. This section provides a blueprint for developing new process metrics or outcomes that may be used in PHM, as summarized in **Fig. 1**.

Conducting a thorough literature review of the topic area of interest is the first step to identify (1) that there is indeed a gap in available measures that can be used for the evaluation and (2) published studies demonstrating an association between

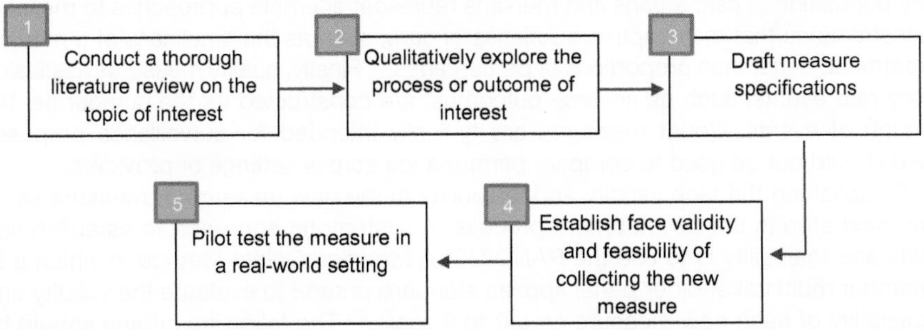

Fig. 1. Process for developing new process and outcome measures for QI research.

processes of care and health outcomes. In the case of process metrics, a stronger association between the process of care and health outcomes will lead to a more valid measure.[21]

If the evidence-base for a process of care or health outcome is weak, the next best step is to conduct a qualitative exploration of the process of care or health outcome of interest.[22] This may include direct observations of the current state (eg, time and motion studies); key informant interviews; or focus groups to elicit stakeholder needs, priorities, and constraints. This will help to establish content validity of the new measure.

The next step is to draft the measure and its specifications, which requires first and foremost identifying the appropriate source for data collection.[23] A variety of different sources of data are available, including administrative (eg, insurance claims reports), medical record (obtained via automated extraction vs manual chart review), patient or provider surveys, and hybrid mechanisms that use a combination of sources. In general, the selection of the appropriate source depends on a variety of factors. For example, in the case of patient and/or family experience measures, the best source is likely a survey-based measure that relies on patient-reported or caregiver-reported data. Alternatively, the best source for a process metric related to narrow-spectrum antibiotic administration for community-acquired pneumonia may be electronic or manual abstraction of medical record data. Additionally, for each measure, the following pieces of information should be clarified to ensure accurate and standardized measurement across patients and populations: (1) inclusion and exclusion criteria (eg, *International Statistical Classification of Diseases and Related Health Problems*, 10th revision, codes), (2) unit of analysis (eg, patient, unit, hospital), (3) condition and severity (eg, mild persistent asthma), (4) assessment time-frame, and (5) a scoring algorithm. Often, a measure set versus a single measure may need to be developed to adequately capture all the important constructs for a given process of care or health outcome.

An important step in the drafting of measure specifications is to consider how the measure will be best constructed. Common measure frameworks include proportions, percentages, ratios, means, medians, and counts.[24] The selection of the approach depends on the specific circumstance and objective of the measure and improvement initiative. Most measures are reported as proportions (typically described as percentages), in which the denominator represents the number of persons treated by a health care provider during a defined time period who were at risk of, or eligible for, the event being described in the numerator. Proportions benefit because they are relatively easy to understand and, therefore, are actionable by providers and improvement leaders. In contrast, in a ratio measure, the denominator represents the best available estimate of the population at risk for the event being measured in the numerator. Ratios are comparatively more difficult to interpret than traditional proportions and it is sometimes unknown to what extent the denominator truly serves as a proxy for measurement of the population at risk. Means and medians represent alternate approaches to measure constructions that may capture subtleties of care, such as the timeliness of a medical treatment, better than proportions or percentages.[24] Finally, quality measures assessing very rare events, such as adverse outcomes, are constructed as the number (ie, the count) of events. Count measures are typically intended for surveillance purposes and should not be used to compare performance across settings or providers.

Establishing the face validity and feasibility of the new measure or measure set is the next step in the development process. A systematic approach to establish validity and feasibility is to use the RAND/UCLA Modified Delphi Method in which a 9-member multistakeholder panel applies standard criteria to evaluate the validity and feasibility of each new measure on a 0 to 9 scale.[25] The following criteria should be applied to assess the validity of a measure: (1) there should be adequate evidence or expert consensus to support the measure, (2) there should be identifiable health benefits associated with receiving the measure-specified care, (3) that providers and provider groups who adhere more consistently to the measure be regarded as providing higher-quality care, and (4) that adherence to the measure is in the control of providers or the health care system. The following criteria should be applied to assess the feasibility of a measure: (1) the measure includes content a typical respondent would be able to correctly identify, recall, and report within the specified time frame, and (2) quality assessments based on the measure would be reliable and unbiased. A standardized scoring system is then used to determine whether the measure or measure set exceeds an acceptable level of face validity and feasibility.

An additional method to strengthen the face validity of new survey-based measures is to conduct cognitive interviews with a representative sample of potential respondents. Cognitive interviews are usually audio-recorded and participants are asked to think aloud as they complete survey items to uncover issues related to the interpretability, understandability, recall, decision processes, and response processes of each survey item, and to provide feedback on the general survey structure.[26] The survey is iteratively revised between rounds of cognitive interviews until participants reveal minimal issues with the survey items and structure.

The final step in measure development is to pilot test the measure in a real-world setting. Operationalization of the measures helps in understanding limitations related to feasibility of data collection (eg, response rates for survey-based measures or time required for medical abstraction) and the integrity of the data (eg, discrepancies in documentation to compute measure scores). Analysis of pilot test data also helps to uncover measurement issues, such as ceiling or floor effects of the measure, limited variation, and sample size requirements. For survey-based measures, analysis of pilot test data allows for psychometrics, examination of missing data, response biases, or significant differences in scores among subgroups that may require case-mix adjustment. Finally, simultaneous data collection of similar measures during the pilot test may allows for additional analyses to establish construct validity of the new measure, further strengthening the quality of subsequent evaluations that will use the new measure or measure set.

PRESENTATION AND DISSEMINATION OF MEASURES TO MAXIMIZE IMPACT

Although the process of measure development is critical, it is just as important to give careful consideration to how the outputs of measurement efforts will be achieved and ultimately presented and disseminated to key stakeholders. To maintain consistency of measurement over time and to facilitate clarity of communication, it is typically helpful to carefully document all aspects of a measure, such as through the sample measurement plan provided in **Fig. 2**. When considering how to present and display measurement findings, generally it is most common for QI efforts to trend data over time using a graphical display such as a run chart. This methodology is often preferred because this approach offers a timely visual picture of whether the improvement effort is working. Run charts can be modified into control charts (ie, statistical process control charts) by placing control limits of the process on the graph. In this way, data points that fall outside a control line indicate a meaningful change in the process being measured.

Whether presented as a run chart, a control chart, or an alternate means of display (eg, funnel plots, scatter plots, bar charts), visual displays of data should be reviewed regularly with key stakeholder providers to review progress and updated findings. Data can be posted in a visible area that is accessible to providers and can also be

Project Title:

Project Leader(s):

Background / Rationale:

SMART AIM:

Measure(s):

Type: ☐ Outcome ☐ Process ☐ Balance

IOM Domain: ☐ Safety ☐ Efficient ☐ Effective ☐ Equitable ☐ Timely ☐ Patient– Centered

Anticipated Measurement Challenges:

Source / References:

Measure Detail	**Description**	**Technical Specifications**
Measure Definition	**Numerator:** **Denominator:** **Inclusion criteria:** **Exclusion criteria:**	**Numerator:** *List ICD codes that will be used to define the numerator* **Denominator:** *eg admissions in specified time period (ex: 1/1/2014-12/31/2014)* **Inclusion criteria:** *ICD codes (specify primary only or primary and secondary)* **Exclusion criteria:** *All admissions with specific ICD diagnoses codes*
Stratifiers/Risk Adjustment	Describe how data should be grouped *Ex: stratify all admissions by age groups <5 years old, between 5-10, >5 years old*	Age definition: *Ex: clarify if age on date of discharge, date of admission, or according to DOB during measurement period*
Data Source & Sampling Method		*If chart review, how many sampled? Method used?*
Data Analysis		*Describe how often data should be analyzed.*
Data Display	*Eg run chart*	

Fig. 2. Sample quality measurement plan. DOB, date of birth; ICD, *International Statistical Classification of Diseases and Related Health Problems*, 10th revision; IOM, Institute of Medicine; SMART, specific, measurable, achievable, relevant, and time-bound. (*Adapted from* the Quality Measurement Plan developed by members of the Boston Children's Hospital Department of Pediatrics Quality Program including Prerna Kahlon, Taruna Banerjee, and Patty Meleedy-Rey; with permission.)

shared electronically (eg, via email) on a regular basis to enhance awareness and communication. For each measure being evaluated, it is helpful to develop a data collection plan and reporting process for the team that identifies who is responsible for collecting the data, how often it will be collected, how it will be reported to champions and front-line providers, who is responsible for reporting it, and how often it will be reported. A sample data collection and reporting plan template is provided in **Fig. 3**.

Measure (with operational definition)	Who Collects the Data?	Collection Frequency	How is it reported to key stakeholders	Who reports it?	How Often Is It Reported?	Notes
Eg: Readmission rate (the percentage of admissions who are subsequently readmitted to the hospital medicine service within 30 d of discharge)	Quality improvement consultant	Monthly	Display on QI board, incorporation in QI newsletter	Hospital medicine QI directors	Quarterly	Aim to reduce rate by 5% prior to July 2019

Fig. 3. Sample measure collection and communication plan.

SUMMARY

Measurement is a key component of PHM because it drives ongoing improvement across institutions and between providers, with the goal of ensuring higher value care and improved outcomes. When selecting, developing, and implementing measures, it is highly important to ensure that selected measures align with improvement goals. Multiple categories of process and outcome measures are available across an abundance of measure repositories with a variable extent of validation. When it is necessary to develop novel measures, specific steps and frameworks are available to guide the development process and ensure high-quality outputs.

REFERENCES

1. Varkey P, Peller K, Resar RK. Basics of quality improvement in health care. Mayo Clin Proc 2007;82(6):735–9.
2. Barrett DJ, McGuinness GA, Cunha CA, et al. Pediatric hospital medicine: a proposed new subspecialty. Pediatrics 2017;139(3). https://doi.org/10.1542/peds.2016-1823.
3. SECTION ON HOSPITAL MEDICINE. Guiding principles for pediatric hospital medicine programs. Pediatrics 2013;132(4):782–6.
4. Six Domains of Health Care Quality. Available at: https://www.ahrq.gov/talkingquality/measures/six-domains.html. Accessed December 22, 2018.
5. Donabedian A. The quality of care: how can it be assessed? JAMA 1988;260(12):1743–8.
6. House SA, Coon ER, Schroeder AR, et al. Categorization of national pediatric quality measures. Pediatrics 2017;139(4):e20163269.
7. Reyes MA, Paulus E. The landscape of quality measures and quality improvement for the care of hospitalized children in the United States: efforts over the last decade. Hosp Pediatr 2017;7(12):739–47.
8. Epstein RM, Street RL. The values and value of patient-centered care. Ann Fam Med 2011;9(2):100–3.
9. NQF: Quality Positioning System ™. Available at: http://www.qualityforum.org/Qps/. Accessed December 22, 2018.
10. Medicare C for, Baltimore MS 7500 SB, Usa M. CMS Measures Inventory. 2018. Available at: https://www.cms.gov/Medicare/Quality-Initiatives-Patient-Assessment-Instruments/QualityMeasures/CMS-Measures-Inventory.html. Accessed December 22, 2018.
11. HEDIS. NCQA. Available at: https://www.ncqa.org/hedis/. Accessed December 22, 2018.
12. Intro to PROMIS. Available at: http://www.healthmeasures.net/explore-measurement-systems/promis/intro-to-promis. Accessed December 22, 2018.

13. Measures | Joint Commission. Available at: http://www.jointcommission.org/core_measure_sets.aspx. Accessed December 22, 2018.
14. AHRQ - Quality Indicators. Available at: https://www.qualityindicators.ahrq.gov/modules/pdi_overview.aspx. Accessed December 22, 2018.
15. McGlynn EA, Halfon N. Overview of issues in improving quality of care for children. Health Serv Res 1998;33(4 Pt 2):977–1000.
16. Berry JG, Zaslavsky AM, Toomey SL, et al. Recognizing differences in hospital quality performance for pediatric inpatient care. Pediatrics 2015;136(2):251–62.
17. Bardach NS, Vittinghoff E, Asteria-Penaloza R, et al. Measuring hospital quality using pediatric readmission and revisit rates. Pediatrics 2013;132(3):429–36.
18. Institute for Healthcare Improvement: Driver Diagram. Available at: http://www.ihi.org/resources/Pages/Tools/Driver-Diagram.aspx. Accessed June 28, 2018.
19. Byron SC, Gardner W, Kleinman LC, et al. Developing measures for pediatric quality: methods and experiences of the CHIPRA pediatric quality measures program grantees. Acad Pediatr 2014;14(5):S27–32.
20. Juniper EF. Validated questionnaires should not be modified. Eur Respir J 2009;34(5):1015–7.
21. McGlynn EA, Adams JL. What makes a good quality measure? JAMA 2014;312(15):1517.
22. Patrick DL, Burke LB, Gwaltney CJ, et al. Content validity–establishing and reporting the evidence in newly developed patient-reported outcomes (PRO) instruments for medical product evaluation: ISPOR PRO Good Research Practices Task Force report: part 2–assessing respondent understanding. Value Health 2011;14(8):978–88.
23. Understanding Data Sources|Agency for Healthcare Research & Quality. Available at: https://www.ahrq.gov/professionals/quality-patient-safety/talkingquality/create/understand.html. Accessed June 28, 2018.
24. Selecting quality and resource use measures: a decision guide for community quality collaboratives. Available at: https://www.ahrq.gov/sites/default/files/publications/files/perfmeas.pdf. Accessed April 9, 2019.
25. Brook R. The RAND/UCLA appropriateness method. In: McCormick KA, Moore SR, Siegel RA, editors. Methodological perspectives. Rockville (MD): US Department of Health and Human Services; 1994.
26. Willis GB. Cognitive interviewing: a tool for improving questionnaire design. Thousand Oaks (CA): Sage Publications; 2004.
27. Mangione-Smith R, Roth CP, Britto MT, et al. Development and Testing of the Pediatric Respiratory Illness Measurement System (PRIMES) quality indicators. Hosp Pediatr 2017. https://doi.org/10.1542/hpeds.2016-0182.
28. Quinonez RA, Garber MD, Schroeder AR, et al. Choosing wisely in pediatric hospital medicine: Five opportunities for improved healthcare value. J Hosp Med 2013;8(9):479–85.
29. Starmer A, Landrigan C, Srivastava R, et al. I-PASS Handoff Curriculum: Faculty Observation Tools. MedEdPORTAL 2013;(9). https://doi.org/10.15766/mep_2374-8265.9570.
30. Leyenaar JK, Desai AD, Burkhart Q, et al. Quality measures to assess care transitions for hospitalized children. Pediatrics 2016;138(2). https://doi.org/10.1542/peds.2016-0906.
31. Desai AD, Burkhart Q, Parast L, et al. Development and pilot testing of caregiver-reported pediatric quality measures for transitions between sites of care. Acad Pediatr 2016;16(8):760–9.

32. Parast L, Burkhart Q, Desai AD, et al. Validation of new quality measures for transitions between sites of care. Pediatrics 2017;139(5):e20164178.
33. Desai AD, Zhou C, Stanford S, et al. Validity and responsiveness of the pediatric quality of life inventory (PedsQL) 4.0 generic core scales in the pediatric inpatient setting. JAMA Pediatr 2014;168(12):1114–21.
34. Bates DW, Evans RS, Murff H, et al. Detecting adverse events using information technology. J Am Med Inform Assoc 2003;10(2):115–28.
35. Bates DW, Cullen DJ, Laird N, et al. Incidence of adverse drug events and potential adverse drug events. Implications for prevention. ADE Prevention Study Group. JAMA 1995;274(1):29–34.
36. Toomey SL, Zaslavsky AM, Elliott MN, et al. The development of a pediatric inpatient experience of care measure: child HCAHPS. Pediatrics 2015;136(2):360–9.

Interprofessional Teams
Current Trends and Future Directions

Jennifer Baird, PhD, MPH, MSW, RN[a,*], Michele Ashland, BA[b], Glenn Rosenbluth, MD[c]

KEYWORDS

- Interprofessional teamwork • Interprofessional education
- Measurement of interprofessional practice • Family involvement

KEY POINTS

- Interprofessional teams help decrease traditionally siloed clinical and operational practices within healthcare organizations and can assist in the flattening of hierarchical power structures.
- Interprofessional practice requires a shift away from parallel working structures toward collaborative and synergistic engagement.
- Achievement of interprofessional practice requires an investment in interprofessional education for both trainees and practicing clinicians.
- Organizations should consider opportunities for family involvement on both clinical and operational teams.

INTRODUCTION

Interprofessional has become a popular buzzword in healthcare, espoused by professional organizations, accrediting agencies, and credentialing bodies.[1–3] The push toward interprofessional clinical and operational practice arose from a recognition that the historically siloed approach to care delivery, in which discipline representatives worked in parallel rather than in collaboration, limits the ability of providers to effectively tackle long-standing challenges and to achieve optimal outcomes for patients and families.[4] Siloes within clinical practice may contribute to serious safety consequences, with insufficient communication creating gaps in understanding that in turn create a risk for potentially harmful medical errors.[5,6] Siloing within operational

Disclosure statement: No disclosures.
[a] Institute for Nursing and Interprofessional Research, Children's Hospital Los Angeles, 4650 Sunset Boulevard, MS #74, Los Angeles, CA 90027, USA; [b] Lucile Packard Children's Hospital Stanford, 725 Welch Road, Palo Alto, CA 94304, USA; [c] Office of Graduate Medical Education, Pediatrics Residency Training Program, Department of Pediatrics, University of California, San Francisco, 5th Floor, Mission Hall Box 3214, 550 16th Street, San Francisco, CA 94143, USA
* Corresponding author.
E-mail address: jebaird@chla.usc.edu

Pediatr Clin N Am 66 (2019) 739–750
https://doi.org/10.1016/j.pcl.2019.03.003 pediatric.theclinics.com

practice may foster the maintenance of well-established power structures within healthcare organizations[7] that disadvantage nonphysician providers, patients, and families by limiting their contributions to the work of improving systems of care delivery.

This article discusses 2 types of interprofessional teams: those responsible for clinical care delivery in the inpatient setting and those that engage in operational work to improve care delivery systems. Both types of teams are composed of representatives from 2 or more professions working collaboratively and synergistically to achieve the team's goal, whether that goal is to successfully discharge a patient from the hospital or to redesign the medication ordering and administration process. This collaborative, synergistic work is what differentiates interprofessional teams from multidisciplinary teams. Members of multidisciplinary teams tend to work side-by-side and in parallel, rather than collaboratively, to achieve their goals.[8] The involvement of families as members of both types of teams has gained increasing acceptance in pediatric healthcare settings.[9]

This article identifies the advantages and challenges of working in an interprofessional team; the key components of interprofessional teamwork; and some examples of successful, evidence-based models of interprofessional clinical teams. It also addresses the growing field of interprofessional education (IPE) and strategies for incorporating families as members of the team. The article concludes with a discussion of strategies for assessment of interprofessional teamwork, the clinical and operational outcomes associated with interprofessional teamwork, and the current and future state of interprofessional practice in pediatrics.

ADVANTAGES OF AN INTERPROFESSIONAL TEAM

An interprofessional approach to practice has the potential to overcome many of the issues that arise from siloing by leveraging the unique skills and perspectives of a broader group of team members.[10] Teams composed of representatives from different disciplines can gain a more nuanced understanding of clinical and operational issues and can attend to these nuances when planning and implementing change, whether it is change to the patient's plan of care or a change in workflow within a department. For example, the addition of a case manager to the daily bedside rounding team might help to facilitate earlier discharge for a patient going home with a gastrostomy tube and feeding pump because the case manager's unique knowledge about the sequence of events necessary to obtain the supplies and support for a home feeding regimen will inform the patient's plan of care and the timeline for discharge. Likewise, the addition of a pharmacist to a workgroup on improving the accuracy of allergy documentation within the electronic health record may help physicians and nurses understand when and where this information is being used and the workflow consequences of missing and/or incomplete data. This information will, in turn, inform the creation of processes for documentation and standards for the timeliness of data capture.

WHAT MAKES A TEAM INTERPROFESSIONAL?

Ensuring appropriate team composition is a critical component of interprofessional practice. Hospital-based interprofessional teams are ideally composed of representatives from all relevant clinical services, with team composition varying based on the clinical or operational case at hand. At a minimum, most teams require physician, nurse, and patient or family involvement; however, rarely are these core members sufficient to create a full interprofessional team. For example, the clinical care team for a ventilator-dependent, developmentally delayed toddler admitted for pneumonia whose parents have limited English proficiency will be composed not only of physicians, nurses, and the parents but also a respiratory therapist, a pharmacist, and an interpreter. Depending on the length of stay and the other clinical and/or psychosocial concerns, the team may additionally involve physical and/or occupational therapists, a child life specialist, a chaplain, and a social worker. Similarly, an operational team charged with improving the timeliness of discharges on a medical unit will necessarily involve physicians, nurses, and pharmacists but may also involve representatives from social work, therapies, and the transport team, depending on the issues that arise. Organizations that have developed the culture and capacity to support consistent patient or family involvement will also have strong family involvement on such operational teams. (See Jennifer L. Everhart and colleagues' article,"Patient- and Family-Centered Care: Leveraging Best Practices to Improve the Care of Hospitalized Children," in this issue.) However, having the right team composition is not sufficient to make a team interprofessional. The hallmark of interprofessional team practice is the ability of the team to work collaboratively by eliciting, understanding, and synthesizing different professional perspectives into a cohesive whole that guides decision-making.[8] Interprofessional practice requires a shift in approach that gives value to diverse voices and perspectives, and that attempts to consistently integrate those perspectives into decision-making.[11] Therefore, it requires that the team come together with some regularity with a goal of listening to understand, and then turning the understanding into practice. **Table 1** contrasts interprofessional teamwork with traditional ways of working within the healthcare system.

The most successful interprofessional teams are deliberate in their work together, even when that work is time-limited to a specific project. They identify team roles, discuss preferred working patterns, and create an understanding of how decisions will be made. Most teams, for example, need a leader who is responsible for convening the team meetings, keeping the work of the team moving forward, and serving as a spokesperson for the team.[11–13] In the traditional paradigm, a physician would have served in this leadership role.[10] However, an interprofessional team could have a leader from any professional background. In the inpatient clinical setting, the team might be most effectively led by a provider who has a longitudinal relationship with the patient and who can, therefore, provide context to care planning and clinical decision-making.[14] Team members also need to decide how they can be most productive as a team, including the frequency, length, and format of meetings, and the value of using meeting times to provide updates versus completing work together.

The work of teams looks quite different for clinical versus operational teams. Clinical teams, particularly those providing care in the inpatient setting, rarely take the time necessary to define roles, working patterns, and decision-making. This is in part due to existing structures and processes that dictate roles and the work of these

Table 1
Traditional versus interprofessional teamwork

Traditional Teamwork	Interprofessional Teamwork
Discipline representatives work in parallel	Discipline representatives work collaboratively
Physician leadership	Expert leadership, regardless of discipline
Family as recipient of care	Family involvement in team discussions and decision-making
Hierarchical decision-making	Respect and incorporation of diverse viewpoints

teams, and in part due to the fluid nature of the team. Frequent rotations of team members on inpatient teams and varied workflows make it difficult to negotiate and establish team norms.[1] Operational teams may have the luxury of a more stable team composition and often try to set aside dedicated time for formal team meetings. These teams may need to spend time defining roles and the assigned work of each team member because existing structures and processes may not be present.

EVIDENCE-BASED MODELS OF INTERPROFESSIONAL TEAMS

Despite increased awareness of the value of interprofessional teamwork, practice in pediatrics still skews heavily toward a multidisciplinary approach wherein professionals work alongside, rather than in collaboration with, each other. There are, however, emerging models of interprofessional practice that point the way toward an evolution in care that better reflects the collaborative and synergistic impact of interprofessional teamwork.

One example of interprofessional teamwork in clinical practice is the pediatric palliative care (PPC) model. PPC teams, which are charged with providing supportive care and advanced care planning for children with complex and likely fatal conditions, have embraced an interprofessional approach.[15] These teams are typically staffed by a diverse group of clinicians, including physicians, advanced practice nurses, nurse care managers, social workers, chaplains, and (at times) expressive arts therapists and/or child life specialists. PPC teams work collaboratively to identify the patient and family's most significant needs, which can range from medical oversight and symptom management to spiritual support at the end of life, and then assign the appropriate team member or members to offer the needed level of support.[15,16] When functioning in the inpatient setting, the PPC team works alongside the primary team to complement and enhance the existing plan of care, and to offer support to primary team members who may struggle with how best to help families facing the decline and/or death of their child. Although formal evaluations of this interprofessional team-based approach as a model of care have yet to be conducted, the available evidence suggests that families find benefit from PPC services and report satisfaction with the team's care.[17,18] There is also limited evidence to suggest that initiation of PPC services may reduce healthcare utilization among certain groups of patients.[19–21]

An example of interprofessional teamwork in operational practice is the emergence of interprofessional quality improvement teams. These teams are charged with identifying gaps in the quality of care delivery and with designing, implementing, and refining interventions to close those gaps. For example, Cincinnati Children's Hospital has developed and implemented a multitiered quality improvement education curriculum designed to create interprofessional teams equipped with the knowledge and skills necessary to conduct quality improvement activities. This initiative has been successful in establishing improvement teams in divisions and departments across the organization, generating improvements to the quality of care delivery that otherwise would have taken much longer to achieve.[22] Other organizations have reported a similar approach to fostering interprofessional operational teamwork and are beginning to see the gains from these investments in time and resources.[23,24]

INTERPROFESSIONAL EDUCATION

Creating a healthcare system in which interprofessional practice is the norm requires extensive education across disciplines. IPE has, therefore, become an area of focus in clinical training programs. IPE, as defined by the World Health Organization (2010), occurs "when students from two or more professions learn about, from, and with each other to enable effective collaboration and improve health outcomes."[25(p13)] Guided by the Core Competencies for Interprofessional Collaborative Practice,[26] educators in programs across the United States are working to provide students with early and frequent exposure to opportunities for cross-disciplinary learning. These IPE activities take a variety of forms, including interprofessional course offerings, workshops and conferences, and simulation experiences.[27] Exposure to IPE enables students to understand diverse professional perspectives, identify the unique contributions and specialized roles of each profession, and begin to experiment with collaborative practice.

Healthcare organizations with training programs have an opportunity to build on students' early IPE exposure in the classroom setting by fostering IPE in the clinical setting for their trainees. Trainees in clinical residency programs (eg, physicians, nurses, pharmacists) can benefit from regularly scheduled IPE opportunities, often composed of a mixture of seminars, discussion sessions, and simulation and debriefing experiences. These types of events help to reinforce interprofessional practice among groups for whom regular clinical contact is likely during the course of their training.

Interprofessional practice should be highlighted to trainees as an opportunity to reinforce knowledge and skills in situ. Although learners on clinical rotations may not experience the technical definition of IPE if they are the only learners, faculty can reinforce opportunities to learn from other professions. For example, medical residents may learn about discharge medication reconciliation from a pharmacist, or a pharmacy student may learn about medication preparation and administration from a nurse. The term faculty should be used broadly to highlight all of the team members who may contribute to learners' educational experience.

Student and trainee IPE should be supplemented with ongoing IPE for practicing clinicians to fill knowledge and skills gaps that exist among those trained before the advent of IPE as an area of focus in professional curricula and to reinforce desired professional practice behaviors. The Agency for Healthcare Research and Quality's TeamSTEPPS (Team Strategies & Tools to Enhance Performance and Patient Safety) program provides a comprehensive curriculum that centers on interprofessional communication for clinical teams, with a focus on reducing error and improving patient safety by ensuring clear, consistent communication and the development of a shared mental model among members of the clinical care team.[28] **Table 2** outlines examples of IPE for different learner groups.

INCORPORATING FAMILIES AS PART OF THE TEAM

Continued evolution of the movement toward patient-centered and family-centered care delivery has created opportunities for families to engage as members of interprofessional teams.[1,9,14] There are a variety of ways in which families can engage as team members, ranging from participation with their child's clinical care team during an

Table 2
Example of interprofessional education

Learner Group	Example of Interprofessional Education
Prelicensure students	Interprofessional courses on patient and family communication, pharmacology, or pathophysiology
Postlicensure trainees	Role shadowing, residency seminars
Practicing clinicians	Simulation using TeamSTEPPS curriculum[28]

inpatient admission to membership on an organizational team charged with reviewing the quality and safety of care delivery across the hospital. (See Jennifer L. Everhart and colleagues' article,"Patient- and Family-Centered Care: Leveraging Best Practices to Improve the Care of Hospitalized Children," in this issue.)

Whatever the level of engagement, working with families as members of the interprofessional team requires an awareness of some practical considerations (**Fig. 1**).[29,30] First, respect for family members' time should be considered when planning team meetings. When feasible, meetings should be timed to accommodate family members' schedules such that participation on the team does not create an unnecessary burden for the family member. Second, if the family member's participation is on a team that affords a benefit to the organization (eg, an operationally focused team), the family member should be compensated for their time when possible. Third, thoughtful attention must be given to incorporating families onto the team, ensuring that clinicians' use of technical language and familiarity with existing clinical processes do not intimidate family members or make it difficult for them to share alternative perspectives. Similarly, clinicians should be prepared to listen to and thoughtfully evaluate ideas that may at first seem unrealistic or unfeasible. The generation of new ideas, some of which may be out of the box, is among the benefits of including family members on interprofessional teams[31] because family members are not as anchored in the structures and processes of the healthcare system and can, therefore, often offer a fresh perspective.

When families are provided an opportunity to fully participate, benefits accrue to team members, to the organization, and to the family participants. Among these benefits is the development of a shared understanding of the causes of clinical and/or

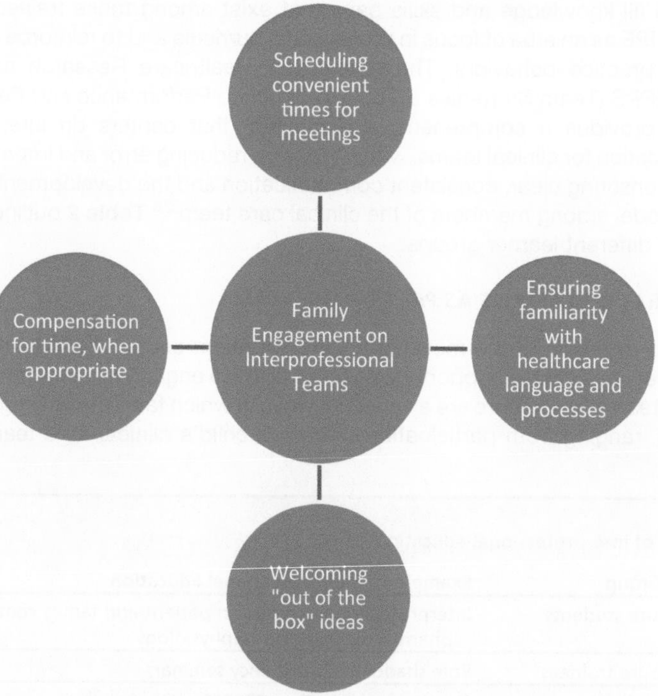

Fig. 1. Considerations for incorporating families into interprofessional teams.

operational problems and the potential solutions to these problems.[29,30] Without family participation, achievement of this shared understanding can be difficult, creating opportunities for misunderstanding that can impede progress and undermine relationships. Engagement of the family as part of the interprofessional team can additionally help to flatten the hierarchical power structures that typically exist within healthcare organizations. These power structures can make it difficult for patients and family members to question clinicians' decision-making and to advocate for their needs. When clinicians are given an opportunity to work alongside families as equal members of the team, they can develop a new appreciation for families' perspectives and an awareness of how best to engage them to promote optimal clinical outcomes. Finally, incorporating families into the interprofessional team can help families recognize both their power to affect change and their responsibility to play an active role in their child's care and in shaping the healthcare system to better meet families' needs. When families are invited and encouraged to show up as active participants, it creates a space for them to take ownership of their own care and to serve as advocates for others. The entire system can benefit as a result of this activation, and it can help to elevate the patient and family role to that of professional.

CHALLENGES AND STRATEGIES

Despite all of the exciting benefits that can occur from the work of interprofessional teams, there are nevertheless numerous challenges that these teams encounter. Although time is often cited as the most significant challenge, effective interprofessional work may actually save time. However, scheduling time for the team to be together is no small feat. Given the hectic nature of the inpatient care environment, it can be difficult to find a mutually agreeable time for a team meeting, whether the team is clinically or operationally focused. Scheduling times for the team to meet can be even more challenging when trying to incorporate family members, many of whom have work responsibilities that supersede their commitment to the team. As healthcare organizations expand to meet growing clinical needs, it is increasingly common for teams to work across campuses of the organization, making it also difficult to gather the team in 1 place for meetings or ongoing work. Technology can play an important role in lowering barriers.[1] Video conferencing creates opportunities for providers to be virtually present on rounds. Speaker phone calls on mobile devices enable family members and other caregivers to participate in discussions that they might otherwise miss.

Clinical teams also have the unique challenge of frequently changing team composition due to the rotating work schedules of physicians, nurses, and other clinical members of the team. These teams may find it difficult to establish roles and norms that enable the team to work in a truly interprofessional nature. Instead, the default may be to return to traditional ways of practice wherein discipline representatives work alongside each other without the full benefit of collaboration. This can be ameliorated through the development of standardized roles and workflows.[12] When every team member knows and follows their role on rounds, individual preferences and styles have less impact on the overall workflow. Team members may know, for example, that the nurse always presents the overnight events and the pharmacist always reviews the medications. In this scenario, new team members are aware of the expectations for their roles and require less orientation.

Patients and family members may require the greatest amount of orientation to their role, especially if the patient has not been previously hospitalized or has previously been admitted to a unit where interprofessional teamwork with family involvement was not the norm.[32] Orientation can be provided via brochures in an admission packet, in-person discussion with a provider, Web-based videos, and more. If expectations and opportunities for engagement are provided, patients and families can be empowered to speak up and take an active role on rounds and in other aspects of the patient's care.

MEASUREMENT OF INTERPROFESSIONAL TEAMWORK

The development of measures to capture the effectiveness of interprofessional teamwork has lagged behind efforts to incorporate interprofessional practice into healthcare organizations. Nevertheless, a variety of measures have been developed for use in both clinical and educational settings. The TeamSTEPPS Teamwork Perceptions Questionnaire (T-TPQ) is a 35-item survey designed to capture perceptions of teamwork across 5 domains: team structure, leadership, situation monitoring, mutual support, and communication.[33] The T-TPQ was developed by experts in teamwork and the TeamSTEPPS curriculum, and underwent cognitive interview, small group trial, and field testing phases. It was subsequently validated in a larger study of US Army medical personnel, generating evidence for both its reliability and validity.[34,35] A 20-item Brief T-TPQ has also been developed and has been validated for use with nurses in acute care settings.[36] Both the T-TPQ and the Brief T-TPQ rely on clinician report rather than direct observation and, therefore, provide perceptions of the teamwork environment rather than objective data about the presence or absence of characteristics associated with high-functioning interprofessional teams.

A second tool to measure perceptions of teamwork, the Assessment for Collaborative Environments (ACE)-15, was developed for rapid assessment of so-called teamness in clinical environments.[36] This tool was designed to facilitate quick identification of strong interprofessional teams with whom it would be beneficial to place learners needing exposure to interprofessional practice. It has 15 items and has undergone initial reliability and validity testing with clinicians in an urban academic medical center.[36]

The Individual Teamwork Observation and Feedback Tool (iTOFT) focuses on IPE and has 2 forms: an 11-item behavioral checklist for beginning students and a 10-item checklist for more advanced students and novice practicing clinicians. The checklist for beginning students assess teamwork behaviors in 2 domains: shared decision-making and working in a team. The checklist for advanced students and novice clinicians adds 2 additional domains: leadership and patient safety. It was developed by faculty from 7 universities across Australia, Canada, and the United Kingdom, and emphasizes the development of behaviors associated with strong interprofessional teamwork in the clinical setting.[37]

OUTCOMES OF EFFECTIVE INTERPROFESSIONAL TEAMWORK

Effective interprofessional teamwork can yield a variety of positive outcomes for patients, families, and healthcare organizations. It creates unique opportunities to identify problems before they occur and to create innovative solutions to current issues. On clinical teams, for example, having a pharmacist present when discussing a care plan may lead to the identification of drug–drug interactions or the need for therapeutic monitoring. Nurses may be able to cohort treatments and procedures (eg, phlebotomy) more effectively if they are given a voice in developing plans for patients. Perhaps most importantly, if the patient and/or family members participate as active team members, they may identify opportunities to improve care or to avoid potential errors and adverse events. On operational teams, the involvement of an interprofessional group of clinicians can help identify unique strategies for workflow improvements and may help the organization avoid trialing changes that are not clinically feasible or that are perceived to be unsustainable.

Patient and family satisfaction with care may also be affected by the extent to which teams demonstrate interprofessional collaboration. Family-centered rounds are among the most tangible ways that families can observe interprofessional teamwork in action, and they represent 1 of the few venues that families have for interacting with the team. Numerous studies have established the positive impact of interprofessional team involvement on rounds on patient and family satisfaction with inpatient care delivery.[32] Additionally, a recent study demonstrated that implementation of interprofessional family-centered rounds was associated with decreased rates of adverse events and improvements in family experience, suggesting that interprofessional teamwork can have multiple and varied positive effects on care delivery.[38]

Strong interprofessional teamwork can also foster employee engagement and may contribute to staff perceptions about the culture of safety within the organization. Many standardized engagement surveys include 1 or more questions on interprofessional teamwork, allowing staff to rate the extent to which they feel a part of a team and offering organizations the opportunity to identify opportunities for improvement in particular work areas. A variety of studies have demonstrated a positive association between interprofessional teamwork and employee wellbeing, including engagement with the organization.[39,40]

WHAT IS NEXT FOR INTERPROFESSIONAL PRACTICE?

As healthcare practitioners' understanding of the value of interprofessional practice continues to develop, driven in large part by the ability to quantify the outcomes of optimal interprofessional teamwork, so too will the sophistication of this type of practice. It is likely that interprofessional teams will increasingly incorporate quality improvement and/or human factors systems engineers, individuals who will help to facilitate continuous evaluation of practice and who will ensure a consistent focus on strategies for improvement.[41,42] The addition of these members to teams will bring a particular emphasis on mechanisms for enhancing the patient and family-centeredness of the care environment and the associated processes of care.

Additionally, it is likely that there will be a further shift of the power structure away from traditional hierarchies and toward patients and families, such that families may define or determine team composition, particularly for the clinical teams charged with their child's care. This shift will be accompanied by an evolution of the healthcare system's understanding of the role of the family, such that family members will be considered as vital professional members of the team, with a defined skill set and a unique body of knowledge that is central to optimal team functioning.

Interprofessional practice is increasingly moving away from buzzword status and into the formal lexicon of the healthcare system. As increasing numbers of clinicians gain experience learning from and working collaboratively with colleagues from a variety of professional backgrounds, the shift from multidisciplinary to interprofessional care delivery is occurring. The incorporation of families into the interprofessional team is also gaining traction, requiring thoughtful and deliberate efforts to flatten traditional hierarchies and accommodate new and diverse viewpoints. These efforts will collectively yield a healthcare delivery system that is more responsive to the needs of patients and families and that more consistently delivers safe, high-quality care.

REFERENCES

1. Mitchell PM, Wynia R, Golden B, et al. Core principles & values of effective team-based health care. Washington, DC: Institute of Medicine; 2012.
2. American Nurses Credentialing Center. Magnet recognition program: 2019 Magnet application manual. Silver Spring (MD): American Nurses Credentialing Center; 2017.
3. Accreditation Council for Graduate Medical Education, American Board of Pediatrics. The pediatrics milestone project. Chicago: ACGME; 2017.
4. Khalili H, Hall J, DeLuca S. Historical analysis of professionalism in western societies: Implications for interprofessional education and collaborative practice. J Interprof Care 2014;28:92–7.
5. Joint Commission. Inadequate hand-off communication. Sentinel Event Alert 2017;(58):1–6.
6. Leonard M, Graham S, Bonacum D. The human factor: The critical importance of effective teamwork and communication in providing safe care. Qual Saf Health Care 2004;13:i85–90.
7. Meleis AI. Interprofessional education: a summary of reports and barriers to recommendations. J Nurs Scholarsh 2016;48:106–12.
8. Choi B, Pak A. Multidisciplinarity, interdisciplinarity, and transdisciplinarity in health research, services, education, and policy: 2. Promoters, barriers, and strategies of enhancement. Clin Invest Med 2007;30:E224–32.
9. Katkin JP, Kressly SJ, Edwards AR, et al. Guiding principles for team-based pediatric care. Pediatrics 2017;140:1–7.
10. Wright D, Brajtman S. Relational and embodied knowing: Nursing ethics within the interprofessional team. Nurs Ethics 2011;18:20–30.
11. Hewitt G, Sims S, Harris R. Evidence of communication, influence, and behavioral norms in interprofessional teams: A realist synthesis. J Interprof Care 2015;29:100–5.
12. World Health Organization. Being an effective team player. Multiprofessional patient safety curriculum guide. Geneva (Switzerland): World Health Organizaition; 2011.
13. Ezziane Z, Maruthappu M, Gawn L, et al. Building effective clinical teams in healthcare. J Healthc Manag 2012;26:428–36.
14. American College of Physicians. Principles supporting dynamic clinical care teams. Philadelphia: American College of Physicians; 2013. Policy Paper.
15. Section on Hospice and Palliative Medicine and Committee on Hospital Care. Pediatric palliative care and hospice care commitments, guidelines, and recommendations. Pediatrics 2013;132:966–72.
16. Stayer D. Pediatric palliative care: a conceptual analysis for pediatric nursing practice. J Pediatr Nurs 2012;27:350–6.
17. Van der Geest IM, Darlington AE, Streng I, et al. Parents' experiences of pediatric palliative care and the impact on long-term parental grief. J Pain Symptom Manage 2014;47:1043–53.
18. Sheetz MJ, Bowman MA. Parents' perceptions of a pediatric palliative care program. Am J Hosp Palliat Care 2013;30:291–6.
19. Schmidt P, Otto M, Hechler T, et al. Did increased availability of pediatric palliative care lead to improved palliative care outcomes in children with cancer? J Palliat Med 2013;16:1034–9.

20. Friedrichsdorf SJ, Postier A, Dreyfus J, et al. Improved quality of life at end of life related home-based palliative care in children with cancer. J Palliat Med 2015;18: 143–50.
21. Smith AG, Andrews S, Bratton SL, et al. Pediatric palliative care and inpatient hospital costs: A longitudinal cohort study. Pediatrics 2015;135:694–700.
22. Kaminski GM, Schoettker PJ, Alessandrini EA, et al. A comprehensive model to build improvement capability in a pediatric academic medical center. Acad Pediatr 2014;14:29–39.
23. Bartman T, Heiser K, Bethune A, et al. Interprofessional QI training enhances competence and QI productivity among graduates: findings from Nationwide Children's Hospital. Acad Med 2018;93:292–8.
24. Larson DB, Mickelsen J, Garcia K. Realizing improvement through team empowerment (RITE): A team-based, project based multidisciplinary improvement program. Radiographics 2016;36:2170–83.
25. World Health Organization (WHO). Department of Human Resources for Health framework for action on interprofessional education and collaborative practice. Geneva (Switzerland): World Health Organization; 2010.
26. Interprofessional Education Collaborative Expert Panel. Core competencies for interprofessional collaborative practice: report of an expert panel. Washington, DC: Interprofessional Education Collaborative; 2011.
27. Fox L, Onders R, Hermansen-Kobulnicky C, et al. Teaching interprofessional teamwork skills to health professional students: A scoping review. J Interprof Care 2018;32:127–35.
28. Agency for Healthcare Research and Quality. TeamSTEPPS 2.0. Rockville (MD): Agency for Healthcare Research and Quality; 2018.
29. Agency for Healthcare Research and Quality. Working with patient and families as advisors: implementation handbook. Rockville (MD): Agency for Healthcare Research and Quality.
30. Institute for Patient and Family-Centered Care. Partnering with patients and families to enhance safety and quality: a mini toolkit. Bethesda (MD): Institute for Patient and Family-Centered Care; 2011.
31. Laurance J, Henderson S, Howitt PJ, et al. Patient engagement: four case studies that highlight the potential for improved health outcomes and reduced costs. Health Aff (Millwood) 2014;33:1627–34.
32. Rea KE, Rao P, Hill E, et al. Families' experiences with pediatric family-centered rounds: A systematic review. Pediatrics 2018;141:2–13.
33. American Institutes for Research. TeamSTEPPS® teamwork perceptions questionnaire (T-TPQ) manual. Washington, DC: American Institutes for Research; 2010.
34. Keebler JR, Dietz AS, Lazzara EH, et al. Validation of a teamwork perceptions measure to increase patient safety. BMJ Qual Saf 2014;23:718–26.
35. Castner J. Validity and reliability of the brief TeamSTEPPS teamwork perceptions questionnaire. J Nurs Meas 2012;20:186–98.
36. Tilden VP, Eckstrom E, Dieckmann NF. Development of the assessment for collaborative environments (ACE-15): A tool to measure perceptions of interprofessional "teamness. J Interprof Care 2016;30:288–94.
37. Thistlethwaite J, Dallest K, Moran M, et al. Introducing the Individual Teamwork Observation and Feedback Tool (iTOFT): Development and description of a new interprofessional teamwork measure. J Interprof Care 2016;30:526–8.

38. Khan A, Spector ND, Baird JD, et al. Patient safety before and after implementing a co-produced family-centered communication program: a multicenter pre-post intervention study. BMJ 2018;363:k4764.
39. Kaiser S, Patras J, Martinussen M. Linking interprofessional work to outcomes for employees: A meta-analysis. Res Nurs Health 2018;41:265–80.
40. Havens DS, Gittell JH, Vasey J. Impact of relational coordination on nurse job satisfaction, work engagement, and burnout: achieving the quadruple aim. J Nurs Adm 2018;48:132–40.
41. Carayon P, Wetterneck TB, Rivera-Rodriguez AJ, et al. Human factors systems approach to healthcare quality and patient safety. Appl Ergon 2014;45:14–25.
42. Salas E, Zajac S, Marlow SL. Transforming health care one team at a time: ten observations and the trail ahead. Group Organ Manag 2018;43:357–81.

Communication at Transitions of Care

Shilpa J. Patel, MD[a,*], Christopher P. Landrigan, MD, MPH[b]

KEYWORDS

• Handoffs • Transitions of care • Handovers • Patient safety • Culture of safety
• Structured communication

KEY POINTS

- Applying high-reliability principles to communication during transitions of care improves patient safety and culture of safety.
- Structured communication programs, such as the evidence-based I-PASS handoff bundle, are effective at standardizing processes to decrease adverse events.
- Structured handoff communication has added beneficial effects for the medical team beyond transitions of care.
- Workplace-based assessments with feedback aid in behavior change.
- Implementation of a successful and sustained handoff improvement program requires planning, high-level leadership support, and frontline provider input.

INTRODUCTION/ROLE OF COMMUNICATION IN MEDICAL ERRORS

Caring for patients in the hospital setting requires expertise, skill, and the seamless interplay of numerous intricate and delicately balanced processes. Health care workers undergo years of intensive training to obtain the knowledge and skills required to use the vast amount of evolving information available to them to best perform in their areas of expertise. This expertise is essential to clinicians seeking to diagnose

Disclosures: Drs C.P. Landrigan and S.J. Patel hold equity in and have consulted with the I-PASS Patient Safety Institute. The I-PASS Patient Safety Institute is a company that seeks to train institutions in best handoff practices and aid in their implementation. Dr S.J. Patel holds stock options in the I-PASS Patient Safety Institute. Dr C.P. Landrigan has received monetary awards, honoraria, and travel reimbursement from multiple academic and professional organizations for teaching and consulting on sleep deprivation, physician performance, handoffs, and safety, and has served as an expert witness in cases regarding patient safety and sleep deprivation.
[a] John A. Burns School of Medicine, Kapi'olani Medical Center for Women & Children, Hawaii Pacific Health, 1319 Punahou Street, 7th Floor, Honolulu, HI 96826, USA; [b] Boston Children's Hospital, Brigham & Women's Hospital, Harvard Medical School, 300 Longwood Avenue, Enders 1, Boston, MA 02115, USA
* Corresponding author.
E-mail address: Shilpa.patel@kapiolani.org

Pediatr Clin N Am 66 (2019) 751–773
https://doi.org/10.1016/j.pcl.2019.03.004
pediatric.theclinics.com

illnesses, develop and execute treatment plans, and ultimately improve patients' well-being. Doing so also requires tremendous coordination between teams of skilled individuals. Nurses, physicians, pharmacists, therapists, social workers, case managers, and a myriad of behind-the-scenes hospital workers must interact effectively in order for patients to receive high-quality care when hospitalized. Historically, however, health care provider training has been focused primarily on individual knowledge and skill development. Far less attention has been devoted to ensuring that health care workers are skilled in teamwork and communication skills, and have robust processes and tools in place to ensure optimal coordination. The manner in which information is transferred is critical to ensuring that desired outcomes are achieved. As one patient safety improvement–focused insurance organization has put it, "information is the currency of safe care, and communication is the vehicle by which that currency moves."[1]

When adequate communication does not occur in hospitals, patients often have poor outcomes[2] and incur large financial costs.[3] In response to data between 1995 and 2006[4] showing communication errors as the leading root cause of sentinel events, the Joint Commission established a National Patient Safety Goal that specifically addressed handoffs in the hospital. More recently, the Joint Commission has again highlighted the critical importance of communication failures as a root cause of sentinel events[5] and has begun to focus on this problem during periodic accreditation reviews of hospitals.

Miscommunications are a leading cause not only of sentinel events in hospitals but of malpractice claims.[1] The Controlled Risk Improvement Company Strategies' Comparative Benchmarking System represents the medical professional liability experience of more than 400 diverse hospitals and 165,000 physicians.[1] It found that communication was a factor in 30% of nearly 24,000 cases contributing to patient harm; 44% of these were in the inpatient setting and 37% of 8445 high-severity cases involved a communication failure.[1] Provider-to-provider communication errors accounted for 57% of all cases and provider-to-patient communication error cases comprised 55%, with a 12% overlap of causes.[1] Communication lapses occurred across all provider types (physicians of all specialties and nurses).[1] Investigations into these malpractice cases confirmed that miscommunication, noncommunication, or the assumption of communication not only triggers harm, it also fails to prevent harm.[1] As numerous as these cases are, malpractice claims represent only the tip of the iceberg because not all medical errors related to communication lapses are recognized or result in a claim.

Communication errors in the inpatient setting occur for a host of reasons. Within the complex environment of health care delivery, numerous process vulnerabilities and failures exist and contribute to so-called latent errors that can lead to patient harm,[6] despite the best of intentions and efforts. Vulnerabilities and process failures that may potentially contribute to communication failures include:

- Suboptimal workplace culture
- Excessive workload and work compression
- Distractions and interruptions in situations that require attention to detail
- Complex and suboptimally designed electronic health record (EHR) systems and processes
- Competing demands on health care providers during a clinical shift (eg, hospital, educational, clinical, or administrative meetings; teaching sessions; academic or research-based demands; quality improvement/patient safety initiatives)

- Siloing of responsibilities within hospital departments or divisions
- Work flow that precludes different groups of providers meeting in person
- Provider fatigue, burnout, and depression
- Increasing medical complexity of patients who have inadequate resources and support in the community setting

Transitions of care, such as when patients move from one hospital unit to another, or at shift changes, represent a particular vulnerability to communication failures. At transitions of care, providers typically hand off or hand over or sign out a patient to a receiving provider or team of providers; that is, they communicate with the receiving provider information about the patient. If not handled well, critical information can be lost or miscommunicated during these transitions, creating the potential for downstream medical errors.

However, it is important to point out that well-managed transitions can conversely provide an opportunity to improve patient safety and quality of care. Discussion of the patient with a provider unfamiliar with the patient can provide opportunities to avoid fixation bias, to uncover erroneous assumptions and thereby avoid errors, or to provide a fresh perspective on diagnosis or treatment. When done well, these interactions can promote a positive workplace culture and provide a time to learn clinical information and share clinical pearls.[7–10] The overall physical and cultural milieu of communication in general and for handoffs specifically reveals much about the culture of the workplace, which in turn is an important contributor to patient safety.[11]

In the current health care environment of compressed lengths of stay for patients, shortened duty hours for medical residents, and transfer of patient care between and within large care teams whose members have varying levels of formal handoff training, the potential for communication errors at transitions of care increases dramatically. Communication errors include omissions, miscommunications, incomplete or confusing communication, and misunderstandings. A surprising fact is that communication gaps have been found to occur more often among people who know each other well than those who do not, perhaps because familiarity leads to shortcuts in either the handoff process or the use of tools, or because overly colloquial or nonspecific language was used.[12,13]

Although communication errors may take many different shapes, the final common pathway is that there is a disconnect between the information the giver of a handoff intended to convey and what was actually received or comprehended by the receiver; that is, the giver and receiver of the handoff did not have the same understanding of the patient and plans after the handoff: they lacked a shared mental model.

EVIDENCE THAT IMPROVED HANDOFFS LEAD TO IMPROVED PATIENT SAFETY

As the health care system has become more attuned to concerns about patient safety in general and communication-related safety problems in particular, it has looked for solutions to other industries in which the consequences of communication failure are also high, such as nuclear power, aerospace, and transportation.[9,14] Lessons learned from these nonmedical industries combined with a growing body of patient safety/health services research show that improving communication reliability to improve patient outcomes requires using evidence-based interventions in the context of a receptive culture.[11,15,16] Evidence-based handoff systems that improve patient outcomes contain specific practices that promote and confirm a shared mental model between the giver and receiver of the handoff.[9,16–19] Providing information in a consistent and predictable manner improves communication[7,20,21] and can be facilitated by use of standardized tools and processes that support a structured format and a defined content for the handoff. Face-to-face communication with minimal interruptions and low ambient noise allows for clarifications, bidirectional information sharing, and a clear transfer of responsibility. In addition, maximizing team effectiveness by nurturing and modeling a culture of learning and transparency allows concerns to be raised, questions answered, and the development of a supportive team environment.[11,16]

From 2010 to 2011, the Children's Hospital Association implemented a 23-site children's hospital handoff collaborative that included a change package encompassing some of the elements described earlier and achieved a significant reduction in handoff-related care failures.[16] Notably, the collaborative studied a diverse group of providers (physicians of different disciplines, nurses) and handoff types (shift to shift, emergency department [ED] to inpatient, perioperative to inpatient, inpatient to radiology, inpatient to different inpatient unit).[16] They concluded that the 4 key handoff elements in the change packet (defined handoff intent, content, process, and maximized team effectiveness) led to standardized communication processes and increased reliability, regardless of the type of unit or provider, resulting in overall reduction in handoff errors and, therefore, likely a reduction in patient harm, although this was not directly measured.[16]

The I-PASS Handoff Study went a step further. Following a single-center pilot study that showed a reduction in medical errors after implementation of a handoff bundle,[22] the I-PASS Handoff Study was conducted from 2010 to 2013.[18] This study measured the effects of a resident handoff bundle implemented in 9 children's hospitals on medical errors and preventable adverse events; that is, injuries caused by medical errors.[18] The bundle included a series of complementary interventions designed to improve the handoff process: introduction of a novel mnemonic for oral and written handoffs to structure communication (I-PASS: illness severity, patient summary, action list, situation awareness, synthesis by receiver); changes to the verbal handoff process; introduction of a written handoff tool; teamwork and handoff training; faculty development; a campaign to raise awareness of the intervention; and a robust observation, feedback, and sustainability program.[18] Following implementation of I-PASS medical errors decreased 23% and, most importantly, preventable adverse events decreased by 30%.[18] Process measures such as inclusion of key elements in verbal handoff communication and in the written/printed documents showed significant improvements as well, with no significant change in the duration of handoff or in resident workflow.[18]

These studies provide evidence that structuring communication to facilitate development of a shared mental model allows health care workers of all types to communicate more reliably; to reduce medical errors; and, most importantly, to prevent harm to patients. Ideally, achievement of a shared mental model allows a comprehensive view of the patient that travels with the patient, across multiple providers and settings (**Fig. 1**).

CURRENT STATE OF HANDOFFS IN GRADUATE MEDICAL EDUCATION

The number of handoffs between resident physicians that a patient may experience is important to consider. After the 2003 and 2011 Accreditation Council for Graduate Medical Education (ACGME) duty hour changes, the average number of resident physicians caring for a patient and the number of transitions of care increased, prompting the investigators in one study to make a plea for increased supervision and training in handoffs.[23] The ACGME, recognizing this vulnerability, made care transitions one of its 6 key Clinical Learning Environment Review (CLER) topics, specifically addressing

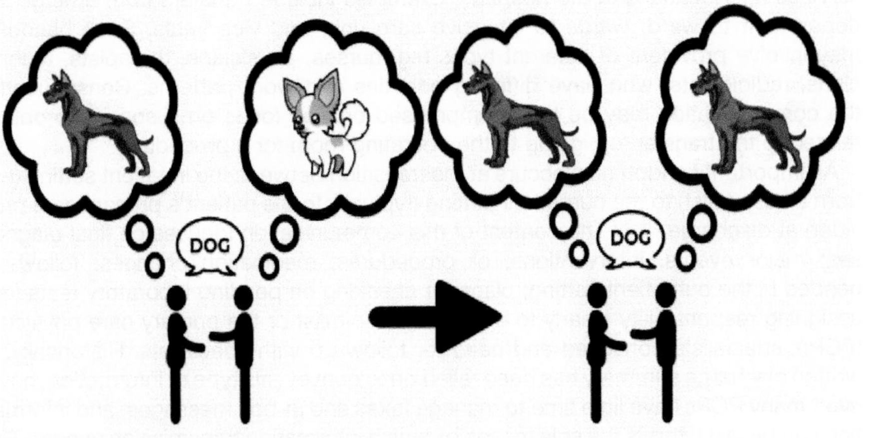

Fig. 1. Shared mental model. (*Courtesy of* Jensen Tabil.)

inpatient transition processes and change of duty transitions as 2 of the 4 major areas of focus. Three years of formative CLER visits revealed that resident physicians report using standardized processes for handoffs but there is not a standardized approach across programs within most institutions.[24] They also report that in most learning environments, when resident handoffs were observed, a standardized format (processes/tools/structure) was not confirmed and the handoffs did not include essential elements of reliable transitions of care.[24] In addition, they report that programs did not engage faculty members in performing resident/fellow observations with feedback, nor were the transitions of care inclusive of other team members such as nurses or pharmacists.[24] The report recommended the use of structured communication models such as the I-PASS program.[17,24] The CLER committee also recommended workplace-based assessments of both verbal handoff communication and of the written/printed handoff tool to ensure learning and reliable use of effective communication skills.[24] Of note, the I-PASS handoff program provides an evidence-based curriculum for residents and faculty that has been associated with reductions in medical errors and adverse events.[18,25–27]

VARIOUS TYPES OF HANDOFFS IN THE INPATIENT SETTING

The precise information transferred during a handoff varies according to the type of handoff, provider type, and unit or service. The most common handoffs in the inpatient setting are shift-to-shift handoffs among providers of the same type (eg, resident to resident, attending to attending, physician to physician, nurse to nurse). These handoffs occur when one provider is transferring care for a period of time to another provider, such as at the end of a day shift with plans to return the next morning. If the outgoing provider is transferring care for a longer period, the content of the handoff varies accordingly, with more attention to longer-term plans, discharge planning and goals, social issues, changes in care routine or medications from the care provided at home on admission, and caretaker/parental expectations.

Handoffs also occur when a patient moves from one location to another within the hospital. Transfers between locations include transient moves (eg, a patient going to radiology for a test) as well as more permanent ones (eg, a patient changing teams/

services and locations in the hospital). Examples include transfers from emergency department to ward, wards to intensive care unit, and vice versa. Such handoffs may involve providers of different types (eg, nurses, physicians, therapists, technicians, radiologists) who have differing priorities and work patterns. Consequently, the communication may be time compressed or may focus on a specific problem related to the transfer (eg, going to the operating room for a procedure).

An important handoff also occurs at the transition between the inpatient setting (eg, from a hospitalist) to the outpatient setting (typically to the patient's primary care provider) at discharge.[28–30] The content of this communication focuses on final diagnoses; major events, interventions, or procedures; medication changes; follow-up needed in the outpatient setting; plans for checking on pending laboratory tests (eg, assigning responsibility clearly to either the hospitalist or the primary care physician [PCP]); specialists consulted and need for follow-up with specialists. Historically, a written discharge summary has been relied on to convey this type of information; however, many PCPs have little time to manage faxes and in-box messages, and information can be lost if this is the sole means by which information transmission occurs. The discharge summary is a necessary and important document but can be laden with excess information that does not highlight the most salient points. A phone call from the inpatient team to the outpatient provider that allows for questions and clarifications supplements the discharge summary, just as the written/printed handoff complements the verbal handoff in a shift-to-shift handoff during hospitalization. In addition, including how the PCP can reach the discharging physician or a covering hospitalist is a key component of communication because issues may arise when the PCP sees the patient for the posthospitalization follow-up appointment.

Interprofessional communication (eg, during morning clinical rounds) can be considered yet another type of handoff in which hospitalists routinely engage. These handoffs may include hospitalists, subspecialists, nurses, case managers, child life, social workers, and pharmacists, as well as patients and families themselves. Transitions between individuals with different clinical backgrounds and perspectives can be particularly challenging, because it can be more difficult to ensure that all are on the "same page" following an exchange (See Jennifer Baird and colleagues' article, "Interprofessional Teams: Current Trends and Future Directions," in this issue). Principles of health literacy become particularly important in handoffs that involve patients and families directly, who may have varying levels of understanding of health and health care. Confirming a shared mental model by sharing information explicitly or by asking for a read back ensures that everyone is on the same page. Some early data suggest that efforts to improve these handoffs may also have a beneficial effect on patient safety (See Alexander F. Glick and colleagues' article, "Health Literacy in the Inpatient Setting: Implications for Patient Care and Patient Safety," in this issue).[31,32]

ELEMENTS OF EFFECTIVE HANDOFFS

An effective handoff develops and confirms a shared mental model of a patient and the treatment plans required to best fulfill the patient's needs. It should include both a verbal and a written component, consistently use a standardized format (the written/printed handoff structure should match the verbal structure, although the level of detail provided verbally and in writing may differ), and include essential processes to promote effective communication. The structured format provides the scaffolding on which content specific to unit, provider, or handoff type is organized and delivered. The unique elements should be informed by frontline providers in that workplace area and undergo tests of change in the clinical environment to ensure usability and inclusion of essential elements.[33]

All handoffs must have certain elements, which can be organized into environmental, process, verbal, and written communication categories.[33–37] (**Table 1** shows a list of essential elements for an effective handoff.) Some of these are global elements that include the environment in which the handoff takes place (eg, noise level, interruption potential) or involve the handoff process or work flow (eg, face to face, overlap of outgoing and incoming providers, expectation that the patient information has been updated by afternoon rounds, and "touching base" with other team members). Elements related to the actual verbal and written communication involve a structure (eg, I-PASS) as well as granular logistical and identifying patient information (eg, name, location).

Mnemonics for handoffs are abundant. Nasarwanji and colleagues[37] analyzed the literature from 1987 to 2008 and found more than 30 different mnemonics purportedly used for handoffs. They found that none of the published mnemonics contained all the important identified themes; however, there was agreement on 12 key themes of information that should be communicated.[37] One commonly used mnemonic, SBAR (situation, background, assessment, recommendation), was developed to communicate efficiently regarding a specific situation during which quick decisions must be made

Table 1
Elements of effective handoffs

Category	Elements to Consider/Include
Environmental	• Consistent location • Dedicated time • Limited interruptions • Limited noise levels
Process	• Face to face • At patient bedside • Overlap of outgoing and incoming providers • Clear transfer of responsibility • Appropriate pace • Updated written/printed handoff document • Recent information about patient (eg, recent examination of patient/check in with bedside nurse)
Verbal communication	• High-level overview (hospital level and team level) • Illness severity • Patient summary • To-do list • Contingency plans • Read back • Consideration of learning style of receiver
Written communication	• Location • Code status • Name • Weight • Allergies • Pertinent past medical history • Lines/drains/devices/airways • I-PASS mnemonic elements (illness severity, patient summary, action items, situation awareness, synthesis) • Consulting providers • Discharge goals for hospitalization

with limited key points of information.[17] Although the use of SBAR has been adopted for handoffs, it does not provide the structure needed to transfer information about complex patients or a panel of multiple patients. Multiple other mnemonics have been described, several of which are listed in **Table 2**.[16] **Table 3** describes the I-PASS mnemonic structure with description and rationale for the elements required for an effective handoff. **Table 4** provides an example of how the I-PASS mnemonic might be populated for a typical hospitalized pediatric patient.

An effective handoff can improve clinical reasoning and patient care skills. For example, the I-PASS mnemonic component patient summary typically includes 5 subsections (summary statement, events leading to admission, hospital course, ongoing assessment, overall plan) that can contribute to an articulated patient summary and link to illness scripts.[38,39] Likewise, the action list and the situation awareness components of the mnemonic can also help to promote discussion and a shared mental model with the interprofessional team during bedside rounds with the patient and family: reviewing the to-do items and the contingency plans during clinical work rounds helps to promote a shared mental model with all team members, including the patient/family and bedside nurse. The synthesis by receiver component of the I-PASS mnemonic also ensures a shared mental model: it allows the giver to confirm that they actually relayed what they wanted to relay. It requires practice and feedback to learn to provide a cogent read back that includes only the relevant elements and, when done well, the read back can provide a sort of reflection for givers that not only confirms their original understanding but illuminates new aspects that may not have been explicitly recognized.

THE PRINTED HANDOFF TOOL

Retention of verbally conveyed information is enhanced when supported by written/printed tools.[40,41] In addition, printed handoff tools can improve provider work flow and satisfaction, increase adherence to essential elements of standardized verbal communication structure,[33,35,42–44] and are associated with improved patient safety.[45] As such, most experts recommend a written/printed component to support and

Table 2
Examples of verbal handoff mnemonics in literature

Mnemonic	Description
HANDOFFS[79]	Hospital location, allergies, name, do not attempt resuscitation, ongoing medical/surgical problems, facts about this hospitalization, follow-up, scenarios
SIGNOUT[80]	Sick or do not resuscitate, identifying data (patient), general hospital course, new events of the day, overall health/clinical conditions, upcoming possibilities with plan, tasks to complete
IPASSTHEBATON[81]	Introduction (team), patient (identifiers), assessment, situation (eg, current medical status), safety concerns (eg, allergies), background (eg, comorbidities), actions, timing, ownership, next (eg, anticipatory guidance)
SBAR,[82] SBARR[83–85]	Situation, background, assessment, recommendation; response or read back
5Ps/6Ps[81,86]	Patient, plan, purpose, problems, precautions, progress
I-PASS[17]	Illness severity, patient summary, action list, situation awareness/contingency plans, synthesis or read back

Data from Refs.[37,77,78]

Table 3
An I-PASS handoff with high-level overview and rationale

Abbreviation	Element Title	Element Description	Rationale
I	Illness severity • Stable • Watcher • Unstable	• Describes how clinically active the patient's medical condition might be over next shift	• Hones the receiver's attention to the sickest patients
P	Patient summary	• One or 2 sentences that describe the patient: age, pertinent past medical history, active problems, overall treatment goals	• Develops a picture of the patient from which to consider primary problems and treatment goals • Provides framework for understanding this specific patient (pneumonia in a PH toddler vs an ex–24-wk preemie with VPS, GT, tracheostomy)
A	Action list	• What needs to be done for the next shift • To-do items that include timeline and ownership	• Highlights nonroutine items • Allows receiver to plan activities of shift • Specificity and ownership prevent duplicate or extraneous work and misunderstandings
S	Situation awareness/ contingency plans	• If/then statements that plan for events if patient has unexpected clinical status changes	• Allows receiver to anticipate, plan, and prepare for things that might go wrong • Gives receiver quick access to information that might be difficult to glean quickly from medical record • Shares contingency plans about interventions that were reviewed with patient/family
S	Synthesis by receiver	• Cogent synopsis of patient, active problems, action items • Clarifying questions asked	• Ensures giver and receiver have a shared mental model about patient, active medical problems, action items, contingency plans

Abbreviation: GT, gastrostomy tube; PH, previously healthy; VPS, ventriculoperitoneal shunt.

augment the verbal handoff structure for effective transitions of care communication.[4,46,47] When the elements in the printed tool include detail beyond the structure of the verbal handoff, the printed document can be used not only as a tool for transitions of care but also as a reference tool for routine workflow.[33]

Table 4
Example of I-PASS mnemonic used for verbal handoff for a specific patient

Overview	We have 16 patients on the team, 3 watchers, no one is unstable; there are 2 stable patients waiting to be admitted from the ED, 1 discharged patient waiting for ride home with nothing to do. Let's start with the first watcher…
I = illness severity	• Watcher
P = patient summary	• Johnny in room 222 is a 4-y-old previously healthy, immunized boy admitted with hypoxia, respiratory distress, and dehydration in setting of a right lower lobe community-acquired pneumonia with large pleural effusion • Blood culture resulted today with *Streptococcus pneumoniae* so switched from ceftriaxone and vancomycin to ampicillin. Today is day 2 of antibiotics • On 2-L nasal cannula with respiratory rates in the 40–60/s, highs with fevers only, overall trending down slowly. Of note, he has no breath sounds from midback down, +egophony • Still consistently febrile but C-reactive protein and white blood cell count down trending • On maintenance D5 normal saline with electrolytes and with good urine output but not eating or drinking, mostly because he has been sleeping for most of the day, although he is easily arousable. On intravenous ranitidine
A = action list	• Check respiratory status after sign out to get an idea of baseline work of breathing. • Check I + O at 2300 (see situation awareness)
S = situation awareness	• If increased respiratory distress or increased oxygen requirement, get chest radiograph with Nighthawk read to rule out worsening of effusion or empyema. If present, consider ultrasonography to see whether the effusion is loculated. Suggest calling surgery to discuss need for emergent chest tube • If fluid balance at 2300 is negative more than 300 mL, consider 20 mL/kg fluid bolus (because of large insensible losses); if fluid positive more than 300 mL, low urine output, and increased weight, consider SIADH • If concern for SIADH, order sequential metabolic panels and weights, fluid restrict
S = synthesis by receiver	• Should include key points from patient summary, action list, and situation awareness: ○ Concern for a pneumonia possibly evolving into an empyema ○ Concern for possible fluid status issues and with poor baseline oral intake, poor activity level ○ Action items include assessing respiratory status after sign out and I + O check ○ Contingency plans include considering need for chest tube or for SIADH

Abbreviations: I + O, ins and outs; SIADH, syndrome of inappropriate antidiuretic hormone.

Elements included in the printed tool vary based on handoff and provider type; however, essential elements across specialties and disciplines include patient identifiers, hospital service identifiers, admission date, allergies, medications, illness severity, patient summary, action items, and contingency plans. Recommended elements include items such as code status, primary care provider, access or devices, and primary language (see **Table 1**).[33,48]

The role of the EHR in supporting the use of the printed handoff tool is well documented.[33,35,42–44] Autopopulation of the printed tool by the EHR minimizes transcription and typographical errors and the need for manual duplication of information, and can reduce the amount of time spent recording some types of data about the patient.[43] The handoff communication is often not memorialized in the patient chart on discharge because it is considered a transient and evolving communication. Instead, information about patient progress and treatment plans are traditionally contained in the daily documentation, such as physician or nursing progress notes. An interesting cultural shift caused by documentation within the EHR is that it is increasingly considered by providers to be primarily for administrative, medical-legal, or billing purposes[49] instead of the traditional purpose of documenting the narrative about the patient's conditions, clinical decision making, treatment plans, and clinical progress.[50] As such, during an acute event, many providers are relying more and more on the handoff tool in the EHR to glean information needed for clinical decisions or the patient's story instead of the traditional sources such as physician and nursing progress notes, admission notes, or discharge summaries, from which it may be difficult to discern pertinent information to answer clinical questions quickly.[35,51] Studies examining the quality of printed handoffs maintained by resident physicians find that they contain some essential elements but not all, and they often lack key components such as clinical condition, tasks, and anticipatory guidance despite training and templating of the tool.[52,53] In one attending-focused study, although the handoff tool used by nighttime hospitalists was the first source of information for 74% of inquiries, it was considered sufficient to answer the question at hand in isolation only 30% of the time because of lack of contingency plans and action items.[51] Handoff curricula aimed not only at trainees but also at attending physicians (and nurses), with a component of just-in-time training can improve this, as shown by one quality improvement effort aimed at pediatric hospitalists. This project implemented a modified-for-attending-physicians I-PASS handoff bundle, and found significant improvement in written handoff tool elements, including accurateness of reason for admission, patient summary, medications, action items, contingency plans, and lines/devices. These improvements were sustained 12 months after initial implementation for all elements except patient summary.[10]

Most handoff tools within the EHR are designed for use by a single provider type and are often only visible in the EHR by that particular provider type. A study examining essential elements of handoffs for physicians and nurses found a 46% overlap between handoff elements, suggesting that interdisciplinary handoff element lists for key information types within the EHR could facilitate interdisciplinary communication, thereby reducing loss of information and errors of omission.[54] This form of asynchronous communication would be a particularly useful adjunct for transitions of care for short periods of time out of the primary unit, such as for procedures or therapies or diagnostics (eg, inpatient unit to perioperative services or to interventional radiology) or within a patient care unit where the patient undergoes frequent transfers to multiple different provider types (eg, for a procedure, a patient may be under the care of preoperative then intraoperative then postanesthesia providers of various types, including nurses, advanced practice providers, physicians, and technicians). Elements of inclusion relevant for interdisciplinary providers encompass practical information (eg, code status, allergies, laterality for procedures), background information (eg, comorbidities), planning information (eg, medications or laboratory tests needed while anesthetized, postprocedure instructions/limitations/medications, postprocedure unit and accepting physician), and safety information (eg, fall risk, internal or medical devices).

Aside from serving as an adjunct to the verbal handoff to achieve high-reliability communication, the printed/written handoff tool provides beneficial practical work flow enhancements for inpatient providers. It allows the nighttime provider to populate significant overnight events in areas that are immediately visible on the incoming provider's patient list, thereby allowing incoming physicians to triage their attention even before the verbal handoff has occurred as well as avoiding errors of omission caused by fatigue after a busy overnight shift. It can house information that might otherwise get lost after multiple provider changes, such as a primary subspecialist's name or psychosocial information that would not be documented in the progress notes. Contingency plans for medically complex patients, such as complicated medication plans for status epilepticus, fluid/electrolyte abnormalities, or agitation, are easy to access and less susceptible to ordering/dosing errors or to delays while the team attempts to find the same information in a sea of documents in the EHR. When used during the verbal handoff process, the printed handoff document can serve as a cross-check for medications, which is especially important for patients with long hospital stays who are at risk for medication orders expiring and "falling off" the medication administration record.

Time spent manually populating the handoff tool is a significant challenge.[43,55] Another challenge in maintaining an effective written/printed handoff tool is the degradation in accuracy over time. One study determined that the information in the printed handoff tool would be outdated within 6 hours for 50% of a 20-patient service.[56] Even for autopopulated elements, the mere act of printing the handoff starts a clock for certain elements becoming progressively more out of date, making the information difficult or even dangerous to rely on for clinical decision making, depending on the precise element. Understanding which elements are vulnerable to this in a particular patient's case is essential to ensure clinicians are not inappropriately relying on the printed document for that information.

HANDOFF SKILLS IMPROVEMENT: THE ROLE OF WORKPLACE-BASED ASSESSMENT AND FEEDBACK

Formal handoff communication training is a fairly new idea that has become more widespread after the ACGME began to incorporate into the common program requirements the importance of teaching, monitoring, and evaluating resident physician handoff skills in order to reduce communication failures.[30,57,58] Before this time, skills related to handoff communication were relayed on the job by role modeling, and varied greatly across hospitals, units, and specialties, driven in many cases by variation in teamwork culture.

Initial curricula published regarding handoffs focused mainly on handoff structure and implementation of standardized processes for frontline providers.[46,59] However, it has become clear over time that curricula are also needed for supervising nurses and faculty physicians, to aid them in overseeing implementation of handoff programs. Because assessment alone is not adequate for learning and feedback is essential for improvement, supervisor training should be both in assessment of handoffs and in how to effectively give feedback.

The concept of workplace-based assessment is already embedded in medical education and trainees of all types are observed for competency in structured communication in clinical settings.[60] Presentations by trainees about patients help supervising faculty understand the skill level of the trainee's communication, physical examination, and clinical reasoning skills, and feedback on these elements helps them improve not only their presentation skills but also their understanding of the clinical information.[8,38] Similarly, workplace-based assessment of handoff communication provides an opportunity for feedback and improvement. When performed consistently and well, it also provides an opportunity to improve workplace culture.[8,11,16]

Feedback regarding the verbal or written/printed handoff communication is focused on the key elements of the handoff structure. For instance, the I-PASS handoff assessment tool rates adherence to the mnemonic elements (as well as the quality of communication, such as engagement, prioritization of key information, miscommunication, omissions, tangential conversation and pace; rating quality is discussed further later) (**Figs. 2–4**).[61] This structure provides a format for observers to provide specific information regarding consistent use of the handoff elements; this in turn not only reiterates to the persons being assessed the importance of adherence to these high-reliability processes but also allows them to improve performance by targeting specific aspects of the communication.[62–64]

When using a validated assessment tool such as the I-PASS handoff observation tools, structured clinical assessments of verbal handoffs can be performed by people with different experience levels, including peers. Peer-to-peer assessment, a powerful technique used in high-reliability industries, promotes a culture of safety.[65,66] Peer coaching is another powerful technique that promotes an environment conducive to

Appendix B.1 - I-PASS Handoff Assessment Tool - GIVER

I-PASS Handoff Assessment Tool: GIVER

Observation Start: hh:mm _:___AM/PM **Observation End:** hh:mm_____: _AM/PM **Date:**____/____/____*(mm/dd/yy)*

Specialty (circle): Pediatrics / Medicine / Surgery / Other: ________________ **Specific Service /Unit Name:** ________________

Type of service: ICU / general inpatient ward / specialty inpatient ward / other (specify):______________

Learner (Giver) Information: Provider/Resident ID number:__________ PGY Level:____

Observer Information: I-PASS Champion / Faculty ID number:__________Number of individual patient handoffs observed: ________

Situational Overview:		**YES**	**NO**
1	Was a situational overview provided by the provider giving the handoff (eg, description of the "big picture" of what will need to be prioritized by the receivers of the handoff):		

Frequency **of I-PASS Mnemonic Elements (Items 2-6): Indicate the frequency that each element of the mnemonic is present:**

	I-PASS Mnemonic	**Description**	**Never**	**Rarely**	**Some-times**	**Usually**	**Always**
2	Illness Severity	Identification as stable, "watcher" or unstable; must occur at beginning of each patient handoff					
3	Patient Summary	Might include summary statement, events leading up to admission, hospital course, ongoing assessment, plan					
4	Action List	To-do list (must be separated from patient summary)					
5	Situation Awareness/ Contingency Planning	Know what's going on; plan for what might happen					
6	Synthesis by Receiver	Ensures receiver verbally summarizes what he/she heard					

Indicate the frequency with which the provider who gave the handoff did the following:		**Never**	**Rarely**	**Some-times**	**Usually**	**Always**
7	*Actively engages* receiver to ensure shared understanding of patients (e.g. encouraged questions, asked questions, considers learning style of receiver)					
8	*Appropriately prioritizes* key information, concerns or actions					

Quality **of Handoff Information Transferred (Items 9-17): Only complete if sufficient clinical knowledge of patients to evaluate:**

	Rate the frequency with which the provider who gave the handoff included the following:	**Unable to evaluate**	**Never**	**Rarely**	**Some-times**	**Usually**	**Always**
9	Patient summary includes clearly specified plan for remainder of admission						
10	To-do items with clear if/then format when appropriate						
11	To-do list restricted to items that should be accomplished on next shift						
12	High-quality contingency plans with clear if/the format						
13	Miscommunications or transfer of erroneous information						
14	Omissions of important information						
15	Tangential or unrelated information						

Rate the following:		**Unable to evaluate**	**Poor**	**Fair**	**Good**	**Very Good**	**Excellent**
16	Accuracy of Illness Severity Assessments						
17	Quality of Patient Summaries						

18. Circle the phrase that BEST describes the *pace* of the handoff (circle one):

Very slow pace / Very inefficient — Slow pace / Inefficient — Optimally paced / Efficient — Fast / Pressured pace — Very fast / Very pressured pace

19. What was especially effective about the handoff?	**20. What aspect(s) of the handoff could be improved?**	**21. Additional comments:**

60

Fig. 2. Observation tool for giver of handoff. (*From* O'Toole JK, Starmer AJ, Calaman S, et al; for I-PASS Study Education Executive Committee. I-PASS Mentored Implementation Handoff Curriculum: implementation guide and resources. MedEdPORTAL. 2018;14:10736. https://doi.org/10.15766/mep_2374-8265.10736.)

Appendix B.2 - I-PASS Handoff Assessment Tool - RECEIVER

I-PASS Handoff Assessment Tool: RECEIVER

Observation Start: hh:mm _:___AM/PM **Observation End:** hh:mm_: _ AM/PM **Date:**____/____/____*(mm/dd/yy)*
Specialty (circle): Pediatrics / Medicine / Surgery / Other :__________ **Specific Service /Unit Name:**__________
Type of service: ICU / general inpatient ward / specialty inpatient ward / other (specify):__________
Learner (Receiver) Information: Provider/Resident ID number:__________ PGY Level:____
Observer Information: I-PASS Champion / Faculty ID number:__________Number of individual patient handoffs observed: ________

	How *frequently* did the provider receiving the handoff do the following:	Never	Rarely	Some-times	Usually	Always
1	Verbalizes a synthesis of each patient (i.e., check back or read back of patient handoff)					
2	Appear focused, engaged and demonstrate active listening skills					

	Rate the frequency with which the provider who received the handoff included the following:	Never	Rarely	Some-times	Usually	Always
3	Tangential or unrelated information					

	Rate thefollowing:	Unable to evaluate	Poor	Fair	Good	Very good	Excellent
4	Quality of syntheses by receiver						

5. What phrase listed below **BEST** describes your impression of the appropriateness of the length and degree of detail of the syntheses by the receiver (circle one)?

Insufficient length and detail Appropriate length and detail Excessive length and detail

6. What phrase listed below **BEST** describes your impression of the appropriateness of the number of pertinent and clarifying questions asked by the receiver in this handoff (circle one)?

Insufficient number of questions Appropriate number of questions Excessive number of questions

7. What aspects of the receiver's role in this handoff were especially effective?	8. What aspect(s) of the receiver's role in this handoff could be improved?	9. Additional comments:

61 Society of Hospital Medicine (SHM) I-PASS Mentored Implementation Guide

Fig. 3. Observation tool for receiver of handoff. (*From* O'Toole JK, Starmer AJ, Calaman S, et al; for I-PASS Study Education Executive Committee. I-PASS Mentored Implementation Handoff Curriculum: implementation guide and resources. MedEdPORTAL. 2018;14:10736. https://doi.org/10.15766/mep_2374-8265.10736.)

high-functioning teams in which members feel comfortable bringing up concerns and asking questions.[63,67]

Peer coaching is particularly important for improving the performance of senior physicians and nurses. After implementing a modified I-PASS handoff bundle to improve pediatric hospitalist handoffs, not only did adherence to the mnemonic and satisfaction with handoff process improve significantly but, importantly, the perceived quality of the most vulnerable handoff (ie, from a so-called swing shift hospitalist who takes sign out from the day hospitalists and relays to the overnight hospitalist) significantly improved and hospitalists reported an increased level of confidence in giving peers feedback. The improvement in handoff communication also promoted a supportive work environment and hospitalists felt more comfortable asking questions and bringing up concerns, all resulting in greater satisfaction with handoff processes.[10]

In addition, although adherence to elements of structured communication is an essential element of high-reliability communication, evaluating the quality of the communication is also essential. A robust workplace-based assessment of handoffs should provide an opportunity to promote clinical learning by evaluating the clinical content of the handoff. To that goal, Feraco and colleagues[68] developed and validated a verbal handoff assessment tool to measure the quality of verbal handoffs and found

Appendix B.3 - I-PASS Handoff Assessment Tool: WRITTEN

I-PASS Handoff Assessment Tool: WRITTEN

Date:____/____/____*(mm/dd/yy)*

Specialty (circle): Pediatrics / Medicine / Surgery / Other :__________ **Specific Service /Unit Name:**____________

Type of service: ICU / general inpatient ward / specialty inpatient ward / other (specify):____________

Observer Information: I-PASS Champion / Faculty ID number:__________Number of individual patient handoffs observed: ________

***Frequency* of I-PASS Mnemonic Elements (Items 1-5): Indicate the frequency that each element of the mnemonic is present:**

	I-PASS Mnemonic	Description	Never	Rarely	Some-times	Usually	Always
1	Illness Severity	Identification as stable, "watcher" or unstable; must occur at beginning of each patient handoff					
2	Patient Summary	Might include summary statement, events leading up to admission, hospital course, ongoing assessment, plan					
3	Action List	To-do list (must be separated from patient summary)					
4	Situation Awareness/ Contingency Planning	Know what's going on; plan for what might happen					
5	Synthesis by Receiver	Written reminder to prompt receiver to summarize what was heard during verbal handoff					

***Quality* of Handoff Information Transferred (Items 6-14)**
Note: Questions 7-14 should only be completed for those with sufficient clinical knowledge of patients to evaluate.

	Rate the frequency in which the written handoff document had the following:	Unable to evaluate	Never	Rarely	Some-times	Usually	Always
6	Patient summary includes clearly specified plan for remainder of admission						
7	To-do items with clear if/then format when appropriate						
8	To-do list clearly specifies or is restricted to items that should be accomplished on next shift						
9	High-quality contingency plans documented with clear if/then format						
10	Miscommunications or transfer of erroneous information						
11	Omissions of important information						
12	Tangential or unrelated information						

	Rate the following:	Unable to evaluate	Poor	Fair	Good	Very good	Excellent
13	Accuracy of Illness Severity Assessments						
14	Quality of Patient Summaries						

15. What term **BEST** describes your impression of the length of the written handoff document (circle one):

Very abbreviated length / Abbreviated length / Appropriate length / Excessive length / Very excessive length

16. What was especially effective about the handoff document?	17. What aspect(s) of the handoff could be improved?	18. Additional comments:

62

Fig. 4. Observation tool for written document. (*From* O'Toole JK, Starmer AJ, Calaman S, et al; for I-PASS Study Education Executive Committee. I-PASS Mentored Implementation Handoff Curriculum: implementation guide and resources. MedEdPORTAL. 2018;14:10736. https://doi.org/10.15766/mep_2374-8265.10736.)

significant improvement of the content of verbal handoffs after implementation of a resident handoff bundle. Development and validation of other handoff assessment tools will further promote patient safety and the culture of safety.

IMPLEMENTING A HANDOFF PROGRAM

Implementing any quality improvement program that requires behavioral change, be it hand washing or handoff communication, begins with identifying, defining, and assessing the scope of opportunity posed by the problem in order to create a sense of urgency.[69] Specifically, defining the type of handoff to be improved (eg, resident, attending, nursing, all providers) and the scope (eg, 1 unit or multiple units) guides the gathering of baseline data, which can be brought to all levels of leadership to garner support. Types of information helpful to bring to leadership describe the patient safety gap that the handoff improvement will address (eg, unit-specific or hospital-specific reports of adverse events, malpractice claims, patient-specific stories, culture of safety results, or patient experience data).[61]

Building the Team

Creating a team to design, implement, measure, coordinate, and communicate the various aspects of handoff bundle implementation, and assigning specific responsibilities to the members of the team, is also essential at the outset. Such a team must include key stakeholders who practice in the clinical environment to be targeted. An organizational chart is useful in helping team members understand their roles and for all team members to see who is working on each aspect of the improvement effort (**Fig. 5**).[61] An advisory board oversees implementation of the whole project and helps to formulate the vision of the work, which should be informed by input from all levels of stakeholders, especially frontline providers. The vision includes the scope of the project, timeline, and goals and aligns with institutional goals. The advisory board also secures resources needed for successful implementation (eg, time for leaders/core team members to work on improvement efforts; information technology (IT) support; technical/hardware resources; campaign materials).

Process Mapping and Preparing for Implementation

Because it is difficult to improve something that is not well understood, mapping out the baseline handoff processes and tools is a necessary next step to successful implementation. Ideally, baseline and ideal handoff process maps are formulated and informed by frontline providers and include consideration of processes, tools, the workplace environment, and challenges.[34] Review by multiple providers and managers/supervisors achieves a full picture and helps identify gaps left by narrow views.

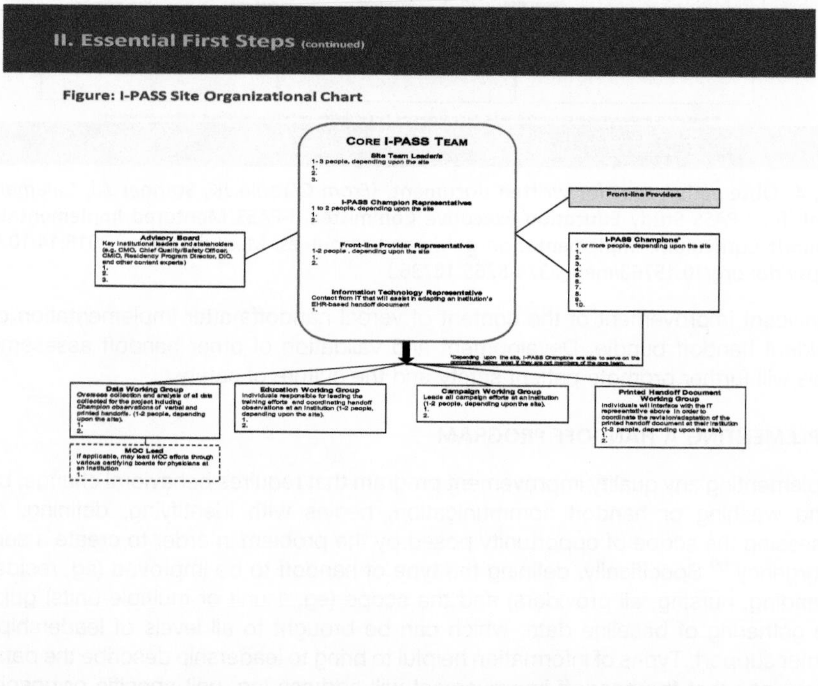

Fig. 5. Organizational chart for implementation. (*From* O'Toole JK, Starmer AJ, Calaman S, et al; for I-PASS Study Education Executive Committee. I-PASS Mentored Implementation Handoff Curriculum: implementation guide and resources. MedEdPORTAL. 2018;14:10736. https://doi.org/10.15766/mep_2374-8265.10736.)

As part of the ideal process mapping, attention given to global elements of effective handoffs (eg, environmental factors, interruptions, computerized resources, which individuals are involved in various handoff types) as well as the specific needs/workflows of the target provider types assists in formulating successful new processes and tools.[28] The concept of structuring flexibility allows system-wide handoff structure and expectations to remain intact while adapting details for provider-specific or unit-specific needs.[70] Development of the printed/written handoff tool and key elements of both the verbal and printed tools for workflow-specific/unit-specific use requires so-called champion/superuser training and time to undergo multiple tests of change by a small group of frontline providers before widespread implementation.[47]

Communication about the results of small tests of change (plan-do-study-act cycles) and the baseline observations should be widely disseminated to maintain a sense of urgency and heighten awareness and importance about the project. This communication should be designed to target the provider type that is the focus of initial improvement efforts but should also be messaged on a larger scale, all the way to executive leadership, in order to promote the program and facilitate future program spread.[69]

Training

Training of supervisors and frontline providers must be considered early so as to secure resources (eg, training rooms, conference or meeting time). Several layers of training must take place: an orientation for team leaders that teaches them handoff bundle content as well as addressing plans and needs for implementation; training of handoff observers and those determining the required elements and ideal work flow (champions); and training of frontline providers. Some individuals may play more than 1 of these roles.[71]

Champion Development, Observation, and Feedback

Recruiting and supporting champions who will conduct observations needs to be carefully considered because this role must be sustained over a long period of time. If using resources such as chief residents or senior residents, then expectations regarding observations and feedback should be set forth from the outset and memorialized in job descriptions or rotation expectations. Embedding handoff observations with feedback into a teaching resident or quality improvement rotation can serve multiple purposes, because it provides an avenue for teaching residents to learn and practice workplace-based assessment skills, use feedback skills, and observe a variety of clinical reasoning and handoff styles. In addition, from the perspective of the handoff improvement program, the use of teaching residents provides an expanded group of observer champions to help teach handoffs to medical students, incoming interns, and even faculty. Of note, handoff observations of residents or hospitalists by observers who are working clinically is fraught with problems (eg, during handoff it is cognitively taxing to focus both on clinical care and providing feedback regarding handoff structure and quality) and should not be encouraged.[27,61,71–73]

If conducting observations of unionized frontline providers (eg, nurses in many hospitals), it is important to recognize that such staff are typically paid for nonclinical work time, a consideration when determining postimplementation goals and project budgets. For pediatric hospitalists and residents, a project designed to obtain part 4 Maintenance of Certification (MOC) points for the American Board of Pediatrics (ABP) is an effective motivator for improvement efforts and can be used for more points when a refresher is needed; in addition, the ABP allows residents to bank part 4 MOC points from projects completed in residency.

Data Tracking

The data collection team can establish goals for baseline and postimplementation workplace-based assessment in order to determine the number of observation champions needed. A communication plan regarding the data should be determined with input from the frontline providers and their managers and brought to leadership at all levels on a regular basis. Using a data-driven improvement approach to data collection and continued quality improvement contributes to sustainability.[73]

Campaign

A campaign to increase visibility (and promote sustainability) includes items such as posters, badge pulls and cards, tips of the day, screen savers, computer frames, articles in newsletters, updates in staff meetings, and booths at conferences.[74]

SUSTAINING EFFECTIVE HANDOFF COMMUNICATION

It is important to recognize that sustainable improvements in handoff communication require transformational change and, as such, they require time to plan, develop, and mature. Leaders at the highest levels must help set realistic change goals and timelines, which are informed by an understanding of the magnitude of resources required. The initial steps for ensuring sustainable change are often lost amid the enthusiasm to begin implementation. Sustainment requires assessing readiness for change, understanding the current handoff environment and communication culture in not only target units but also hospital-wide/program-wide/institution-wide, to prepare for program spread; developing a sense of urgency and setting realistic goals with input from frontline providers and high-level leadership; garnering institutional support and securing resources, with attention given to sometimes overlooked or underestimated requirements, such as the time project leaders will need to fulfill their roles and the IT resources required to develop and adapt an EHR handoff tool for use across settings, specialties, and disciplines.

Engagement of early adopters in the planning and development stages is useful. These people are described as those who welcome experimenting with change, who have the tolerance to test new things, and who are watched by others.[68] Those for whom change is less welcome or who do not understand the impact of the gap on patient safety or have lack of awareness for a need for improvement[75] should be engaged by highlighting quick wins (eg, increased efficiency of communication, which may lead to improved on-time end of shift, or data that show uptake by other members of the unit or improved communication processes). Sustainability efforts should also include plans for just-in-time refreshers, training of new providers, training of new champions, and periodic tool maintenance and process mapping.

Barriers to implementation and sustainment include those commonly encountered with behavioral and cultural change initiatives.[69,71,73,75,76] These barriers can be overcome by securing institutional support, engaging frontline providers of varying opinions at all stages of implementation in order to identify potential barriers and tailor the intervention to work across sites, and communicating clearly about goals, timelines, and outcomes throughout the improvement effort.

Committing to a data-driven improvement approach from the outset helps to hardwire new behaviors through continued workplace-based assessment. Ideas for embedding these assessments are listed earlier and are best deployed when considered/planned preemptively. Sharing culture-of-safety survey results, focus group feedback, unit-based surveys, and patient experience information are all powerful positive reinforcement of the idea that improving handoff communication can improve workplace culture.

In summary, handoff-related communication problems are a leading cause of medical errors and adverse events in hospitals. A growing body of data shows that implementation of comprehensive handoff improvement programs can greatly decrease the risk of handoff-related errors and harms. With careful attention to principles of behavioral and cultural change, engagement of leadership and frontline providers, adaptation to meet the needs of diverse clinicians, and efforts to iteratively refine and sustain improvements, implementation of a handoff program can lead to major, long-lasting improvements in patient safety.

REFERENCES

1. CRICO Strategies. Malpractice risks in communication failures: 2015 annual benchmarking report 2015. Available at: https://www.rmf.harvard.edu/Malpractice-Data/Annual-Benchmark-Reports/Risks-in-Communication-Failures. Accessed June 18, 2018.
2. Croteau R. JCAHO comments on handoff requirement. OR Manager 2005;31(8):8.
3. Agarwal R, Sands DZ, Schneider JD. Quantifying the economic impact of communication inefficiencies in U.S. hospitals. J Healthc Manag 2010;55(4):265–81 [discussion: 281–2].
4. The Joint Commission Center for Transforming Healthcare. Improving transitions of care: hand-off communications 2014. Available at: https://www.centerfortransforminghealthcare.org/assets/4/6/handoff_comm_storyboard.pdf. Accessed June 18, 2018.
5. The Joint Commission. Inadequate hand-off communication. Sentinel Event Alert 2017;(58):1–6. Available at: https://www.jointcommission.org/sentinel_event_alert_58_inadequate_handoff_communications/. Accessed May 1, 2018.
6. Reason J. Understanding adverse events: human factors. Qual Health Care 1995;4(2):80–9.
7. Staggers N, Blaz JW. Research on nursing handoffs for medical and surgical settings: an integrative review. J Adv Nurs 2013;69(2):247–62.
8. Patterson ES, Wears RL. Patient handoffs: standardized and reliable measurement tools remain elusive. Jt Comm J Qual Patient Saf 2010;36(2):52–61.
9. Patterson ES, Roth EM, Woods DD, et al. Handoff strategies in settings with high consequences for failure: lessons for health care operations. Int J Qual Health Care 2004;16(2):125–32.
10. Patel SJ, Di Rocco JR, Okado C, et al. Improvement of patient handoffs between attending hospitalists utilizing the I-PASS handoff bundle and direct peer observation. Institute for Healthcare Improvement 20th Annual Scientific Symposium on Improving the Quality and Value of Healthcare. Orlando, FA, December 8, 2014.
11. Pronovost PJ, Berenholtz SM, Goeschel CA, et al. Creating high reliability in health care organizations. Health Serv Res 2006;41(4):1599–617.
12. Savitsky K, Keysar B, Epley N, et al. The closeness-communication bias: increased egocentrism among friends vs. strangers. J Exp Soc Psychol 2011;47:269–73.
13. Wu S, Keysar B. The effect of information overlap on communication effectiveness. Cogn Sci 2007;31:169–81.
14. De Korne DF, van Wijngaarden JDH, Hiddema UF, et al. Diffusing aviation innovations in a hospital in the Netherlands. Jt Comm J Qual Patient Saf 2010;36(8):339–47.

15. Weick KE, Sutcliffe KM. Managing the unexpected: assuring high performance in an age of complexity. 1st edition. San Francisco (CA): Jossey-Bass; 2001.
16. Bigham MT, Logsdon TR, Manicone PE, et al. Decreasing handoff-related care failures in children's hospitals. Pediatrics 2014;134(2):e572–9.
17. Starmer AJ, Spector ND, Srivastava R, et al. I-PASS, a mnemonic to standardize verbal handoffs. Pediatrics 2012;129(2):201–4.
18. Starmer AJ, Spector ND, Srivastava R, et al. Changes in medical errors after implementation of a handoff program. N Engl J Med 2014;371(19):1803–12.
19. McKeon LM, Oswaks JD, Cunningham PD. Safeguarding patients: complexity science, high reliability organizations, and implications for team training in healthcare. Clin Nurse Spec 2006;20(6):298–304 [quiz: 305–6].
20. Zhang J, Johnson TR, Patel VL, et al. Using usability heuristics to evaluate patient safety of medical devices. J Biomed Inform 2003;36(1–2):23–30.
21. Shneiderman B, Plaisant C, Cohen M, et al. Designing the user interface: Strategies for effective human-computer interaction. 5th edition. Boston: Addison-Wesley; 2009.
22. Starmer AJ, Sectish TC, Simon DW, et al. Rates of medical errors and preventable adverse events among hospitalized children following implementation of a resident handoff bundle. JAMA 2013;310(21):2262–70.
23. Desai SJ, Feldman L, Brown L, et al. Effect of the 2011 vs 2003 duty hour regulation-compliant models on sleep duration, trainee education, and continuity of patient care among internal medicine house staff. JAMA Intern Med 2013; 173(8):649–55.
24. Wagner R, Koh N, Bagian JP, Weiss KB, for the CLER Program. CLER 2016 National Report of Findings. Issue Brief #5: Care Transitions. Chicago: Accreditation Council for Graduate Medical Education; 2017.
25. Starmer AJ, O'Toole JK, Rosenbluth G, et al. Development, implementation, and dissemination of the I-PASS handoff curriculum: a multisite educational intervention to improve patient handoffs. Acad Med 2014;89(6):876–84.
26. Spector ND, Starmer AJ, Allen AD, et al. I-PASS handoff curriculum: core resident workshop. MedEdPORTAL 2013;9:9311.
27. O'Toole J, Sectish T, Starmer A, et al. I-PASS handoff curriculum: faculty development resources. MedEdPORTAL 2013;9:9540.
28. Johnson JK, Barach P, Vernooij-Dassen M. Conducting a multicenter and multinational qualitative study on patient transitions. BMJ Qual Saf 2012;21:i22–8.
29. Marcotte L, Kirtane J, Lynn J, et al. Integrating health information technology to achieve seamless care transitions. J Patient Saf 2015;11(4):185–90.
30. Philibert I. Supervision, preoccupation with failure, and the cultural shift in patient handover. J Grad Med Educ 2010;2(1):144–5.
31. Dykes PC, Rozenblum R, Dalal A, et al. Prospective evaluation of a multifaceted intervention to improve outcomes in intensive care: the Promoting Respect and Ongoing Safety Through Patient Engagement Communication and Technology study. Crit Care Med 2017;45(8):e806–13.
32. Khan A, Spector ND, Baird JD, for the Patient and Family Centered I-PASS Study Group. Patient safety after implementation of a coproduced family centered communication programme: multicenter before and after intervention study. BMJ 2018;363:k4764.
33. Rosenbluth G, Bale JF, Starmer AJ, et al. Variation in printed handoff documents: results and recommendations from a multicenter needs assessment. J Hosp Med 2015;10(8):517–24.

34. Arora V, Johnson J. A model for building a standardized hand-off protocol. Jt Comm J Qual Patient Saf 2006;32(11):646–55.
35. Borowitz SM, Waggoner-Fountain LA, Bass EJ, et al. Resident sign-out: a precarious exchange of critical information in a fast-paced world. In: Henriksen K, Battles JB, Keyes MA, et al, editors. Advances in patient safety: new directions and alternative approaches (vol. 2: Culture and Redesign). Rockville (MD): Agency for Healthcare Research and Quality; 2008. p. 1–21.
36. Jewell JA. Standardization of inpatient handoff communication. Pediatrics 2016; 138(5). https://doi.org/10.1542/peds.2016-2681.
37. Nasarwanji MF, Badir A, Gurses AP. Standardizing handoff communication: content analysis of 27 handoff mnemonics. J Nurs Care Qual 2016;31(3):238–44.
38. Bordage G. Prototypes and semantic qualifiers: from past to present. Med Educ 2007;41(12):1117–21.
39. Bowen JL. Educational strategies to promote clinical diagnostic reasoning. N Engl J Med 2006;355(21):2217–25.
40. Bhabra G, Mackeith S, Monteiro P, et al. An experimental comparison of handover methods. Ann R Coll Surg Engl 2007;89(3):298–300.
41. Pothier D, Monteiro P, Mooktiar M, et al. Pilot study to show the loss of important data in nursing handover. Br J Nurs 2005;14(20):1090–3.
42. Nelson B, Massey R. Implementing an electronic change-of-shift report using transforming care at the bedside processes and methods. J Nurs Adm 2010; 40(4):162–8.
43. Palma JP, Sharek PJ, Longhurst CA. Impact of electronic medical record integration of a handoff tool on sign-out in a newborn intensive care unit. J Perinatol 2011;31(5):311–7.
44. Van Eaton EG, Horvath KD, Lober WB, et al. A randomized, controlled trial evaluating the impact of a computerized rounding and sign-out system on continuity of care and resident work hours. J Am Coll Surg 2005;200(4):538–45.
45. Petersen LA, Orav EJ, Teich JM, et al. Using a computerized sign-out program to improve continuity of inpatient care and prevent adverse events. Jt Comm J Qual Improv 1998;24(2):77–87.
46. Arora VM, Manjarrez E, Dressler DD, et al. Hospitalist handoffs: a systematic review and task force recommendations. J Hosp Med 2009;4(7):433–40.
47. Wohlauer MV, Arora VM, Horwitz LI, et al. The patient handoff: a comprehensive curricular blueprint for resident education to improve continuity of care. Acad Med 2012;87(4):411–8.
48. Van Eaton EG, Horvath KD, Lober WB, et al. Organizing the transfer of patient care information: the development of a computerized resident sign-out system. Surgery 2004;136(1):5–13.
49. Rosenbloom ST, Grande J, Geissbuhler A, et al. Experience in implementing inpatient clinical note capture via a provider order entry system. J Am Med Inform Assoc 2004;11(4):310–5.
50. Gillum RF. From papyrus to the electronic tablet: a brief history of the clinical medical record with lessons for the digital age. Am J Med 2013;126(10):853–7.
51. Fogerty RL, Schoenfeld A, Al-Damluji MS, et al. Effectiveness of written hospitalist sign-outs in answering overnight inquiries. J Hosp Med 2013;8(11):609–14.
52. Bump GM, Jovin F, Destefano L, et al. Resident sign-out and patient hand-offs: opportunities for improvement. Teach Learn Med 2011;23(2):105–11.
53. Schoenfeld AR, Al-Damluji MS, Horwitz LI. Sign-out snapshot: cross-sectional evaluation of written sign-outs among specialties. BMJ Qual Saf 2014;23(1). https://doi.org/10.1136/bmjqs-2013-002164.

54. Collins SA, Stein DM, Vawdrey DK, et al. Content overlap in nurse and physician handoff artifacts and the potential role of electronic health records: a systematic review. J Biomed Inform 2011;44(4):704–12.
55. Poissant L, Pereira J, Tamblyn R, et al. The impact of electronic health records on time efficiency of physicians and nurses: a systematic review. J Am Med Inform Assoc 2005;12(5):505–16.
56. Rosenbluth G, Jacolbia R, Milev D, et al. Half-life of a printed handoff document. BMJ Qual Saf 2016;25(5):324–8.
57. Accreditation Council for Graduate Medical Education. ACGME Common Program Requirements. Available at: https://www.acgme.org/Portals/0/PFAssets/ProgramRequirements/CPRs_2017-07-01.pdf. Accessed June 17, 2018.
58. Philibert I. Use of strategies from high-reliability organizations to the patient handoff by resident physicians: practical implications. Qual Saf Health Care 2009; 18(4):261–6.
59. Horwitz LI, Schuster KM, Thung SF, et al. An institution-wide handoff task force to standardise and improve physical handoffs. BMJ Qual Saf 2012;21(10):863–71.
60. Miller A, Archer J. Impact of workplace based assessment on doctors' education and performance: a systematic review. BMJ 2010;341:c5064.
61. O'Toole JK, Starmer AJ, Calaman S, et al. I-PASS mentored implementation handoff curriculum: implementation guide and resources. MedEdPORTAL 2018;14: 10736.
62. Duff B. Creating a culture of safety by coaching clinicians to competence. Nurse Educ Today 2013;33(10):1108–11.
63. Maynard L. Using clinical peer coaching for patient safety. AORN J 2012;96(2): 203–5.
64. Sekerka LE, Chao J. Peer coaching as a technique to foster professional development in clinical ambulatory settings. J Contin Educ Health Prof 2003;23(1): 30–7.
65. Hudson DW, Holzmueller CG, Pronovost PJ. Toward improving patient safety through voluntary peer-to-peer assessment. Am J Med Qual 2012;27(3):201–9.
66. Pronovost PJ, Hudson DW. Improving healthcare quality through organisational peer-to-peer assessment: lessons from the nuclear power industry. BMJ Qual Saf 2012;21(10):872–5.
67. Agency for Healthcare Research and Quality. TeamSTEPPS Instructor Guide. Available at: http://www.ahrq.gov/teamsteppstools/insructor/index.html. Accessed March 30, 2012.
68. Feraco AM, Starmer AJ, Sectish TC, et al. Reliability of verbal handoff assessment and handoff quality before and after implementation of a resident handoff bundle. Acad Pediatr 2016;16(6):524–31.
69. Small A, Gist D, Souza D, et al. Using Kotter's change model for implementing beside handoff: a quality improvement project. J Nurs Care Qual 2016;31(4): 304–9.
70. Patterson ES. Structuring flexibility: the potential good, bad and ugly in standardisation of handovers. Qual Saf Health Care 2008;17(1):4–5.
71. Shahian DM, McEachern K, Rossi L, et al. Large-scale implementation of the I-PASS handover system at an academic medical centre. BMJ Qual Saf 2017; 26(9):760–70.
72. Starmer AJ, Landrigan C, Srivastava R, et al. I-PASS handoff curriculum: faculty observation tools. MedEdPORTAL 2013;9:9570.
73. Starmer AJ, Spector ND, West DC, et al. Integrating research, quality improvement, and medical education for better handoffs and safer care: disseminating,

adapting, and implementing the I-PASS program. Jt Comm J Qual Patient Saf 2017;43(7):319–29.
74. Rosenbluth G, Patel SJ, Destino LA, et al. I-PASS handoff curriculum: campaign toolkit. MedEdPORTAL 2013;9:9397.
75. Grol R, Grimshaw J. From best evidence to best practice: effective implementation of change in patients' care. Lancet 2003;362(9391):1225–30.
76. Kotter JP. Leading change: why transformation efforts fail. Harv Bus Rev 2007;(1): 96–103.
77. Riesenberg LA, Leitzsch J, Little BW. Systematic re- view of handoff mnemonics literature. Am J Med Qual 2009;24(3):196–204.
78. Cohen MD. Hilligoss Brian. Handoffs in Hospitals: a review of the literature on information exchange while transferring patient responsibility or control 2009. Available at: https://deepblue.lib.umich.edu/handle/2027.42/61498. Accessed December 2, 2018.
79. Brownstein A, Schleyer A. The art of HANDOFFS: a mnemonic for teaching the safe transfer of critical patient information. Available at: www.MDMag.com. Accessed December 2, 2018.
80. Horwitz LI, Moin T, Green ML. Development and implementation of an oral sign-out skills curriculum. J Gen Intern Med 2007;22(10):1470–4.
81. Department of Defense Patient Safety Program. Healthcare Communications Toolkit to Improve Transitions in Care 2005. Available at: https://www.oumedicine.com/docs/ad-obgyn-workfiles/handofftoolkit.pdf?sfvrsn=2. Accessed December 2, 2018.
82. Denham CR. SBAR for patients. J Patient Saf 2008;4(1):38–48.
83. Committee on Patient Safety and Quality Improvement. ACOG Committee Opinion No. 367: communication strategies for patient handoffs. Obstet Gynecol 2007;109(6):1503–6.
84. Guise JM, Lowe NK. Do you speak SBAR? J Obstet Gynecol Neonatal Nurs 2006; 35(3):313–4.
85. Vidyarthi AR, Arora V, Schnipper JL, et al. Managing discontinuity in academic medical centers: strategies for a safe and effective resident sign- out. J Hosp Med 2006;1(4):257–66.
86. Ellis D, Mullenhoff P, Ong F. Back to the bedside: patient safety and handoff report. Clin Nurse Spec 2007;21(2):109.

Section 2: Patient Centered Care

Patient- and Family-Centered Care

Leveraging Best Practices to Improve the Care of Hospitalized Children

Jennifer L. Everhart, MD[a,*], Helen Haskell, MA[b], Alisa Khan, MD, MPH[c]

KEYWORDS

- Patient-centeredness • Patient- and family-centered care
- Patient and family engagement • Coproduction

KEY POINTS

- Patient-centered care is defined as "respectful of and responsive to individual patient preferences, needs, and values and ensuring that patient values guide all decisions" (Institute of Medicine, 2001).
- Patient-centered care and patient- and family-centered care (PFCC) improve patient and family satisfaction, patient self-management, and physical and mental health outcomes.
- Coproduction is an emerging PFCC framework that has the potential to transform the delivery of health care such that it better matches the ideals of patients and improves outcomes.
- Coproduction in hospital medicine consists of cocommissioning (eg, patient-centered outcomes research), codesign (eg, shared decision making), codelivery (eg, patient as educator), and coassessment (eg, quality and process improvement, patient safety).
- Foundational principles that enable coproduction include valuing patients and families as members of the health care team, ensuring inclusive communication, and harnessing technology to promote access to health information.

INTRODUCTION

Many pediatric hospital medicine providers would intuitively agree that patient- and family-centeredness is at the heart of their inpatient pediatric practice. As pioneers in revolutionary interventions such as patient- and family-centered rounds (PFCRs),

Disclosure Statement: The authors have no relevant financial relationships to disclose.
[a] Department of Pediatrics, Division of Pediatric Hospital Medicine, Stanford University School of Medicine, 300 Pasteur Drive MC 5776, Stanford, CA 94305-5776, USA; [b] Mothers Against Medical Error, 155 South Bull Street, Columbia, SC 29205, USA; [c] Division of General Pediatrics, Boston Children's Hospital, 21 Autumn Street, Room 200.2, Boston, MA 02215, USA
* Corresponding author.
E-mail address: JEverhar@stanford.edu

Pediatr Clin N Am 66 (2019) 775–789
https://doi.org/10.1016/j.pcl.2019.03.005
pediatric.theclinics.com

they have championed, modeled, and taught effective communication with patients and families. Patient- and family-centered care (PFCC) is more than just effective communication, however, and it extends beyond morning rounds and even beyond individual patient encounters to the health care system at large.

This article aims to broaden pediatric hospital medicine providers' understanding of PFCC and equip them to both implement and advance the art and science of PFCC. The article begins with a discussion of the origins and history of PFCC and a review of selected relevant literature. The article shares an overview of several existing frameworks for patient-centeredness, emphasizing an emerging concept called coproduction. The article then reviews several attitudes, skills, and infrastructure components, which are considered essential prerequisites for effective coproduction. With this foundation in place, the article highlights several strategies for promoting coproduction in Hospital Medicine, organized around 4 key tenets of coproduction (cocommissioning, codesign, codelivery, and coassessment).

BACKGROUND

Origins of Patient-Centered Care

The term "patient-centered care" (PCC) was coined by the Picker Institute, a foundation dedicated to making patients full partners in health care. Picker originally concentrated on learning the patient's perspective through focus groups and surveys of thousands of patients, family members, and hospital staff. Using information derived from these sources, Picker defined 8 dimensions of health care, which it considered important to patients and that could be called "patient centered." These were as follows:

- Respect for patients' values, preferences, and expressed needs
- Coordination and integration of care
- Information, communication, and education
- Physical comfort
- Emotional support and alleviation of fear and anxiety
- Involvement of family and friends
- Transition and continuity
- Access to care[1]

Other organizations also did significant early work in PCC. Among these were the Institute for Patient- and Family-Centered Care, whose 4 principles of dignity and respect, information sharing, participation, and collaboration are a widely cited definition of PCC, and Planetree, Inc, which has organized hospitals along patient-centered principles since the 1970s.[2,3]

Historical Perspective

PCC took its place on the national agenda in 2001, when the Institute of Medicine (IOM) followed up its highly publicized medical error report, *To Err is Human*, with a second publication laying out a roadmap for quality solutions. This second report, *Crossing the Quality Chasm*, named patient-centeredness as 1 of the 6 primary aims of care. The report's definition of PCC as "respectful of and responsive to individual patient preferences, needs, and values and ensuring that patient values guide all clinical decisions" was derived from the Picker principles, with 6 of Picker's 8 dimensions (ie, all but transition and access) quoted and discussed directly in the report. Patient-centeredness was noted to be integral to the IOM's "agenda for improvement," whose goals were to "reduce the burden of illness, injury, and disability, and to improve the health and functioning of the people of the United States." Citing the work of Picker, Planetree, and others, the authors of *Crossing the Quality Chasm* paid close attention to problems reported by patients and focused their 10 "rules to redesign and improve care" on patients' needs: individualization, control, information, science, safety, transparency, anticipation, value, cooperation, and care that extends beyond individual patient visits.[4]

Patient-Centeredness Versus Patient Engagement

Over the years, the term "patient-centered care" has often been eclipsed by "patient engagement," the implication being a somewhat greater self-efficacy on the part of the patient. In this model, patient engagement can be viewed as an expansion or evolution of PCC. It is important to note that this health care–specific use of the term "patient engagement" is distinct from its use in manufacturing and technology, in which "patient engagement" is often synonymous with customer relations, and the interests of patients are not always in the forefront.

Making the Case for Patient- and Family-Centered Care: A Review of the Evidence

Translating the IOM's aspirations into practice has been a slow but steady process, and PCC/PFCC interventions vary in the degree to which they help achieve this goal.

A systematic review of adult PCC literature in 2012 found significant relationships between certain elements of PCC and outcomes but no relationship between others. Satisfaction and self-management were most positively influenced by PCC.[5] For example, adult patients who received a list of necessary medical assessments and personalized self-management action plans and goals had higher levels of self-management goal setting and received more diabetes-related preventive care after 6 months.[5,6] Of note, none of the studies in this review included family (a key distinction when considering PFCC in pediatrics), and many included only outpatient interventions.[5]

Regarding the impact of PCC in the inpatient setting, 1 study found poorer health and more chest pain 12 months after discharge in patients who reported lower levels of PCC during their index hospitalizations.[7] Another found a significant association between lower PCC in the hospital and increased mortality 6 months and 1 year after discharge for patients hospitalized for acute myocardial infarct.[8]

In the adult intensive care unit (ICU) setting, a systematic review and meta-analysis of PFCC intervention outcomes found improved family satisfaction scores in 55% of qualifying studies (eg, with implementation of novel communication strategies, liberalized visitation policies, and/or involvement of family members in patients' care). Patient satisfaction scores similarly increased with interventions such as noise reduction, daylight exposure, and liberalized visitation policies.[9] Patients were more likely to achieve their medical care goals with incorporation of an ethics consult.[9,10] All 6 studies examining the relationship between PFCC interventions (such as early end-of-life conferences and palliative care rounding) and mental health outcomes reported an improvement in 1 or more symptoms of depression, anxiety, or posttraumatic stress disorder.[9] PFCC's impact on morbidity and mortality was less convincing: only 1 of 13 studies showed a significant improvement in mortality (ie, 8.6% decrease in mortality over 4 years with implementation of a communication intervention).[9,11] Similarly, only 1 study showed improvement in morbidity: stable infection rate and decreased cardiovascular complications with implementation of a more liberal cardiovascular intensive care unit visiting policy.[9,12]

Although the pediatric literature on the impact of PFCC is evolving, it shows that PFCC is highly prevalent in pediatrics but subject to multiple threats. A review of pooled data from more than 22,000 Medical Expenditure Panel Surveys found that 94% to 97% of parents "usually or always" thought their child's provider respected their input, listened carefully, provided easily understood explanations, and spent sufficient time with their child, behaviors the investigators thought represented PFCC. Public insurance, racial and ethnic minority status, low socioeconomic status, special health care needs, poorer parent-perceived health status, and increased number of annual visits were all associated with lower prevalence of PFCC.[13]

Review of Existing Frameworks and Resources for Patient- and Family-Centered Care

There are several existing frameworks and accompanying resources for learning and implementing PFCC, summarized in **Table 1**.

Coproduction: an Emerging Framework for Patient- and Family-Centered Care

Probably the most disruptive PFCC framework to emerge in recent years is coproduction, a concept borrowed from community services that maintains that services are enhanced by greater involvement of the recipient. This model carries the implicit assumption that health care is a service, not a product, and that like all services it can only be produced, or coproduced, through the efforts of both patients and health care professionals embedded within a larger social context (**Fig. 1** shows a proposed conceptual model of coproduction in health care).[20] By promoting the value of each side's lived experiences and encouraging communication and decision making centered on patient preference, coproduction has the potential to redesign the delivery of health care in a way that better matches the ideals of patients and improves outcomes across all levels of care. The challenge for health care systems and leaders is to create circumstances that encourage all parties to take an active role in order to allow strong, mutually beneficial coproduction to flourish. The remainder of this article explores how the pediatric hospital medicine community can promote effective coproduction in the pediatric inpatient setting for the benefit of patients and providers alike.

FOUNDATIONAL PRINCIPLES ENABLE COPRODUCTION

Patients and Families Valued as Members of Health Care Team

In order for health care providers to engage in coproduction with patients and families, patients and families must be seen as valued members of the team. This principle can be modeled for learners and interprofessional team members by the attending physician, who is often seen as the team leader. Simple actions such as giving patients and families a meaningful role on rounds, having patients and families share their concerns first during medical discussions, and thanking patients and families for their contributions to medical care and decision making can reinforce the value of patients and families on medical teams.

Communication Is Inclusive of Patients and Families

Patients and families must also be equipped to participate in health care discussions and decisions in order to coproduce effectively. It is imperative that communication be inclusive and patient- and family-centered. Conducting rounds discussions according to a patient's or parent's preferences is a first step toward inclusive communication (eg, formal PFCRs or one-on-one updates later in the day, inside the room or in the hallway, at a time that is convenient for the patient and family). Incorporating health literacy techniques, such as choosing patient- and family-appropriate language, limiting the use of unclarified medical terms, providing accompanying written

Table 1
Existing frameworks and resources for patient- and family-centered care

Organization	Frameworks & Resources	Descriptions/Comments
Agency for Healthcare Research and Quality (AHRQ)	Guide to Patient and Family Engagement in Hospital Quality and Safety (2012)[14]	A system of tools and implementation strategies for family advisory councils, enhanced patient communication, bedside change of shift, and the AHRQ IDEAL (Include, Discuss, Educate, Assess, Listen) discharge process
	Comprehensive Unit-based Safety Program toolkit (2012)[15]	A modular and modifiable toolkit to support unit level change. Includes slides, tools, and videos for various modules, including one on patient and family engagement that emphasizes making sure patients and families understand what is happening during a hospitalization, actively participate in the patient's care, and prepare for discharge
	Guide to Improving Patient Safety in Primary Care Settings by Engaging Patients and Families (2017)[16]	Materials and tools promote collaboration between primary care providers and patients
American Institutes of Research (AIR)	Multidimensional Framework for Patient And Family Engagement in Health and Health Care (2013)[17]	Portrays patient engagement in health care as a matrix, with the continuum of engagement on 1 axis (from consultation to involvement to partnership and shared leadership) and levels of engagement on the other (from direct care to organizational design and governance to policy making). Patient engagement is measured by the amount of information flowing between patient and provider, the degree of patient activity in care decisions, and the level of involvement of patients in health organization decisions and policy making. Interdependence of different areas of engagement is highlighted
	Roadmap for Patient and Family Engagement in Healthcare Practice and Research (2014)[18]	An evolution of the AIR's Multidimensional Framework into an online roadmap composed of 8 strategies (patient and family preparation, clinician and leadership preparation, care and system redesign, organizational partnership, measurement and research, transparency and accountability, legislation and regulation, and partnership in public policy) for advancing patient engagement, each with its own tactics and milestones specific to the anticipated level of impact

(*continued on next page*)

Table 1 (*continued*)		
Organization	**Frameworks & Resources**	**Descriptions/Comments**
National Academy of Medicine	Evidence and Experience to Change Culture: A Guiding Framework for Patient and Family Engaged Care (2017)[19]	Examines both the evidence base and the experience of patients and providers and expands the concept of patient engagement to include external drivers, such as workplace culture, physical environment, and the quality of interactions and communication

communication, and engaging the patient and family in bidirectional communication via teach-back, is important as well.

Supervising physicians have an opportunity to both model and teach inclusive, patient- and family-centered communication. Residents have been shown to overestimate their use of recommended patient- and family-centered communication techniques: for example, reporting frequent use of plain language (88%) and teach-back (48%) but being observed to actually use jargon an average of 2 times a minute and

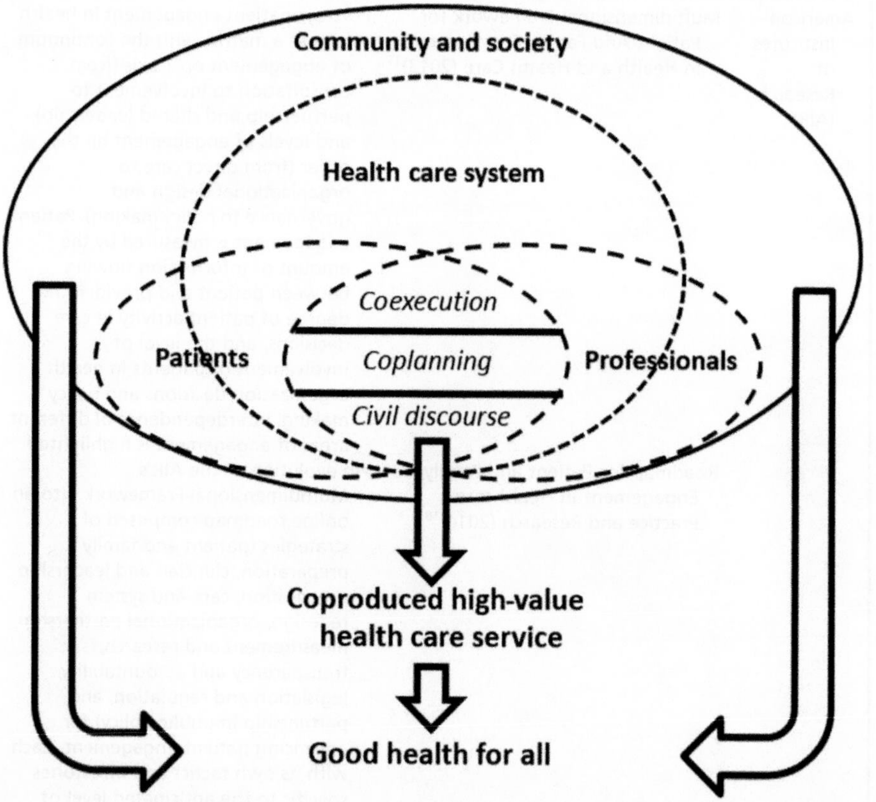

Fig. 1. Conceptual model of coproduction in health care. (*From* Batalden M, Batalden P, Margolis P, et al. Coproduction of healthcare service. BMJ Qual Saf. 2016;25(7):509–17. https://doi.org/10.1136/bmjqs-2015-004315; with permission.)

use teach-back only 22% of the time.[21] Although medical students more commonly underestimate patients' understanding of medical jargon, they do overestimate at times, and this has the potential to hinder communication with patients and families.[22] A supervising physician is well positioned to model effective communication (ideally priming learners in advance and debriefing encounters after they occur) and provide real-time formative feedback during and after patient interactions.

Technology Promotes Access to Health Information

Technology can also be harnessed to allow patients and families better access to their health information in order to more effectively coproduce. Patients desire information transparency, including access to physicians' notes and operative reports, radiology results, and billing and general hospital information. Parents able to access information about their child's hospitalization on an inpatient portal reported that they thought it improved care (94% of respondents) by giving them access to information that helped them better track and understand their child's care and make relevant decisions. Sixty percent of parents thought access to the portal improved communication with the health care team; 89% thought it reduced errors in care, and 8% reported identification of actual medication list errors.[23]

COPRODUCTION IN HOSPITAL MEDICINE

Overview of the 4 Components of Coproduction in Hospital Medicine

Coproduction in health care can be broken down into 4 key tenets: (1) cocommissioning, (2) codesign, (3) codelivery, and (4) coassessment, as illustrated in **Fig. 2**.[24,25]

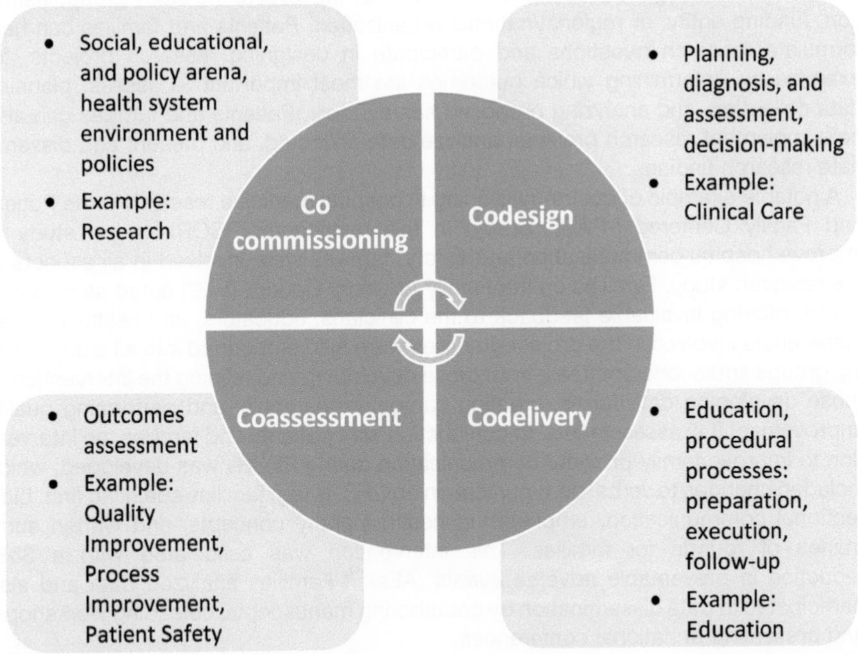

Fig. 2. Aspects of coproduction in hospital medicine. (*Adapted from* Haskell H, Lord T. Patients and Families as Coproducers of Safe and Reliable Outcomes. In: Sanchez JA, Barach P, Johnson J, Jacobs JP, eds. *Surgical Patient Care: Improving Safety, Quality and Value*. Springer; 2017:101–20; Figure 8.3; with permission.)

Cocommissioning refers to planning policies and prioritizing agendas. Codesign refers to planning services. Codelivery refers to managing and performing services. Coassessment refers to monitoring and evaluation. To further enhance PFCC in hospital medicine, the authors propose the following strategies for incorporating these 4 principles of coproduction.

Cocommissioning: Research

Cocommissioning can be applied to hospital medicine via patient-centered outcomes research (PCOR). The Patient-Centered Outcomes Research Institute (PCORI), established under the 2010 Patient Protection and Affordable Care Act to fund patient-centered comparative clinical effectiveness research, extends patient-centeredness from health care delivery to health care research.[26] PCOR considers the preferences and needs of patients, focusing on their desired health care outcomes (eg, symptom reduction, survival, health-related quality of life) and emphasizing autonomy. It seeks to study diverse settings and populations and balance stakeholder concerns, including individual burden and resource availability. This variety and diversity help address individual differences and dissemination/implementation barriers, including availability of services, technology, and personnel. It can be applied to diagnostic, preventative, palliative, therapeutic, and health care delivery–based interventions and health care choices. PCOR ultimately strives to help patients, families, and stakeholders at all levels make better-informed decisions about health and health care options, highlighting comparisons and outcomes that matter to individuals.[27]

PCOR principles call for including patients and families throughout the research process. This inclusion can be accomplished first by ensuring that patients and families help set research agendas and priorities, at either the level of the study group, institution, funding entity, or regional/national organization. Patients and families can help formulate research questions and participate in designing research projects, for example by determining which outcomes are most important to assess, planning data collection, and analyzing proposed survey tools. Patients and families can also help implement research projects, analyze data collected, and present and disseminate research findings.

A notable example of cocommissioning in hospital medicine research is the Patient and Family Centered I-PASS Study. In this multicenter PCORI-funded study to improve hospital communication and safety, families were involved in all aspects of the research study. Families on the Family Advisory Council (FAC) acted as a soundboard, offering invaluable feedback to the clinicians, educators, and health services researchers involved in the project. Families were also embedded into all study working groups and subcommittees, from those developing and refining the intervention to those developing data forms, creating campaign materials, and performing quality improvement (QI) assessments. In conjunction with patients and families, an intervention to improve family-provider communication during PFCRs was developed, which included changes to verbal communication on PFCRs (eg, families speaking first, bidirectional communication, emphasizing health literacy concepts) and written summaries of rounds for families. This intervention was associated with a 38% reduction in preventable adverse events (AEs).[28] Families analyzed data and also participated in data dissemination by coauthoring manuscripts, coleading workshops, and presenting at national conferences.

Codesign: Clinical Care

Partnering with patients and families in shared decision making (SDM) is an example of codesign in the clinical setting. SDM has been defined as "an approach where clinicians and patients make decisions together using the best available evidence" and share ownership for those decisions.[29,30] Patients communicate their preferences by weighing the likely benefits and harms of each option.[29]

A systematic review of SDM synthesized the data from 39 studies that measured both clinical SDM and its relationship with patient outcomes. Of the 97 assessments of unique patient outcomes, 43% showed positive relationships between SDM and the outcome of interest. Affective-cognitive patient outcomes were most often significantly positively affected, followed by behavioral and health outcomes.[31]

Most of the existing SDM literature looks at SDM in the context of adult medicine, where an adult patient is participating in decision making regarding his or her care. SDM in pediatrics is fundamentally different in several ways. The parent or family member often acts as a surrogate decision maker, since pediatric patients generally cannot participate in discussions regarding their values, beliefs, and self-identified best interests. It is the parent's or family member's responsibility to make decisions in what he or she deems is the patient's best interest. There is often scrutiny as to whether these preferences are indeed in the patient's best interests, and this can undermine the team's ability to build consensus with the family. SDM-appropriate decisions in pediatrics are also more restricted. A competent adult patient retains the right to do nothing, for example, regardless of the potential harm this decision may cause. Parents whose decision has the potential to significantly harm their child are often superseded. This paradox is confounded by the fact that degrees of risk and harm can be subjective, certain decisions affect the health of others (eg, the decision whether to vaccinate), and decisions in pediatrics often do not involve disease but rather focus on preventive care (eg, supine sleep position, breastfeeding).[32]

There are several published toolkits aimed at supporting and teaching SDM. AHRQ's SHARE Approach is a 5-step process that promotes a meaningful dialogue between the patient and health care provider regarding the potential benefits, risks, and harms of each option as they relate to the patient's individual values. Steps include seeking the patient's participation in decision making, helping the patient explore and compare options, assessing the patient's values and preferences, reaching a decision with the patient, and evaluating the decision made. The AHRQ provides accompanying training tools, a workshop curriculum, and webinars.[33] The Ottawa Hospital Research Institute has published 2 decision guides to help patients weigh the benefits and risks of treatment choices as they relate to their individual values. The Ottawa Personal Decision Guide shepherds patients through the decision-making process, beginning with clarifying the decision to be made, exploring arguments for and against available options, identifying sources of support, identifying necessary resources, and planning next steps. The Ottawa Personal Decision Guide for Two guides 2 decision makers through this process.[34] Finally, "Shared Decision-Making (SDM) Toolkit: Train-the Trainer Tools for Teaching SDM in the Classroom and Clinic" was published by the Association of American Medical College's MedEdPORTAL in 2013 and includes self-study materials and tools for in situ provider training in SDM.[35]

Codelivery: Education

Actively involving patients and family members in medical education is an example of codelivery. When developing, describing, and monitoring patient-learner encounters, some important factors to consider include patient culture, educational setting (community vs hospital), type of participation (passive vs active role), and scope of participation (general vs specific).[36] Patient and family member involvement can be conceptualized as a spectrum ranging from paper-based or electronic clinical scenarios, to standardized patient encounters, to real patients and families sharing their experiences within a faculty-directed curriculum, to patients and families teaching and/or evaluating students, to patients and families acting as equal partners with other educators in education, evaluation, and curriculum development in a time-limited fashion, to patients and families filling this role longitudinally.[37]

Bedside teaching is a common component of inpatient encounters at academic medical centers, allowing trainees to simultaneously learn provider-patient communication, physical examination skills, clinical reasoning, professionalism, and empathy. In bedside teaching, the patient (and/or family member), learner (eg, medical student, resident), and teacher (eg, senior resident, attending physician) form a learning triad in which all members contribute and participate.[38] An example of this triad in action might be the learner sharing what he read about a recent development in the treatment of the patient's disease, the attending physician modeling giving relevant anticipatory guidance, and the patient teaching the team about a specific aspect of her disease (such as how it first presented) or treatment (such as how she monitors for side effects at home). The patient and family may also provide feedback to learners on their communication skills and patient care via informal or formal (eg, 360°) evaluations. It is important to note that although learners may worry they are inconveniencing or worrying patients by involving them in bedside teaching, the vast majority of patients (77%) enjoy it. Only 17% of patients report it causing anxiety.[39]

Patient narratives have also been found to be an effective way for patients and families to asynchronously teach learners. Radiology residents who reviewed deidentified letters from patients and specialty-specific cases found both tools helped them think differently about their patient interactions (64% for the letters, and 73% for the cases), specifically encouraging them to be more patient-centered and enhancing their understanding of professional physician behavior.[40] After completing a multimodal curriculum that consisted of assigned reading and related discussions (eg, journal excerpts, book), meeting with a veterans outreach coordinator, and participating in the Veterans History Project, nurse residents reported better understanding of the veteran patient population and the ability to provide more appropriate, personalized patient care.[41]

Finally, by incorporating patients and families into teaching roles that have traditionally been reserved for clinicians, organizations can tap into patients' and families' valuable expertise and encourage an institutional culture of coproduction. Inviting patients and family members to share their narratives in a large-group setting, such as noon conference or grand rounds, for example, allows their message to be received by a broader audience.[42] Patients and family members can facilitate educational sessions, such as coleading PFCR training workshops or facilitating small group role plays on giving bad news. Patients and family members can also act as coaches, observing residents on rounds and giving formative feedback on their communication techniques.

Coassessment: Quality Improvement, Process Improvement, and Patient Safety

Coassessment involves partnering with patients and families in monitoring and evaluating and can be applied to many aspects of hospital medicine, including research, education, clinical care, hospital operations, QI, process improvement (PI), and patient safety.

Clinically, patients and families can help monitor and assess the quality of care occurring at both the patient and system levels. They can serve as "vigilant partners"[43] at the bedside, given their availability, proximity, knowledge of the patient's history, and motivation for a good outcome. If effectively counseled for this role, they can help monitor and assess inpatient progress (eg, meeting oral intake goals, notifying the nurse if breathing becomes worse). Operationally, patients and families can be embedded at all levels of the organization, from executive committees to working groups tackling unit-level clinical problems (eg, helping formulate a clinical practice guideline to shorten hospital length of stay for febrile neonates). They can partner in hospital QI and PI initiatives, from their design to execution. As an example, in the Patient and Family Centered I-PASS Study, families participated in QI observations of PFCRs to inform rapid cycles of improvement and ensure adherence to PFCR best practices.

Patients and families provide unique information about hospital safety, and their inclusion in hospital safety activities has the potential to improve both the quality and the safety of care. Patients and families can participate in root cause analyses and morbidity and mortality conferences for hospital safety events after they occur, providing valuable insight and ensuring that proposed improvement solutions work for patients and families. They can also participate in committees responsible for overseeing and evaluating hospital safety policies in order to help assess, monitor, and improve the safety of hospital care processes while maintaining patient- and family-centeredness.

Organizations can also involve patients and families in hospital safety reporting. Strategies include involving them in voluntary event reporting, embedding safety reporting questions in patient experience surveys, and encouraging patients and families to speak up about safety during rounds, at admission, at discharge, and during transitions of care. Hospitals typically do not include patients and families in their safety surveillance processes; however, growing research shows that patients and families are reliable reporters of hospital safety incidents who provide otherwise undetected safety information. In 1 multicenter study, families of hospitalized pediatric patients were administered brief Family Safety Interviews weekly and before discharge. More than 1 in 4 families of hospitalized pediatric patients reported experiencing safety concerns, most of which were potential errors or AEs (**Fig. 3**). Families were as good as providers at detecting errors and AEs. Moreover, families reported 5 times the rates of errors and 3 times the rates of AEs as hospital safety reporting systems. Rates of errors were 16% higher and rates of AEs were 10% higher with family reporting than without.[44]

Challenges

Although promising, coproduction is not without its challenges. In order to ensure effective coproduction, institutions must invest resources in families. This investment includes commitments to meaningfully engage families as partners across the organization in research, education, clinical care, hospital operations, QI, PI, and patient safety. It involves being mindful of families' competing needs (eg, caring for ill children, caring for siblings, work commitments, travel, and time and money costs of participating). Many hospitals are hiring paid family partners beyond the FAC, which is an important start. In addition, lack of diversity continues to be a challenge in effective coproduction in hospital settings. Many FACs do not include underrepresented and minority groups or those from more disadvantaged backgrounds (eg, with respect to race/ethnicity, language, education, and socioeconomic status). Therefore, hospitals can take care to actively recruit patients and families of varying backgrounds, and to also adequately compensate families for their time and effort to address some of the material barriers to engagement.

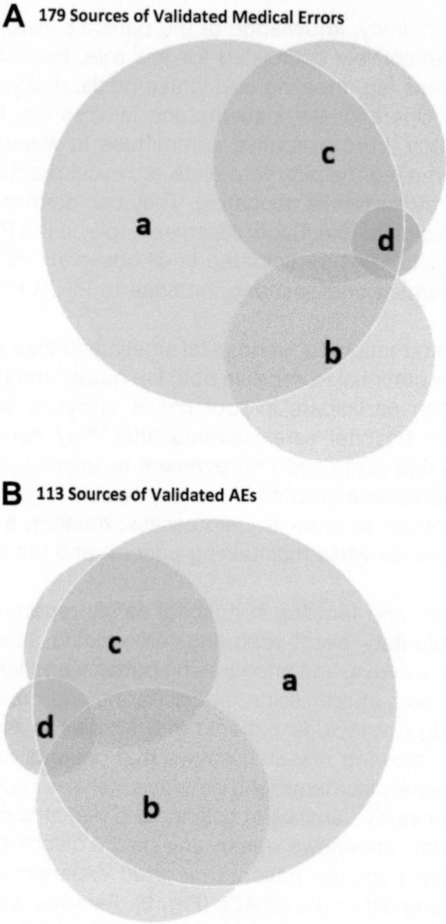

a	Chart Review	137
b	Family	39
c	Provider	50
d	Hospital Incident Report	5

a	Chart Review	137
b	Family	39
c	Provider	50
d	Hospital Incident Report	5

Fig. 3. Sources of errors and AEs. (*A*) Sources of medical errors validated through 2-step methodology. (*B*) Sources of AEs validated through 2-step methodology. For both medical errors and AEs, families reported unique incidents that were not otherwise reported by chart review, providers, or hospital incident reports. (*Adapted from* Khan A, Coffey M, Litterer KP, et al. Families as partners in hospital error and adverse event surveillance JAMA Pediatr. 2017;171(4):372–81. https://doi.org/10.1001/jamapediatrics.2016.4812; with permission.)

SUMMARY

PFCC that respects patients' and families' preferences, needs, and values has the potential to improve patient and family satisfaction, patient self-management, and health outcomes, and truly transform health care. By engaging in the various elements of coproduction (cocommissioning, codesign, codelivery, and coassessment), pediatric hospital medicine providers and educators can lead this change in their units, training programs, institutions, and the health care system as a whole. A solid foundation in which patients and families are valued as members of the health care team, communication is inclusive, and technology is harnessed to promote access to health information is critical. It is hoped the strategies outlined in this article will serve as inspiration for the field moving forward, with the ultimate goal of improving the care of hospitalized children.

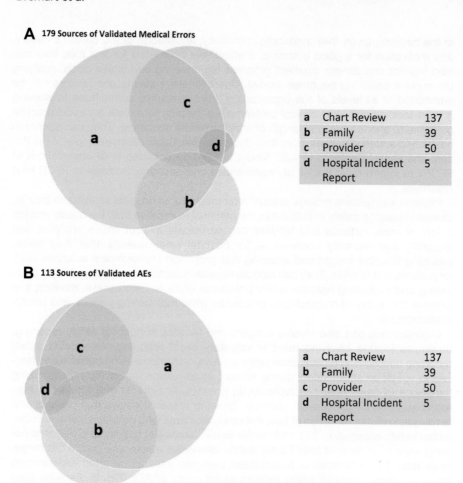

REFERENCES

1. Improving Healthcare through the Patient's Eyes: Principles of Patient-Centered Care. Picker Institute Web site. Available at: http://pickerinstitute.org/about/picker-principles/. Accessed May 31, 2018.
2. What is PFCC? Institute for Patient- and Family-Centered Care Web site. Available at: http://www.ipfcc.org/about/pfcc.html. Accessed May 31, 2018.
3. Planetree History. Planetree, Inc. Web site. Available at: https://planetree.org/reputation/. Accessed May 31, 2018..
4. Institute of Medicine Committee on Quality of Health Care in America. Crossing the quality chasm: a new health system for the 21st century. Washington, DC: National Academies Press; 2001.
5. Rathert R, Wyrwich MD, Boren SA. Patient-centered care and outcomes: a systematic review of the literature. Med Care Res Rev 2013;70(4):351–79.
6. Glasgow RE, Nutting PA, King DK, et al. A practical randomized trial to improve diabetes care. J Gen Intern Med 2004;19(12):1167–74.
7. Fremont AM, Cleary PD, Hargraves JL, et al. Patient-centered processes of care and long-term outcomes of myocardial infarction. J Gen Intern Med 2001;16(12):800–8.
8. Meterko M, Wright S, Lin H, et al. Mortality among patients with acute myocardial infarction: the influences of patient-centered care and evidence-based medicine. Health Serv Res 2010;45(5 Pt 1):1188–204.
9. Goldfarb MJ, Bibas L, Bartlett V, et al. Outcomes of patient- and family-centered care interventions in the ICU: a systematic review and meta-analysis. Crit Care Med 2017;45(10):1751–61.
10. Chen YY, Chu TS, Kao YH, et al. To evaluate the effectiveness of health care ethics consultation based on the goals of health care ethics consultation: a prospective cohort study with randomization. BMC Med Ethics 2014;15:1.
11. Lilly CM, De Meo DL, Sonna LA, et al. An intensive communication intervention for the critically ill. Am J Med 2000;109:469–75.
12. Fumagalli S, Boncinelli L, Lo Nostro A, et al. Reduced cardiocirculatory complications with unrestrictive visiting policy in an intensive care unit: Results from a pilot, randomized trial. Circulation 2006;113:946–52.
13. Bleser WK, Young SI, Miranda PY. Disparities in patient- and family-centered care during US children's health care encounters: a closer examination. Acad Pediatr 2017;17:17–26.
14. Guide to Patient and Family Engagement in Hospital Quality and Safety. Agency for Healthcare Research and Quality Web site. Updated February 2017. Available at: http://www.ahrq.gov/professionals/systems/hospital/engagingfamilies/index.html. Accessed May 19, 2018.
15. Patient and Family Engagement. Agency for Healthcare Research and Quality Web site. Updated July 2018. Available at: http://www.ahrq.gov/professionals/education/curriculum-tools/cusptoolkit/modules/patfamilyengagement/index.html. Accessed May 19, 2018.
16. Guide to Improving Patient Safety in Primary Care Settings by Engaging Patients and Families. Agency for Healthcare Research and Quality Web site. Updated July 2018. Available at: http://www.ahrq.gov/professionals/quality-patient-safety/patient-family-engagement/pfeprimarycare/index.html. Accessed May 19, 2018.
17. Carman KL, Dardess P, Maurer M, et al. Patient and family engagement: a framework for understanding the elements and developing interventions and policies. Health Aff (Millwood) 2013;32(2):223–31.

18. Carman KL, Dardess P, Maurer ME, et al. A roadmap for patient and family engagement in healthcare practice and research. Palo Alto (CA): Gordon and Betty Moore Foundation; 2014.
19. Frampton S, Guastello S, Hoy L, et al. Harnessing evidence and experience to change culture: a guiding framework for patient and family engaged care. 2017. Available at: https://nam.edu/wp-content/uploads/2017/01/Harnessing-Evidence-andExperience-to-Change-Culture-A-GuidingFramework-for-Patient-and-Family-Engaged-Care.pdf. Accessed May 31, 2018.
20. Batalden M, Batalden P, Margolis P, et al. Coproduction of healthcare service. BMJ Qual Saf 2016;25(7):509–17.
21. Howard T, Jacobson KL, Kripalani S. Doctor talk: physicians' use of clear verbal communication. J Health Commun 2013;18(8):991–1001.
22. LeBlanc TW, Hesson A, Williams A, et al. Patient understanding of medical jargon; a survey study of U.S. medical students. Patient Educ Couns 2014;95(2):238–42.
23. Kelly MM, Hoonakker PLT, Dean SM. Using an inpatient portal to engage families in pediatric hospital care. J Am Med Inform Assoc 2016;24(1):153–61.
24. Bovarid T, Loeffler E. The role of co-production for better health and wellbeing; why we need to change. In: Loeffler E, Power G, Bovaird T, et al, editors. Co-production of health and wellbeing in Scotland. Birmingham (United Kingdom): Governance International; 2013. p. 20–8.
25. Haskell H, Lord T. Patients and families as coproducers of safe and reliable outcomes. In: Sanchez JA, Barach P, Johnson J, et al, editors. Surgical patient care: improving safety, quality and value. Cham (Switzerland): Springer; 2017. p. 101–20.
26. Compilation of Patient Protection and Affordable Care Act: Extracted sections concerning Patient-Centered Outcomes Research and Authorization of the Patient-Centered Outcomes Research Institute (PCORI). Patient-Centered Outcomes Research Institute Web site. 2018. Available at: https://www.pcori.org/document/authorizing-legislation. Accessed June 1, 2018.
27. Research We Support. Patient-Centered Outcomes Research Institute Web site. 2014. Updated July 25, 2018. Available at: https://www.pcori.org/research-results/research-we-support. Accessed June 1, 2018.
28. Khan A, Spector ND, Baird JD, et al. Patient safety after implementation of a coproduced family centered communication programme: multicenter before and after intervention study. BMJ 2018;363:k4764.
29. Elwyn G, Laitner S, Coulter A, et al. Implementing shared decision making in the NHS. BMJ 2010;341(7780):971–3.
30. Moumjid N, Gafni A, Bremond A, et al. Shared decision making in the medical encounter: are we all talking about the same thing? Med Decis Making 2007;27(5):539–46.
31. Shay LA, Lafata JE. Where is the evidence? A systematic review of shared decision making and patient outcomes. Med Decis Making 2015;35(1):114–31.
32. Opel DJ. A push for progress with shared decision-making in pediatrics. Pediatrics 2017;139(2). https://doi.org/10.1542/peds.2016-2526.
33. The SHARE Approach. Agency for Healthcare Research and Quality Web site. 2014. Updated August 2018. Available at: http://www.ahrq.gov/professionals/education/curriculum-tools/shareddecisionmaking/index.html. Accessed June 4, 2018.

34. Ottawa Personal Decision Guides. The Ottawa Hospital Research Institute Web site. 2015. Updated April 23, 2018. Available at: https://decisionaid.ohri.ca/decguide.html. Accessed June 4, 2018.
35. Mincer S, Adeogba S, Bransford R, et al. Shared decision-making (SDM) toolkit: train-the-trainer tools for teaching SDM in the classroom and clinic. MedEdPORTAL 2013;9:9413.
36. Spencer J, Blackmore D, Heard S, et al. Patient-oriented learning: a review of the role of the patient in the education of medical students. Med Educ 2000;34:851–7.
37. Tew J, Gell C, Foster S. Learning from Experience: involving service users and carers in mental health education and training. Nottingham (United Kingdom): Higher Education Academy/National Institute for Mental Health in England/Trent Workforce Development Confederation; 2004.
38. Garout M, Nuqali A, Alhazmi A, et al. Bedside teaching: and underutilized tool in medical education. Int J Med Educ 2016;7:261–2.
39. Nair BR, Coughland JL, Hensley MJ. Student and patient perspectives on bedside teaching. Med Educ 1997;31:341–6.
40. Miller MM, Slanetz PJ, Lourenco AP, et al. Teaching principles of patient-centered care during radiology residency. Acad Radiol 2016;23(7):802–9.
41. Vessey JA, Wendt J, Glynn DM, et al. Teaching patient-centered care through the veterans history project. Nurse Educ 2018;43(6):322–5.
42. Weinberger SE, Johnson BH, Ness DL. Patient- and family-centered medical education: the next revolution in medical education? Ann Intern Med 2014;161(1):73–5.
43. Schwappach DLB. Review: engaging patients as vigilant partners in safety: a systematic review. Med Care Res Rev 2010;67(2):119–48.
44. Khan A, Coffey M, Litterer KP, et al. Families as partners in hospital error and adverse event surveillance. JAMA Pediatr 2017;171(4):372–81.

Communication with Diverse Patients

Addressing Culture and Language

Jennifer K. O'Toole, MD, MEd[a,*], Wilma Alvarado-Little, MA, MSW[b], Christy J.W. Ledford, PhD[c]

KEYWORDS

- Limited English proficiency (LEP) • Language assistance • Cultural competency
- Linguistic competency • Patient-provider communication

KEY POINTS

- Communication with patients at baseline is a complex process; cultural and linguistic differences between providers, patients, and their families add another layer of complexity.
- Culture embodies layers of ethnicity, race, nationality, religion, regionalism, family, and group memberships, such as professional or hobby groups. Cultural differences may prompt misunderstandings, because the team and patient family interpret words and actions through different lenses.
- All patients should receive language assistance appropriate to their culture and language when hospitalized. Language assistance refers to the oral and written language services needed to assist patients and their families with limited English proficiency to communicate with health care providers in order to gain meaningful access and an equal opportunity to participate in all aspects of their medical care.
- Training in cultural and linguistic competency should optimally occur well in advance of beginning clinical experiences with patients and should continue throughout an individual's undergraduate and graduate medical education and follow into practice.

Disclosures/Conflicts of Interests: Dr J.K. O'Toole holds stock options in and has consulted for the I-PASS Patient Safety Institute. The I-PASS Patient Safety Institute is a company that seeks to train institutions in best handoff practices and aid in their implementation. Ms W. Alvarado-Little has no relevant financial or nonfinancial relationships to disclose. She contributed to this article based on her experience in the field of health literacy and cultural competency and the opinions and conclusions of the article do not represent the official position of the New York State Department of Health. Dr C.J.W. Ledford contributed to this article as a federal employee. The views expressed are her own and do not necessarily represent the views of the Uniformed Services University of the Health Sciences, the US Department of Defense, or the United States Government.

[a] Departments of Pediatrics and Internal Medicine, Cincinnati Children's Hospital Medical Center, University of Cincinnati College of Medicine, 3333 Burnet Avenue, MLC 5018, Cincinnati, OH 45229-3039, USA; [b] New York State Department of Health, Office of Minority Affairs and Health Disparities Prevention, 9th Floor Corning Tower, ESP, Albany, NY 12237, USA; [c] Department of Family Medicine, Uniformed Services University, 4301 Jones Bridge Road, Bethesda, MD 20814, USA

* Corresponding author.

E-mail address: Jennifer.otoole@cchmc.org

Pediatr Clin N Am 66 (2019) 791–804

https://doi.org/10.1016/j.pcl.2019.03.006

INTRODUCTION

Effective communication is key when providing quality health care.[1] The practice of good communication skills in the medical profession is integral for the development of meaningful and trustworthy relationship between the doctors and patients and, thus, is beneficial to both of them.[2] However, the dynamics of communication within the health care team and the patient and family can be challenging during a situation when emotions are high, whether this involves the delivery or receiving of positive or difficult information. Whether originating from the patient and/or patient's family or that of the provider, it is information that should be communicated clearly and respectfully. Building rapport when all parties speak a common language can at times be difficult.

Adding a linguistic and cultural layer to this exchange can add a level of complexity to the encounter. This section discusses cultural and linguistic challenges; strategies to provide effective communication with limited English speakers and the deaf and hard of hearing communities; an overview of the intersection of interpreting, translation, and health literacy; and finally, how to teach these critical skills to physicians.

CULTURAL AND LINGUISTIC CHALLENGES IN COMMUNICATING WITH PATIENTS IN THE HOSPITAL

A Specialty Environment

Medical professionals who deliver inpatient care are tasked with working together to expedite patient flow while maintaining quality standards.[3] These inpatient teams must attend to patient questions, order and manage medical testing, coordinate treatment plans, and respond to medical emergencies. In this setting, it is critical that health care providers (HCPs) communicate effectively to address patient needs.[4]

The inpatient pediatric environment adds another layer of complexity to the interaction, as the care team communicates with both the patient and the patient's family.[5] Parents add value to the inpatient team, specifically reporting otherwise undocumented safety errors and adverse events.[6,7] However, families and care teams often have a lack of shared understanding of the plan of care.[8] A repeated challenge and a contributing factor to the lack of understanding for patient parents is the shifting composition of the health care team through an admission. Another factor associated with the overall patient experience is their perception of communication with the night physicians and nurses.[9]

Culture is a multifaceted communicative process that influences economic, social, and political structures, which in turn guide attitudes, perception, and behavior.[10] In doing so, culture may be the greatest determinant of knowledge formation, cocreated meanings, and behavioral shifts.[11,12] Culture embodies layers of ethnicity, race, nationality, religion, regionalism, family, and group memberships, such as professional or hobby groups. Each layer of culture can inform how individuals think about health and medicine. Among groups that seem superficially similar, values and attitudes toward health care can vary, such as Amish and Appalachian women—2 distinct groups of White American women—who have culturally bound perspectives of breast and cervical cancer screening.[13]

Cultural differences may prompt misunderstandings, because the team and patient family interpret words and actions through different lenses. Miscommunication can occur at the level of the words and phrases, but also at the deeper level of values and beliefs.[14] Hospital teams can benefit from the expertise both of cultural experts to explain cultural beliefs and customs and of professional interpreters to explain the meaning of words, which together can help the team communicate with a patient and family from a culture different than team members.[15] For example, despite most physicians agreeing that they should pursue religion/spirituality when prompted by the patient,[16,17] physicians rarely reported talking to patients about spiritual topics.[18] These conversations are critical when care teams encounter patients with cultural beliefs that are different from their own or unacceptable within Western ethical norms.[19]

One defining feature of culture that influences communication with patients in the hospital is language. A language difference among the health care team and patient and family presents a common barrier to effective communication. It also affects the health literacy of a patient and their family in understanding one's illness, communicating with providers, and navigating the health care system. Please also see Alexander F. Glick and colleagues' article, "Health Literacy in the Inpatient Setting: Implications for Patient Care and Patient Safety," in this issue for additional information on health literacy. In the United States, this difference is most common when the care team speaks English and the patient or patient's family has limited English proficiency (LEP) or when the provider's English is heavily accented and English is not the patient's family preferred language. Health care teams who work with LEP patients should partner with trained medical interpreters to provide the most complete understanding of what a patient is saying.[20] The alternatives of relying on family members, using untrained bilingual staff, or allowing clinicians to use limited language ability to communicate in the patient's language, can negatively affect the patient's care.[20] The use of professional interpreters improves communication, clinical outcomes, and satisfaction with care.[21] Professional interpreters have more positive influence on clinical outcomes than ad hoc interpreters.[21] However, in adult medicine, care team use of interpreters is highly variable, ranging from 4.8% of teams using an interpreter for LEP patients when a hospitalist is present to 16.8% of teams using an interpreter for LEP patients with a non-physician provider.[22] In pediatrics, interpreter use is increasing, likely due to the availability of telephonic interpreters.[23] About half of LEP parents report that physicians and nurses use an interpreter often; however, the investigators describe this prevalence as "suboptimal."[24] The use of well-prepared multilingual written materials, such as intake and consent forms, in addition to other vital documents such as instructions to prepare for surgery or taking medication, can also improve communication with LEP patients and families.[25]

Integrating the Patient and Family into Family-Centered Rounds

Family-centered rounds are challenging interactions for patient and family members, in which the health care team has 2 (sometimes competing) goals: an educational goal to teach team members and a patient care goal to include the patient and family in their medical care.[26] Family-centered care is identified by 4 key principles: clear and open information sharing with patients and family members, respect for patients and family members, participation of patients and family members, and collaboration with patients and family members.[27,28] **Table 1** presents recommended communicative actions and pitfalls to avoid within this framework. Please also refer to Jennifer L. Everhart and colleagues' article, "Patient- and Family-Centered Care: Leveraging Best Practices to Improve the Care of Hospitalized Children," in this issue for more information on patient- and family-centered care.

EXECUTING CULTURALLY AND LINGUISTICALLY COMPETENT COMMUNICATION WITH PATIENTS

To establish a relationship of trust with the patient and their family, health literacy must be viewed in the context of language and culture.[30] Therefore, it is important to keep in mind the patient's expectation of the health care,[31] along with clinician attitudes that

Table 1
Core concepts and common pitfalls to avoid in the practice of patient- and family-centered care

Recommended Action	Pitfalls to Avoid
Information sharing	
To clearly and openly share information, use unambiguous language and multiple modalities (verbal, written, and action-oriented) to communicate with patients and family members. Using "living room" language. Using plain language also assists the interpreter in providing a clear and accurate conversion.	• The team may slip into medical jargon, particularly as they talk to each other across the patient and family. • When talking with the family and team simultaneously, the team may be tempted to develop a comprehensive differential and plan (verbalize a list of all possible scenarios that may occur). Worst-case scenarios can alarm patients and families unnecessarily, and they may not understand when it does not apply to their own case. • If this is discussed in the interpreter's presence, the interpreter is obligated to interpret this information as well. • Perhaps should not be discussed in their presence or should be discussed outside of the patient's room.
Dignity and respect	
To communicate respect for patients and family members, the team must navigate the physical and social space of a hospital room. • Physically, the team must decide what part of rounds is accomplished outside vs inside the patient room.[29] The furniture, square footage, and number of people in the room all present opportunities and challenges to communicating respect. The team must adapt how they position themselves (standing or sitting; near or far; grouped or individually separated) to each room and each patient-team case. • Teams must also navigate the social space, particularly the emotional context of rounding encounters. Teams must show respect and empathy for patients, while also demonstrating respect for their peers. • The team's positioning will provide valuable cues for the interpreter as to how to position themselves as well.	• Some parents choose to stand during rounds, whereas others may recline due the exhaustion of a prolonged illness. • Hospital cribs present a challenge—they generally dominate the room vertically and horizontally, even interrupting sight lines.
Participation	
Participation of patients and family members requires the team to facilitate that engagement. The physical environment needs attention—the team can facilitate patient participation by decreasing distractions.	• For some attendings, this goal can be particularly challenging, because they try to balance patient participation and medical education. It is important for attending questioning of residents to focus on questions for which the answers directly

(continued on next page)

Table 1
(continued)

Recommended Action	Pitfalls to Avoid
The health care team should identify who is in the room so that the interpreter is aware who they are interpreting for.	address the family's information needs. This method includes the family, while promoting a learning environment. • Team members can turn off televisions and ask patients to pause video games. Patient families will consistently support this effort, because it creates an environment conducive to family-centered rounds.
Collaboration	
Collaboration is a step beyond participation, when the team does not only ask questions to gather information for its own decision-making. Collaboration with family often depends on the family's motivation to interact. Although this is common and expected, it does challenge the team to be more intentional with the passive or quiet parent or patient, who does not more naturally engage.	• Teams may feel confronted when parents express "lay theory," which contradicted the team's plan. This presents an opportunity for the team to address the inaccuracy of the theory while respecting the family member's role in care and teach how the plan would address the issue. This interaction can result in a more knowledgeable and confident parent who will play a critical role in the patient's care after discharge. This scenario can be challenging for the interpreter as 2 cultures intersect. • Engaged parents will likely want to take notes throughout the encounter. Do not discourage this behavior or tell them "not to worry" about writing anything down because it will be in the discharge instructions or in a handout. Patients and parents benefit in 2 ways from taking their own notes: (1) it gives them a kinesic role in the interaction, which may facilitate their learning, and (2) it enables them to take notes in their own plain language and understanding.

can be perceived as a barrier to health care by some groups.[32] Language assistance services provide the health care team with an additional set of skills to continue to provide excellent, patient-centered care.

Language Access and Language Assistance

A point of clarification is presented for the terms "language access" and "language assistance." According to the Department of Health and Human Services Language Access Plan, *language access* is achieved when individuals with LEP can communicate effectively with employees and contractors and participate in programs and activities.[33] *Language assistance* is when all oral and written language services needed to assist individuals with LEP to communicate effectively with staff and contractors. In addition, it allows individuals to gain meaningful access and an equal opportunity to participate in the services, activities, programs, or other benefits. Simply, language access addresses the language access plan in place and language assistance addresses the various methods of service delivery.[33]

Interpretation Services

Addressing language differences involves various methods of delivery. Interpreting, whether signed or spoken, is the process of understanding and analyzing a spoken or signed message and reexpressing that message faithfully, accurately, and objectively in another language, taking the cultural and social context into account. The purpose of interpreting is to enable communication between 2 or more individuals who do not speak each other's languages.[34] LEP patients identify 2 factors that help them decide when they need an interpreter: (1) self-identified level of English proficiency and (2) anticipated complexity of the health care communication.[35]

Often referred to only by the term "translation," written translation is the rendering of a written text in one language in a comparable written text in another language.[36]

A common component of health care communication is the provision of written materials. However, materials are often unavailable in languages other than English. To remedy this pitfall, the interpreter resorts to sight translation, which is providing the oral rendition of text written in one language into another language and is usually done in the moment. Unfortunately, often staff does not realize that a much needed document is not available in the patient or patient's family preferred language. The interpreter will then be handed the document written in English and asked to read it out loud in a language other than English, therefore reading it in English and providing the content out loud in a language other than English. Sight translation is often requested of an interpreter during an interpreting assignment.[34] The interpreter will work from the source language (the language used in the moment) to the target language (the language in which the information needs to be converted). Often the scenario involves an interpreter being handed a document written in English, which describes the side effects of a medication or risks and benefits of a procedure. Often, it is in this moment that the interpreter has seen this document for first time. The interpreter will need to use various cognitive skills to relay the information accurately and completely. She/he will have a moment to have a preliminary view of this document, read the document in English while processing and converting the document into the patient's native language, and provide an oral rendition of document originally written in English. Although this might be appropriate for a very short document, a document longer in length should be translated.

The ability to sight translate and to do written translation is certainly an asset in an interpreter. However, sight translation requires different skills than oral interpreting, and sight translating long documents can consume quite a lot of time, fatigue the interpreter, and increase the risk for error.[36] Health care facilities and providers also need to understand that these different skills require different preparation so that they do not ask interpreters to do what they are not prepared or qualified to do.[36] When it comes to sight translations, the interpreter is at a disadvantage. They have not had an opportunity to review the document and assess it for meaning and terminology, have resources available to decipher words that are unfamiliar, or do not have an equivalent term in the target language. In the absence of a translation of said document, the provider can read the document and the interpreter can interpret what is being said.

Health care services may be available but not accessible for those whose preferred language is one other than English or who are deaf or hard of hearing. This may be due to a lack of awareness of federal,[37] local, or organizational policies that are in place or simply lack of trained interpreters.[38] Providing and receiving services can be complicated by a communication barrier that affects all parties involved. In situations where an individual can benefit from language services, assumptions are made to either support or hinder the provision of language access services.

A common misconception is that exchanges using an interpreter will take more time. As more complex patients need more time, patients for which interpreters are necessary will require additional time. However, to partner effectively and efficiently, it is imperative that a qualified, professional interpreter be used instead of an untrained (ad hoc) interpreter. The professional interpreter has the skills to navigate the flow of the message; provide accurate terminology and vocabulary specific to the encounter and the patient's diagnosis; understand the cultural nuances that could affect clinical care[39]; and most importantly, abide by their code of ethics as health care interpreters to ensure accuracy and completeness with the message delivered by either the patient, the patient's family members, or the provider. A perceived challenge by providers may be the insertion of an individual who may or may not be perceived as part of the health care team. Health care interpreters can provide insight into common sources of communication problems. Their bilingual and often bicultural position and depth of experience means that interpreters contribute to a broader understanding of patient-provider communication problems.[31]

Tips for Working with Interpreters

Interpreter qualifications

A qualified interpreter has participated in an interpreter training program, has undergone an oral language proficiency skills assessment, and abides by their code of ethics and standards of practice.[40] A professional health care interpreter explains his or her role to the patient, patient's family, and the provider in addition to how to partner with an interpreter, whether it be in person, over the phone, or via video relay. When interpreting in a pediatric situation where the patient speaks English and the preferred language of the primary caretaker is one other than English, it is important for the interpreter to communicate their role and purpose to all parties involved in the encounter.

Communicating with patients via an interpreter

When using an interpreter, provide the interpreter with relevant information before the interpreting encounter. In pediatrics, an important piece of information to share is to state for whom the interpreter will be interpreting. If there are issues of confidentiality and/or HIPPA, it is necessary that the interpreter have an awareness of who is "in the room." Often, there is an assumption that culturally, because everybody present in the patient's room is welcomed, the primary caretaker does not have any requests regarding privacy. It is recommended that the providers privately ask the primary caretakers with whom they want their child's information shared and who is to make decisions on the patient's behalf. Culturally, some diagnosis may be perceived as taboo, or, if the cause is not understood, information in the absence of facts generate myth, stereotype, or illness due to lack of adherence to prenatal cultural beliefs from community elders,[39] all of which contribute to judgment toward the family and disempowerment.

In addition, providers should not have side conversations with other staff members or discuss another patient in front of the interpreter. An interpreter is obligated to interpret every utterance, which is presented by either the patient, the patient's family, or the provider. A rule of thumb is if it is not to be interpreted, then it should not be spoken or signed. If this encounter would be taking place between a provider and patient who were both English speaking, certain information or statements would not be shared out loud. Also, remember to ask the patient what questions they have while the interpreter is present. This avoids the provider from attempting to have a conversation once the interpreter has been dismissed from the encounter. If the provider has any questions about the patient or family members understanding of the information provided, do not ask the interpreter, "Do you think they understood that?" Rather, before ending the encounter with the patient and/or family, use a teachback method or ask them, "When you leave here, your other family members might ask about (insert patient name). If you're comfortable sharing information with them, would you tell me what you'll say to them? I know we covered a lot today."

Because interpreters take their cues from the health care team leadership, it is important that they share with the interpreter who is going to be present during this meeting. Because of cultural nuances, there may be a hierarchical structure to the community, independent of family, who are involved in the sharing of information. In addition, sharing of information regarding specific needs such as a family who is perceived to be stressed, combative, or overwhelmed may require a consultation between the provider and the interpreter before meeting with the patient and family members.

Positioning when working with interpreters

Another area to address is that of positioning; this will vary based on the method of interpreting. For example, with a spoken language interpreter, it is important that the provider and the patient face each other and not the interpreter. Often, however, it comes down to the dynamics of the room (room size, number of individuals present, patient's diagnosis, parent's preference, the role of a community elder) as to where an interpreter will position themselves. It can be much like a dance and knowing how to stay put or change positions with staff, knowing when to move so that the interpreter is positioned in a way that benefits the team, the patient, and the patient's family. For sign language, the interpreter is positioned in front of the patient, so the patient and/or family member will not have an obstructed view of the interpreter and the provider.

When using a telephonic interpreter, be aware of background noises, the positioning of the telephone, and your own voice as any of these will affect the volume and range needed to clearly hear the patient and the provider's words. Regardless of the method of service delivery, remember to speak clearly and pause frequently to allow questions or opportunities for clarification if needed by the interpreter.

Special circumstances when working with interpreters

Although there are instances where individuals who are deaf or hard of hearing are communicated with other mechanisms other than a sign language interpreter, it is best to ask the individual for their preferred method of communication. In either case—the utilization of a spoken or sign language interpreter—it is not appropriate to use a minor.[37] This changes the power dynamic, and in some cases, there are cultural nuances that involve a minor asked to interpret information or questions that are sensitive or perceived as disrespectful to an elder or of a different gender. For similar reasons, it is not recommended to use a friend or family member because their primary role is not as interpreter. Previous work has shown that family members and untrained staff who provide ad hoc interpretation can commit many errors of interpretation.[38] A provider can explain that a professional interpreter will convey all the information accurately and completely, that this is a way to provide support to the family during this time and therefore provides the opportunity for the family members to focus on their loved one, and the health care organization provides interpreters at no cost. In addition, the health care provider prefers to use the health care interpreter provided by the organization. Although the provider is taking measures to provide services that are culturally and linguistically appropriate and respectful, this should not be interpreted as a barrier when having to address issues with a discontent patient or family member. Being culturally aware and respectful can provide insight to challenges when questions arise as to whom should or should not receive information, perceptions of noncompliance, lack of adherence, or family decision-making situations.

For situations where the provider is truly bilingual and other members of the health care team are present, the provider should not act as an interpreter. Instead, an interpreter should be present to interpret for the health care team colleagues. During this encounter, the provider's role and focus is that of a health care provider and not as an interpreter. In addition, the provider and interpreter should be aware of nonverbal communication that could be misinterpreted by the family. A sigh or shrugging of shoulders could have an alternate meaning in diverse cultures.

As an interpreter, it is one's ethical responsibility to interpret accurately and completely. To do this, the interpreter's introduction will state their name and title, and provide a synopsis of their role and function, sharing this introduction with the health care team and patient and patient's family. The interpreter will address themselves in third person, interpreting in the first person to remain transparent. An interpreter will request additional information for an utterance that needs clarification. Bottom line, the message is not to be edited, omitted, or altered. If a provider senses this happening, the provider should pause and confirm with the interpreter regarding the content of the message.

HOW TO TEACH CULTURAL AND LINGUISTIC COMPETENCE TO PROVIDERS

The population of the United States of America is becoming more diverse, and it is predicted that by the year 2050 ethnic minorities will become the majority.[41] Despite the increase of ethnic minorities in the US population, the country is still plagued with health care disparities.[42] Some patients delay seeking care, have concerns they will receive lower quality care, and perceive they will be treated poorly.[32,43] Evidence suggests that training physicians in cultural competence will improve communication between patients and physicians, improve patient satisfaction, improve clinical outcomes through improved adherence, and ultimately reduce health disparities.[32,44–46]

Currently, the Liaison Committee for Medical Education and the Accreditation Council for Graduate Medical Education promote training in cultural competence for medical students and residents.[47–49] The US Department of Health and Human Services Office of Minority Health via their National Standards for Culturally and Linguistically Appropriate Services in Health and Healthcare also promotes education of health care providers to ensure culturally and linguistically appropriate practices for all patients and their families.[50] Despite these recommendations, training of physicians during their formal education is lacking. Their cultural competence training often occurs in short intervals during their preclinical years and is not linked with hands-on, real life experiences or targeted feedback from experts in cultural and linguistic competence.[32,44,51] A study of resident physicians in 2003 found that they felt ill prepared to provide cross-cultural care as compared with other clinical tasks.[52] They also noted that there was little time allotted to training in these areas during residency training and no formal evaluation or modeling by faculty members.[52] With the US population becoming more diverse and strong data to support health care disparities, it is imperative for the US medical education system to begin instituting interactive and evidence-based education on cultural competency and linguistics across the medical education continuum.

Table 2
Tips for providing successful cultural and linguistic competence education

Tips	Aspects of Practical Implementation
Provide training across the continuum of medical education and on into practice	• Training should be targeted to fit the needs of learner level and specific skills they will be required to master. • Training should begin during undergraduate medical education and continue through continuing medical education in practice.
Use cutting-edge instructional techniques	• Interactive, hands-on experiences that embrace new educational technologies will help learners gain the critical, real-life skills for patient care. • Instructional techniques recommended include standardized patient encounters, simulation or role play, virtual reality, reflection exercises, and journaling.
Teach practical skills that can be directly applied in real life settings	• Do not focus solely on the acquisition of knowledge about cultural or linguistic competency. • Teach skills that learners can directly apply to real life scenarios. • Do not oversimplify concepts, instead teach knowledge, skills, and attitudes that are applicable to many patients and cultures.
Embrace adult learning theory[54] in curriculum development	• Adult learners prefer to be involved in the planning and evaluation of their learning and their previous experiences should be taken in to account during instruction. • Makes content and activities relevant to their current activities, allow them to apply new knowledge and skills immediately, and share how it will affect their current job. • Make training problem-centered vs content-oriented.
Do not isolate training, instead embed throughout one's training or practice	• Isolated training experiences disconnect learners from seeing opportunities for practical application of knowledge, skills, and attitudes in multiple venues and scenarios. • Attempt to weave cultural and linguistic competency training, daily training if possible.
Training faculty and supervisors is critical	• Many faculty members and supervisors have never received cultural or linguistic competency training. Furthermore, they are uncomfortable providing mentoring and feedback to trainees. • Training for faculty and supervisors in this area will be critical to curriculum roll out, skills modeling, and feedback for learners.

(*continued on next page*)

Table 2
(*continued*)

Tips	Aspects of Practical Implementation
Provide observation and direct assessment	• Direct observation of one's cultural and linguistic competency is key for skill acquisition and advancement. • Faculty and supervisors should provide observation and feedback, including using structured assessment tools.
Train a core group of faculty members as experts in the areas of cultural and linguistic competency	• These faculty members can serve as your team of individuals that will help with training, observation, feedback, and role modeling.
Make training and feedback evidence-based and a "real science"[53]	• Cultural and linguistic competency can often be viewed as a "soft science" that is based more on communication skills and empathy, as compared with the evidence-based fact-oriented rest of medical education. • There is a great deal of emerging evidence that is available regarding cultural and linguistic competency. Weave this evidence into training sessions.
Incorporate quality improvement methodologies into training and feedback	• Often, improving cultural and linguistic competency in a health care system requires major culture and systems change. • Using quality improvement methodologies to invoke uptake and execution of improved knowledge, skills, and attitudes. It also provides a system to provide feedback and small tests of change.

Data from Kripalani S, Bussey-Jones J, Katz MG, Genao I. A prescription for cultural competence in medical education. J Gen Intern Med. 2006;21(10):1116-1120.

Training in cultural and linguistic competency should optimally occur well in advance of beginning clinical experiences with patients and should continue throughout an individual's undergraduate and graduate medical education and follow into practice. Training while in practice is critical because communication and linguistic practices and their associated technology, requirements, and laws are constantly evolving. Furthermore, practitioners may move from one location of practice to another or change their line of work, thus necessitating them to care for populations with varying regional cultural, racial, and linguistic preferences. Evolution of practice and requirements makes on-demand, just-in-time training an efficient and effective way to deliver important training or updates when needed. Additional recommendations for how to provide effective cultural and linguistic education are provided in **Table 2**.

SUMMARY

Although barriers exist to effective communication with patients and families during hospitalizations, evidence-based strategies and policies exist for health care providers and institutions to integrate into practice to improve patient- and family-centered communication. Incorporating the techniques, strategies, and policies discussed in this chapter, both in clinical and educational endeavors, will help ensure patients and families receive safe, equitable, and informed care during hospital stay, according to their own linguistic and cultural practices.

REFERENCES

1. Perloff R, Bonder B, Ray G, et al. Doctor-Patient Communication, Cultural Competence, and Minority Health: Theoretical and Empirical Perspectives. Am Behav Sci 2006;49(6):835–52.
2. Ranjan P, Kumari A, Chakrawarty A. How can doctors improve their communication skills? J Clin Diagn Res 2015;9(3):JE01–4.
3. White HL, Glazier RH. Do hospitalist physicians improve the quality of inpatient care delivery? A systematic review of process, efficiency and outcome measures. BMC Med 2011;9:58.
4. Manojlovich M, Harrod M, Holtz B, et al. The use of multiple qualitative methods to characterize communication events between physicians and nurses. Health Commun 2015;30(1):61–9.
5. Fisher MJ, Broome ME. Parent-provider communication during hospitalization. J Pediatr Nurs 2011;26(1):58–69.
6. Khan A, Furtak SL, Melvin P, et al. Parent-reported errors and adverse events in hospitalized children. JAMA Pediatr 2016;170(4):e154608.
7. Khan A, Coffey M, Litterer KP, et al. Families as partners in hospital error and adverse event surveillance. JAMA Pediatr 2017;171(4):372–81.
8. Khan A, Rogers JE, Forster CS, et al. Communication and shared understanding between parents and resident-physicians at night. Hosp Pediatr 2016;6(6):319–29.
9. Khan A, Rogers JE, Melvin P, et al. Physician and nurse nighttime communication and parents' hospital experience. Pediatrics 2015;136(5):e1249–58.
10. Airhihenbuwa C. Health and culture: beyond the western paradigm. Thousand Oaks (CA): Sage Publications; 1995.
11. Basu A, Dutta MJ. Centralizing context and culture in the co-construction of health: localizing and vocalizing health meanings in rural India. Health Commun 2007;21(2):187–96.
12. Helman C. Culture, health, and illness. Bristol (United Kingdom): Wright; 1986.
13. Documet PI, Green HH, Adams J, et al. Perspectives of African American, Amish, Appalachian And Latina women on breast and cervical cancer screening: implications for cultural competence. J Health Care Poor Underserved 2008;19(1):56–74.
14. Sklar DP. Cultural competence: glimpsing the world through our patients' eyes as we guide their care. Acad Med 2018;93(9):1259–62.
15. Weaver C, Sklar D. Diagnostic dilemmas and cultural diversity in emergency rooms. West J Med 1980;133(4):356–66.
16. Luckhaupt SE, Yi MS, Mueller CV, et al. Beliefs of primary care residents regarding spirituality and religion in clinical encounters with patients: a study at a midwestern U.S. teaching institution. Acad Med 2005;80(6):560–70.
17. Curlin FA, Sellergren SA, Lantos JD, et al. Physicians' observations and interpretations of the influence of religion and spirituality on health. Arch Intern Med 2007;167(7):649–54.
18. MacLean CD, Susi B, Phifer N, et al. Patient preference for physician discussion and practice of spirituality. J Gen Intern Med 2003;18(1):38–43.
19. Cochran D, Saleem S, Khowaja-Punjwani S, et al. Cross-cultural differences in communication about a dying child. Pediatrics 2017;140(5).

20. Jacobs B, Ryan AM, Henrichs KS, et al. Medical interpreters in outpatient practice. Ann Fam Med 2018;16(1):70–6.
21. Karliner LS, Jacobs EA, Chen AH, et al. Do professional interpreters improve clinical care for patients with limited English proficiency? A systematic review of the literature. Health Serv Res 2007;42(2):727–54.
22. Lopez L, Rodriguez F, Huerta D, et al. Use of interpreters by physicians for hospitalized limited English proficient patients and its impact on patient outcomes. J Gen Intern Med 2015;30(6):783–9.
23. DeCamp LR, Kuo DZ, Flores G, et al. Changes in language services use by US pediatricians. Pediatrics 2013;132(2):e396–406.
24. Zurca AD, Fisher KR, Flor RJ, et al. Communication with limited english-proficient families in the PICU. Hosp Pediatr 2017;7(1):9–15.
25. Oshimi T. Effective written communication for patients with limited English proficiency. Chest 2007;132(5):1688–90.
26. Kuo DZ, Sisterhen LL, Sigrest TE, et al. Family experiences and pediatric health services use associated with family-centered rounds. Pediatrics 2012;130(2):299–305.
27. Subramony A, Hametz PA, Balmer D. Family-centered rounds in theory and practice: an ethnographic case study. Acad Pediatr 2014;14(2):200–6.
28. Institute for patient and family-centered care: what is patient and family-centered care?. Available at: http://www.ipfcc.org/about/pfcc.html. Accessed August 24, 2018.
29. Ward DR, Ghali WA, Graham A, et al. A real-time locating system observes physician time-motion patterns during walk-rounds: a pilot study. BMC Med Educ 2014;14:37.
30. Andrulis DP, Brach C. Integrating literacy, culture, and language to improve health care quality for diverse populations. Am J Health Behav 2007;31(Suppl 1):S122–33.
31. Hudelson P. Improving patient-provider communication: insights from interpreters. Fam Pract 2005;22(3):311–6.
32. Flores G, Gee D, Kastner B. The teaching of cultural issues in U.S. and Canadian medical schools. Acad Med 2000;75(5):451–5.
33. The Department of Health and Human Services Language Access Plan. 2013. Available at: http://www.hhs.gov/sites/default/files/open/pres-actions/2013-hhs-language-access-plan.pdf. Accessed May 9, 2018.
34. What's in a word: a guide to understanding interpreting and translation in health care. Available at: http://www.healthlaw.org/publications/search-publications/whats-in-a-word-a-guide-to-understanding-interpreting-and-translation-in-health-care-full-guide#.Wupa0DBrzv8. Accessed May 9, 2018.
35. Schwei RJ, Schroeder M, Ejebe I, et al. limited english proficient patients' perceptions of when interpreters are needed and how the decision to utilize interpreters is made. Health Commun 2018;33(12):1503–8.
36. The National Council on Interperting in Health Care (NCIHC) sight translation and written translation: guidelines for healthcare interpreters. 2010. Available at: https://ncihc.memberclicks.net/assets/documents/translation%20guidelines%20for%20interpreters%20revised%20031710.pdf. Accessed May 9, 2018.
37. Guidance to federal financial assistance recipients regarding title VI prohibition against national origin discrimination affecting limited english proficient persons. Available at: https://www.hhs.gov/civil-rights/for-individuals/special-topics/limited-english-proficiency/guidance-federal-financial-assistance-recipients-title-vi/index.html. Accessed May 14, 2018.

38. Flores G, Laws MB, Mayo SJ, et al. Errors in medical interpretation and their potential clinical consequences in pediatric encounters. Pediatrics 2003;111(1):6–14.
39. Flores G. Culture and the patient-physician relationship: achieving cultural competency in health care. J Pediatr 2000;136(1):14–23.
40. The National Council on interpreting in health care code of ethics and standards of practice. Available at: http://www.ncihc.org/ethics-and-standards-of-practice. Accessed May 14, 2018.
41. Projections of the size and composition of the U.S. population: 2014 to 2060. Available at: https://census.gov/content/dam/Census/library/publications/2015/demo/p25-1143.pdf. Accessed May 18, 2018.
42. CDC health disparities & inequalities report (CHDIR) - US. 2013. Available at: https://www.cdc.gov/minorityhealth/chdireport.html. Accessed May 24, 2018.
43. Martin KD, Roter DL, Beach MC, et al. Physician communication behaviors and trust among black and white patients with hypertension. Med Care 2013;51(2):151–7.
44. Beach MC, Price EG, Gary TL, et al. Cultural competence: a systematic review of health care provider educational interventions. Med Care 2005;43(4):356–73.
45. Carrillo JE, Green AR, Betancourt JR. Cross-cultural primary care: a patient-based approach. Ann Intern Med 1999;130(10):829–34.
46. Brach C, Fraser I. Can cultural competency reduce racial and ethnic health disparities? A review and conceptual model. Med Care Res Rev 2000;57(Suppl 1):181–217.
47. Cultural Competence Education - Association of American Medical Colleges. Available at: https://www.aamc.org/download/54338/data/. Accessed May 24, 2018.
48. Ambrose AJ, Lin SY, Chun MB. Cultural competency training requirements in graduate medical education. J Grad Med Educ 2013;5(2):227–31.
49. ACGME common program requirements. Available at: http://www.acgme.org/Portals/0/PFAssets/ProgramRequirements/CPRs_2017-07-01.pdf. Accessed May 24, 2018.
50. The National CLAS Standards. Available at: https://minorityhealth.hhs.gov/omh/browse.aspx?lvl=2&lvlid=53. Accessed May 24, 2018.
51. Betancourt JR. Eliminating racial and ethnic disparities in health care: what is the role of academic medicine? Acad Med 2006;81(9):788–92.
52. Weissman JS, Betancourt J, Campbell EG, et al. Resident physicians' preparedness to provide cross-cultural care. JAMA 2005;294(9):1058–67.
53. Kripalani S, Bussey-Jones J, Katz MG, et al. A prescription for cultural competence in medical education. J Gen Intern Med 2006;21(10):1116–20.
54. Knowles MS, Holton EF, Swanson RA. The adult learner: the definitive classic in adult education and human resource development. 7th edition. New York: Routledge; 2012.

Health Literacy in the Inpatient Setting

Implications for Patient Care and Patient Safety

Alexander F. Glick, MD, MS[a,*], Cindy Brach, MPP[b],
Hsiang Shonna Yin, MD, MS[c], Benard P. Dreyer, MD[d]

KEYWORDS

• Health literacy • Communication • Patient safety • Patient- and family-centered care • Pediatrics • Inpatient care • Bedside rounds • Discharge

KEY POINTS

- Health literacy plays a role in the events leading up to children's hospitalizations, during hospital admission, and after discharge.
- Hospitals and providers should use a universal precautions approach and routinely incorporate health-literacy-informed strategies in communicating with all patients and families to ensure that they can understand health information, follow medical instructions, participate actively in their own/their child's care, and successfully navigate the health care system.
- Interventions that incorporate health-literacy-informed strategies and that target patients/families and health care systems should be implemented to improve patient outcomes and patient-centered and family-centered care.

HEALTH LITERACY CHALLENGES RELATED TO HOSPITALIZATION

Each year, more than 1.5 million children are hospitalized.[1] Families face many challenges during their child's hospitalization, as well as at the time of hospital discharge. They are tasked with the responsibility of describing their child's symptoms and

---

Disclosure: The authors have no commercial or financial conflicts of interest. Dr A.F. Glick is funded by an institutional K award through the NYU-NYC Health + Hospitals CTSI (KL2TR 001446). Dr H.S. Yin is funded through the following: FDA HHSF223201510148C, NIH/NICHD R01 HD059794, and the USDA - Agriculture and Food Research Initiative.
[a] Department of Pediatrics, NYU School of Medicine, NYU Langone Health, Bellevue Hospital Center, 462 1st Avenue, Administration Building 3rd Floor, New York, NY 10016, USA; [b] Center for Evidence and Practice Improvement, Agency for Healthcare Research and Quality, 5600 Fishers Lane, 5W08, Rockville, MD 20857, USA; [c] NYU School of Medicine, NYU Langone Health, Bellevue Hospital Center, 550 1st Avenue, NBV 8E 14, New York, NY 10016, USA; [d] NYU School of Medicine, NYU Langone Health, Bellevue Hospital Center, 550 1st Avenue, NBV 8E-11D, New York, NY 10016, USA
* Corresponding author.
E-mail address: alexander.glick@nyulangone.org

Pediatr Clin N Am 66 (2019) 805–826
https://doi.org/10.1016/j.pcl.2019.03.007

providing a coherent, detailed history, and are presented with possible diagnoses by health care providers. Families must choose to accept or reject possible treatments, weighing risks and benefits. They are asked to learn how to take care of their child when it is time to go home and what they should watch out for that would warrant renewed medical attention.

Health literacy skills impact the ability of families to handle the hospital demands placed on them. Health literacy has been traditionally defined as "the ability to obtain, process, understand, and use basic health information and services needed to make appropriate health decisions."[2] There is, however, growing support of the construct that health literacy is a product of both the skills and abilities of individuals, and the complexity of health information and health care tasks presented to families by those in the health care system. How effectively families are able to participate in their child's care during and after a hospitalization therefore depends largely on how easy the hospital makes it for them to understand and act on information, and navigate the health care system.[3]

Without realizing it, hospitals frequently make the hospitalization experience difficult for families. Clinicians and other staff use specialized medical terminology that is effectively shorthand among themselves but frequently is incomprehensible to others.[4,5] Members of the hospital staff often provide families with too much information at one time and do not check whether they understood it.[6] They send families home with prescriptions for medicines without determining whether families are able to fill them or know how to administer medicines correctly.[7] Families are often sent home with confusing discharge instructions, without an assessment by hospital staff to ensure that they are able to follow them properly.[8] Providers also make referrals for additional tests and care without providing assistance in making the follow-up appointments or taking into consideration transportation barriers.[9,10] Lack of attention to these health literacy issues creates a patient safety risk. Each time an instruction is misunderstood, a medicine is not taken, or an appointment is not kept is a patient safety event, that is, an event that has the potential to lead to a worse patient outcome.

EPIDEMIOLOGY

According to the most recent health literacy data, 77 million adults, or 36% of adults in the United States, are categorized as having limited health literacy, indicating that they have no more than the most simple and concrete literacy skills[11,12]; this includes nearly 21 million parents (29% of US parents).[13] Notably, only 12% of adults are considered to have "proficient" health literacy skills,[11] which means that the vast majority of individuals experience health literacy challenges. In addition, only 8% of US adults have "proficient" numeracy skills; such skills are often needed in health-related decision-making, including tasks such as understanding the relative risks and benefits of treatment options, and correct administration of medications (amount, frequency, duration).[14] Those from low socioeconomic status backgrounds, low educational attainment, racial/ethnic minority groups, and non-English speakers, are disproportionately affected by limited health literacy.[11] A growing body of research indicates that health literacy is an important contributing factor to income-associated and race/ethnicity-associated health disparities.[13]

Although an individual's overall health literacy skill level is important, another issue to consider is the dynamic nature of health literacy, and the impact of anxiety and stress on an individual's ability to process and act on health information.[15] For example, parents who believe their child is in pain are less likely to understand information provided during encounters with the health care team.[16] Throughout the hospitalization and at the time of hospital discharge, parents are often sleep deprived and are experiencing high levels of stress and fear related to their child's prognosis, which can interfere with their ability to function at their normal level of health literacy. Given that health literacy is dynamic and not static, a "state" rather than a "trait," health care providers should consider *all* individuals to be at risk for limited health literacy. Experts therefore recommend following health literacy universal precautions: assuming that all patients may have difficulty comprehending health information and accessing health services.[17]

Measuring individuals' health literacy is not recommended as part of clinical practice. This is because not only is health literacy dynamic, but all patients benefit from clear communication. Measuring health literacy can be important at the population level, however, and is essential for research purposes. Researchers have used a wide variety of measures to assess individuals' health literacy. Tools used to assess health literacy include both objective measures (eg, Short Test of Functional Health Literacy in Adults,[18] Newest Vital Sign,[19] Parental Health Literacy Activities Test[20]) and subjective measures, focusing on an individual's self-reported ability to understand health information (eg, Single Item Literacy Screener[21]) or work with numbers (Subjective Numeracy Scale[22]). The Health Literacy Toolshed Web site houses a comprehensive listing of health literacy measures (https://healthliteracy.bu.edu).[23]

HEALTH-LITERACY-INFORMED COMMUNICATION STRATEGIES

The Joint Commission has asserted that unaddressed health literacy issues undermine the safety of patients and the ability of health care organizations to comply with accreditation standards, which require hospitals to identify and meet patients' oral and written communication needs.[24] Adopting health literacy universal precautions is a way of meeting those needs that benefits everyone, regardless of their education or literacy level. One of the most important components of health literacy universal precautions is the teach-back method, also known as the teach-to-goal method. In the context of provider-parent communication, providers ask parents to describe the information they have been given using their own words. If the parent teaches back the information inaccurately, or repeats the provider's exact words, the provider re-teaches the information in a different way and again asks for a teach-back of the information. This is repeated until the parent can describe the information correctly in his or her own words. The Agency for Healthcare Research and Quality and the National Quality Forum declared teach-back to be a Safe Practice for informed consent[25,26]; "Always Use Teach-back" is a key component in the Institute for Healthcare Improvement's recommended discharge process.[27] Research studies show that teach-back can increase comprehension, reduce medication errors, and reduce readmissions.[28–30] Best practice calls for using the "chunk-and-check" strategy, whereby teach-back is performed intermittently in a discussion so that each set of information is digested before another is introduced. If the information is an instruction about how to use a medication or equipment, such as how to use an inhaler or administer a medication via a feeding tube, the "Show Me" or "Show-Back" method, in which a provider asks for a demonstration rather than a spoken teach-back (often after first demonstrating the steps of a task), is more effective at detecting misunderstanding than teach-back.[30]

Teach-back is just one of a number of health-literacy-informed strategies for spoken communication. One of the strategies that health care providers find difficult to implement is limiting the amount of information presented at one time. Prioritizing 2 or 3 most important messages requires distinguishing between "need-to-know" and "nice-to-know" information. With large quantities of "need-to-know" information, it is optimal if educators can begin to provide teaching at the beginning of the hospital stay, recognizing that multiple teaching sessions might be needed to ensure learning. Other strategies include speaking distinctly, at a moderate pace, and using common, everyday language, that is, plain language that is free of medical jargon. Listening without interrupting is a highly effective and undervalued skill. Encouraging questions by asking "What questions do you have for me?" recognizes that families are likely to have questions; this strategy is preferred over asking "Do you have any questions?" which is more likely to lead to a response of "no" even when families do have questions. Communication must also be culturally and linguistically competent, showing respect for diverse cultures, customs, and beliefs. Only qualified interpreters should be used when there are language barriers (See Jennifer K. O'Toole and colleagues' article,"Communication with Diverse Patients: Addressing Culture and Language," in this issue).

Use of written information to supplement what is discussed verbally is known to help reduce cognitive load (or the amount of information that working memory can hold and process at one time), making it easier for families to understand and act on the information provided.[31] It is best to use materials that incorporate plain language principles, include simple visual aids, make their purpose evident, focus on a limited number of messages, sequence information logically, break-up information into sections with informative titles, break-up actions into manageable steps and make numbers easy to understand and do not require calculations. Referring to written materials as part of verbal counseling is considered to be especially effective. The American Academy of Pediatrics' *Plain Language Pediatrics: Health Literacy Strategies and Communication Resources for Common Pediatric Topics* is one example of educational materials that are easy to understand and can complement a verbal explanation of many common diagnoses.[32] It is important to keep in mind, however, that many individuals have poor reading skills; 18% of the US adult population scored at the lowest level of an international literacy assessment.[11,12] Others may not learn well by reading. Still others may lack time or concentration to read materials. Technology, such as talking touchscreens or audiovisual presentations, can sometimes overcome literacy barriers; providers could use this as part of verbal counseling to reinforce concepts, but should not assume that the families they care for have access to such technologies for home education. Written handouts are still important memory aids and reference documents. When it comes to written materials, experts give the following advice:

- Choose materials that are easy to understand and act on. You can evaluate materials by using an assessment tool such as the Patient Education Materials Assessment Tool (PEMAT) (note that there is a PEMAT-AV as well, which is helpful for assessing audiovisual information).[33]
- Provide materials in languages your patients read[34] (see Communication with Diverse Patients: Addressing Language and Culture).
- Never assume people are going to read what you give them. Review written materials together. Personalize and highlight important information (eg, circle, underline, star important concepts).[35]
- When reviewing written information, use easy-to-understand words, organized in a logical fashion, and focus on key action items.[36]
- Use of pictures or drawings to support the text is linked to improved understanding and ability to act on medical instructions.[37,38]
- Even when written materials are given to families, teach-back, and show-back should still be used whenever possible to confirm understanding.[7,32]

- To create written materials that are understood by the target audience follow guidance such as that outlined in the Toolkit for Making Written Materials Clear and Effective.[39]

A summary of health-literacy-informed verbal and written communication strategies is presented in **Table 1**.

IMPACT OF HEALTH LITERACY ON MANAGEMENT OF CHRONIC CONDITIONS THAT CAN LEAD TO HOSPITALIZATION

Limited health literacy is associated with poor chronic disease management, contributing to emergency department (ED) visits and hospitalizations. Most of the pediatric research to date has been related to asthma and diabetes. Parents with limited health

Table 1
Health literacy communication strategies and resources

Health Literacy Strategies for Spoken Communication	Health Literacy Strategies for Written Materials
• Use a private, quiet space • Sit down and be at the patient's eye level • Make good eye contact • Ask the patient/family to invite others they want to be part of the conversation • Limit discussion to 2–3 main points • Listen without interrupting • Speak distinctly and at a moderate pace • Use every day, familiar words • Use medical terms only if it is important for the patient to become familiar with a medical term; be sure to explain what the term means and check understanding • Show pictures or use models • Use the teach-back method (Example of provider statement: "I want to make sure I did a good job explaining how to give Carlos the medicine. Can you tell me how much medication you will give each time?"); try to "chunk-and-check" so that teach-back focuses on one topic at a time • Demonstrate how it is done (eg, exercises, taking medicine) and have the patient or family member "show-back" how they would do it; encourage questions and elicit concerns and priorities • Repeat key points • Respect diverse cultures, customs, and beliefs (see Communication with Diverse Patients: Addressing Language and Culture) • Use only qualified interpreters when there are language barriers (See Communication with Diverse Patients: Addressing Language and Culture) • Teach trainees to explain information to families in words they can understand • Speak to and involve the child as appropriate	• Make purpose evident • Focus on a limited number of messages • Sequence information logically • Break-up information into sections with informative titles • Use plain language • Make numbers easy to understand and do not require calculations • Provide clear instructions (eg, Uniform Medication Schedule – UMS; "give medicine in the morning and in the evening" more explicit than "give 2 times a day") • Use simple visuals that enhance understanding rather than distract • Use large font size, bulleted text, and short sentences • Make use of alternatives to print, including talking touch screens, audiovisual, and multimedia materials. • Break-up actions into manageable steps • Review print information verbally, personalizing it by using strategies such as highlighting, circling, starring, and underlining, to draw attention to key information

literacy have poor asthma knowledge and have difficulty following their child's asthma action plan.[40,41] With respect to understanding and management of diabetes mellitus, parents with lower health literacy scores have worse adherence to complex insulin regimens compared with those with adequate health literacy.[42] Children of parents with low numeracy scores have poorer diabetes control as reflected by higher hemoglobin A1C levels.[43]

Limited health literacy is frequently associated with increased health care utilization. ED visits[41,44] and hospitalizations[45] are more likely in children with asthma whose parents have limited health literacy. In addition, children whose parents had limited health literacy have more ED visits overall.[46]

IMPACT OF HEALTH LITERACY ACROSS THE HOSPITALIZATION AND BEYOND: EVIDENCE FOR HEALTH-LITERACY-INFORMED COMMUNICATION STRATEGIES

A patient or parent's health literacy is relevant across the course of a hospitalization, beginning at the time of admission and continuing through discharge. In this section, we review key timepoints during a hospitalization using a health literacy perspective, incorporating information from the pediatric inpatient literature when possible and expanding to other settings and adult literature when relevant. These are summarized in **Table 2**. Pertinent interventions that may help overcome the effects of limited health literacy in the inpatient setting also are discussed.

Taking Complete and Accurate History

Health literacy skills affect the ability of caregivers and patients to report a thorough, accurate, and coherent history. Individuals often do not have a good understanding of their children's chronic medical problems,[40,41,47] which can make it challenging to give detailed information about past medical history and medications. One study found that two-thirds of patients had a poor understanding of their home medications.[48] Several studies have focused on an individual's understanding of their family history; between 20% and 60% of adults inaccurately report their family history of cancer.[49,50] The manner in which the history is taken should be taken into consideration; for example, those with limited health literacy struggle when written screening tools are used to elicit the history of a symptom.[51]

Improving parental understanding of a child's chronic diseases and overall history is important for a parent to be able to report this information on admission. One intervention that targeted parents of children with asthma used low literacy, pictogram-based and photograph-based asthma action plans; parents receiving the low literacy plan were more likely to understand which medications to give every day and when sick; they also made fewer errors regarding spacer use.[52] Although education to improve parent understanding of their child's chronic disease management regimen may begin in the outpatient setting, this teaching should continue during the hospital stay so families can become more comfortable with this information.

Just as families struggle to convey information on a child's medical history, provider history-taking techniques have also been found to be suboptimal. Some studies have shown that more than half of providers use jargon during their initial encounter with families, and many ask lengthy and complex questions.[4,5] If providers use confusing language and do not effectively ask questions that guide patients through the history-taking process, they may not obtain a complete and accurate picture, and diagnosis and treatment may be delayed.

Use of health-literacy-informed communication strategies can improve the likelihood that providers elucidate a clear history. Providers should ask simple questions

Table 2
Health literacy–related challenges for families across the hospitalization and ways to optimize this process[a]

Challenges for Family	Ways Provider/System Can Optimize This Process

Reporting an accurate history
• Chronic medical problems/past medical history
• Medications
• Reporting symptoms
• Family history
	• Acknowledge that what you are asking the parent to do is difficult. They are likely tired or stressed because their child is sick; you may need to return at a later time to clarify key points, especially if you're taking a history in the middle of the night.
	• Stay clear of distractions (eg, looking at computers/tablets, noisy environments)
	• Take a clear and thorough history
	  ○ Start with open-ended questions
	  ○ Progress to more focused questions when needed
	  ○ Ask clarifying questions
	  ○ Ask questions in multiple different ways if families are having trouble (eg, history of medical problems, prior hospitalizations, types of doctors child is being followed by)
	  ○ Use clear language the family can understand
	  ○ Ask one question at a time
	  ○ Summarize the history
	  ○ Take history as a team or share history among the team to eliminate the need for parents to repeat a history multiple times
	• Do not use screening tools that are difficult for parents to navigate

Provider to parent communication at admission • Diagnosis • Reason for admission	• Ensure that families understand their chronic and other medical conditions at the point of diagnosis • Use written or audiovisual materials that use health-literacy-informed strategies to supplement verbal counseling on diagnosis • May need to explain information again if family members are tired, in pain, or experiencing stress/anxiety
Plan of care: tests, treatments, procedures, and informed consent	• Explain risks, harms, and benefits of choices, including the choice to not have a test, procedure, or treatment • Use high-quality decision aids to elicit goals and values • Use easy-to-understand consent documents • Use whiteboards, easy-to-understand written materials, or easy-to-access patient portals to supplement verbal counseling on plan of care • Update the family throughout the hospitalization • Use easy-to-access patient portal to share easy-to-understand explanations of results • Provide written information summarizing results in a way the family can understand • Ensure providers are on the same page, providing one centralized message throughout the hospital stay
Bedside rounds	• Start with the family's concerns first • Review the child's health status in the context of the hospital stay • Summarize what is new and what has changed • Summarize the plan for the day • Discuss things that might happen/change and what family members can do to help and watch out for • Provide an easy-to-understand written summary of the plan for the day

(*continued on next page*)

Table 2
(continued)

Challenges for Family	Ways Provider/System Can Optimize This Process

Discharge	• Start education at the beginning of the hospital stay
	• Use shared decision-making strategies for reaching an agreement about discharge goals and postdischarge treatment
	• Use health-literacy-informed verbal communication strategies (eg, plain language, teach-back, limit information, encourage questions)
	  ○ Use health-literacy-informed written communication strategies (eg, 6th–8th-grade level, understandable and actionable)
	• Make sure verbal and written instructions include all key domains of care
	  ○ Medications (including changes to medication regimen, dosing, side effects)
	  ○ Appointments
	  ○ Return precautions
	  ○ Diet, activity, bathing restrictions
	  ○ Information on return to school/daycare
	  ○ Equipment
	  ○ Additional postdischarge imaging/testing needed
	  ○ Information on who to contact with questions or if problems arise
	• Navigation assistance
	  ○ Make appointments at a convenient time for the family and establish that they have a plan to get to appointments
	  ○ Set up delivery of equipment and ensure family knows how to use it
	  ○ Delivery of medications to bedside if possible, ascertain how medicines will be obtained in the future, and whether financial assistance is needed
	• Postdischarge
	  ○ Send the discharge summary to the outpatient clinician the day of discharge as many children will have appointments the next day. This ensures the outpatient clinician has the information at the follow-up visit and does not have to rely on the parent
	  ○ Conduct a follow-up phone call 2–3 days after discharge to check on the child, ensure instructions have been followed, and that no additional issues have come up
	  ○ Staff and provide a phone number for families to call with questions after discharge

[a] This table contains a list of strategies to use during specific parts of the hospitalization. The general health-literacy-informed strategies mentioned in **Table 1** should be incorporated at every point throughout the hospitalization.

one at a time and ask clarifying questions to obtain all of the necessary details. The interview should start with open-ended questions, followed by more focused questions. The interviewer should also summarize the patient's history to confirm that the health care team has accurately understood the information conveyed.[53] Although self-administered written screening tools can be confusing and difficult to navigate, an intervention that used a multimedia version of such a tool (incorporating color coding, written questions, and a video of someone reading the questions with ability to have the question repeated) led to improved ability to answer the questions in patients across all literacy levels.[51]

Communication of the Diagnosis and Reason for Admission

Discussion of potential diagnoses and plans of care takes place after the initial history and physical and throughout the hospitalization. As part of these conversations, providers must explain the most likely diagnosis, other potential diagnoses being considered, the rationale for hospitalization (for admission or the need for continued inpatient care), and the plan for care of the hospitalized child.

Families frequently misunderstand information related to the diagnosis and reason for admission. Approximately 25% of parents are unable to state their child's diagnosis in the ED, and complex admissions associated with multiple diagnoses are even more confusing.[54] Other studies have shown that up to 50% of individuals misunderstand the reason for admission.[16]

A number of provider behaviors have been identified as contributing to poor understanding of the diagnosis by patients and their families. Physicians often leave out key information related to diagnoses[55] and include jargon in these descriptions.[56] Complaints that physicians do not give enough information about medical conditions are especially common among patients with limited health literacy.[57] These studies highlight the need for provider use of health-literacy-informed communication strategies such as teach-back with patients and families to confirm understanding. Several health-literacy-informed interventions have been developed to improve understanding of the reason for admission. One intervention focused on use of bedside huddles with the nurse, physician, and parents for the 2 most medically active patients on the unit; written update sheets with the plan of care were given to these families. The intervention led to parents' reporting better communication with overnight doctors, improvement in shared understanding between the parent and nurse, and a trend toward improvement in concordance between the reason for admission reported by the parents and what was documented in the written signout.[58]

Understanding the Plan of Care: Tests, Treatment, Procedures, and Informed Consent

Another domain of inpatient care in which health literacy plays a role and in which parent misunderstanding is common is the plan of care, including treatments provided, as well as tests and procedures to be performed. One study found that only one-third of parents completely understood the plan of care, including treatment and potential tests or procedures.[59] Another study found that 38% of patients were unaware of all the tests planned for a given day, and 10% were unaware of planned procedures.[60] Complex plans are more likely to be associated with a lack of shared understanding between the provider and parent.[61] Parents have particular difficulty understanding postoperative pain management plans, with up to one-third having no understanding of risks associated with their child's pain management regimen.[62] In general, patients with limited health literacy are also less likely to ask physicians questions about therapeutic regimens,[63] which may further contribute to poor understanding. Much of the lack of parental understanding may be due to poor communication from the inpatient team. One study by Khan and colleagues[64] have shown that information given to families by providers during the inpatient stay is often conflicting, delayed, or erroneous. Patients with limited health literacy are more likely to rate inpatient communication as poor.[65]

Studies examining patient and family ability to understand care delivered in hospitals indicate that consent, if obtained at all, was frequently not adequately informed. For example, one study found that 76% of parents of children undergoing an endoscopy did not understand alternatives to the procedure and only 14% had a complete understanding of the entire informed consent discussion. Incomplete provider counseling was a key barrier.[66] Even when information is provided to parents, they often misunderstand the risks associated with surgical procedures[67] and anesthesia.[68]

The inpatient team should strive to present clear and timely information to families to ensure understanding of this information. Providing a clear written and verbal summary of events occurring during the hospital course can help. In one study of an intervention that used patient white boards to assist with communication, a greater proportion of patients knew their goals for admission, and nearly all patients wanted the white boards to list upcoming tests and studies.[69] In another intervention, providers wrote patient-directed letters describing the events of the hospitalization. The provider read the letter to the patient and allowed the patient to ask questions. After the intervention, patients had better understanding of the reasons for hospitalization, tests performed in the hospital, and treatments received.[70] However, this after-the-fact communication does not comport with the principles of informed consent, which requires understanding of information about tests, treatment, and procedures before they are administered. The informed consent process can be improved in several ways, including use of supplemental written information, audiovisual materials, and teach-back.[71] Hospitals can use the Agency for Healthcare Research and Quality's Making Informed Consent an Informed Choice: Training Module for Health Care Professionals to help providers learn how to use clear communication strategies.[72] Even when formal written informed consent is not required, providers should use these strategies when explaining the plan of care to ensure a shared understanding with the patient and family. There is also a second module designed for hospital leadership; the purpose of the module is to ensure that informed consent policies are complete and unambiguous and infrastructure supports are in place.

Conducting Bedside Rounds

One of the most important contexts for communication in the inpatient setting is bedside or family-centered rounds. Unfortunately, providers often use complex language on rounds without providing plain language explanations.[73] In addition, key content, such as information about discharge timing and medications, may not be presented on rounds.[74] Unsurprisingly, families often do not understand the information presented on rounds. One study found that only 40% of parents could accurately report the full plan discussed on rounds, and 1 in 4 were unaware of the diagnosis discussed on rounds.[75]

Provider use of health-literacy-informed communication strategies can improve a family's understanding of the information presented on bedside rounds. The Patient and Family-Centered I-PASS model,[76] designed using health literacy principles, gives providers a standard communication framework for rounds to ensure that important domains are covered. It is recommended that families are engaged from the very beginning of rounds, where family concerns are elicited and a shared understanding of the reason for admission and continued hospitalization is achieved. This is followed by information presented in "chunks," including (1) reviewing the child's health status in the context of the hospital stay (I = illness severity), (2) summary of the interval history (P = patient summary), (3) plan for the day (A = action list), and (4) things that might happen/change and what family members can help watch out for (S = situational awareness and contingency planning). All the while, providers use health-literacy-informed strategies (eg, chunk-and-check and simple, clear language). The parents can later synthesize the information (ie, teach-back). A written "rounds report" (on paper or on a white board) that uses health-literacy-informed strategies is provided. This gives parents the ability to more easily digest the information provided on rounds and allows them to have something to reference throughout the day and share with other family members.

Families often find rounds to be intimidating and may not understand what their role is on rounds. Providers can "set the stage" early in the admission to empower families to be actively engaged on rounds, emphasizing the important role that families play in describing concerns, asking questions, and helping to formulate the plan for the day. At admission, the health care team can designate a staff person to discuss this important role with families, and members of the health care team can reinforce this daily before rounds; an easy-to-understand pamphlet or handout clearly describing the rounds process, the family's role, and the role of each team member, can be helpful to supplement the verbal information conveyed by the team. This strategy has been used as part of the Patient and Family-Centered I-PASS model[76] (See Jennifer Baird and colleagues' article, "Interprofessional Teams: Current Trends and Future Directions," in this issue).

Preparing for Discharge

Families eagerly await discharge and do not always understand why the patient is still in the hospital and not yet discharged. One example from the pediatric emergency medicine literature found that one-third of families were not completely aware of the reasons they were still in the ED. Families with lower educational attainment were more likely to have answers discordant from those of the physicians.[73] When the time for discharge arrives, and most children are being prepared to go home, it is often chaotic. Parents are presented with a great deal of information, often right before leaving the hospital, about how to manage their child's care at home. Discharge instructions cover a wide range of domains including medications, appointments, return precautions (the signs and symptoms that must be monitored for at home), restrictions (eg, diet, activity-related), and equipment; these instructions are often confusing for families.[77]

Understanding of medication instructions can be particularly challenging for parents, especially those with limited health literacy,[78] posing a major threat to patient safety. Comprehension of medication duration, frequency, and indication is often poor.[77] More than 40% of parents do not understand medication side effects[79] and dose liquid medications incorrectly.[7] One intervention designed to improve parent ability to understand and follow medication instructions focused on use of health-literacy-informed communication strategies (teach-back, demonstration, medication instruction sheets with a pictographic representation of the amount of medication to be given, dosing tool provision). This intervention led to a reduction in dosing error rates for short-course prescribed medications (eg, antibiotics, steroids) from 48% to 5%, in addition to improvements in medication adherence.[7]

Parents also commonly misunderstand instructions related to their child's follow-up appointments,[79,80] return precautions,[81] activity restrictions,[82] medical equipment,[83] and testing needed after discharge.[84] Overall, patients with limited health literacy are less likely to understand and adhere to discharge instructions.[85]

Although health literacy has been linked to several aspects of postdischarge care, associations with postdischarge hospital utilization are mixed. One study found that patients with limited health literacy were almost twice as likely to have a readmission or ED visit within 30 days of discharge compared with those with adequate health literacy.[86] Although some studies have shown that limited health literacy is associated with readmissions,[87,88] this association was not found in all studies.[89,90]

Studies have found that providers often do not use health-literacy-informed communication strategies to ensure that patients and families understand their discharge instructions. In one study, use of medical terminology in verbal counseling was the factor most likely to contribute to poor understanding.[91] Few providers use health-literacy-informed communication strategies as part of discharge counseling; teach-back, for example, is used less than half of the time.[36] Adult studies have found an increased length of stay in patients with limited health literacy even after controlling for other factors including illness severity[92]; families with limited health literacy may require additional time for discharge counseling and coordination of postdischarge care, which may account for this increased length of stay. This would make sense in the context of patients with limited health literacy having lower scores on readiness for discharge scales.[93] Hospital systems should start discharge education at the beginning of the hospital stay so that families have more time to learn this information. Health-literacy-informed communication techniques such as teach-back can lead to significant improvements in understanding of discharge instructions,[28] and should therefore be incorporated into regular discharge counseling practices.

Another challenge is that families are often provided with suboptimal written instructions. Discharge instructions at one large academic referral center had a mean readability level of 10th grade, had poor understandability scores, and were missing key content (eg, diagnosis, signs and symptoms to watch for).[94] One national study of asthma action plans found that 70% of plans studied were written above the sixth grade level, and many used unsuitable layout and typography or failed to use graphics.[95] Hospital-wide initiatives are needed to prioritize the provision of health-literacy-informed, easy-to-understand written discharge instructions. Health literacy impacts a patient's ability to interact with written information related to their home care. For example, individuals with limited health literacy are more than 3 times as likely to misunderstand warnings on medication bottle labels.[96] For optimal learning by patients and families, it is helpful for written discharge instructions to be referenced as part of verbal counseling, providing a framework for standardized, organized counseling. This will increase the likelihood that parents are aware of the tasks they are responsible for taking care of at home.

Use of technology-based strategies can also be helpful. For example, implementation of video discharge instructions with content at or below the eighth grade reading level improved understandability of discharge instructions for pediatric fever and closed head injury in the ED.[97]

It is also important to keep in mind that families with limited health literacy may have difficulty navigating the health care system. Strategies to make this process easier for families include making appointments before the family leaves the hospital, working with the family to identify convenient times for them, having medications filled and brought to the hospital for review before discharge or ensuring medications are easy to obtain at a pharmacy close to the child's home, and making sure equipment and services are set up appropriately before discharge. Finally, "closing the loop" of communication by quickly sending discharge information to the child's outpatient providers, including the primary care provider within a child's medical home, as well as subspecialists and other caregivers such as home care providers, will limit the information that the family will need to transmit and reduce errors in understanding by the provider team who will take on the child's care after hospital discharge.

A variety of comprehensive health-literacy-informed interventions have been developed with aims to reduce postdischarge hospital use. These interventions include components that both help families understand health information and navigate the health care system. One intervention, RED (Re-Engineered Discharge), uses a discharge educator during the hospital stay to provide patient education, confirm understanding using teach-back, coordinate postdischarge appointments and equipment, and quickly transmit the discharge summary to the outpatient clinician; the patient is provided with an after-hospital care plan and a postdischarge phone call. In a randomized controlled trial, rehospitalization and ED visit rates were lower in the group receiving the intervention.[98] One pediatric-focused intervention known as Project IMPACT included counseling using teach-back, implementation of a transition checklist, a postdischarge phone call, and timely and complete communication with the outpatient pediatrician. Initial pilot data established feasibility and showed improved rates of teach-back, patients being discharged with medications in-hand, and patient satisfaction with education about medication side effects; however, it did not lead to an improvement in hospital utilization rates (eg, readmissions, ED visits, urgent clinic visits).[99] Several other health-literacy-informed resources have been developed that focus on various aspects of the discharge process, ranging from engaging patients and families in discharge planning, to improving communication, to promoting ability to manage discharge instructions.[27,100–102]

PROMOTING SYSTEM-WIDE IMPLEMENTATION OF HEALTH-LITERACY-INFORMED COMMUNICATION STRATEGIES

Adoption of health-literacy-informed strategies will not happen without concerted organizational effort. Health systems often start by conducting health literacy organizational assessments, focusing on written and spoken communication, that can be used to document problems and build support for change.[103] Internal advocates can make arguments for addressing deficiencies by pointing to how health-literacy-informed strategies can help the hospital achieve its goals, such as reducing readmission.[98] Often they start with a quality improvement project, then gradually spread the intervention to the entire hospital and expand it to encompass additional health-literacy-informed strategies.

Training has to be central to any implementation effort. Training should be a recurrent activity that can take the form of online modules augmented by practice sessions, orientation and in-service training, in situ training at bedside, and other methods. Hospitals, however, also need to think through a range of system actions if they are to make the use of health-literacy-informed strategies normative. For example, organizations have used the following policies and standardized processes to reinforce the use of teach-back:

- The charge nurse joins rounds with nurses and ensures the nurses are using the teach-back method correctly.
- Educational information is assigned in the electronic medical record and it is not marked as completed until educators attest to a successful teach-back.
- Daily huddles, e-mails, and posters are used to remind staff to use teach-back.
- Facilities report monthly on observed teach-back for the first 6 months of implementation.
- Members of the care team are designated to follow-up with parents who have difficulty teaching back information during rounds to continue to re-teach and confirm understanding.
- Staff members are required to sign a pledge committing themselves to use teach-back.

Table 3
Health literacy resources

Agency for Healthcare Research and Quality (AHRQ) Health Literacy Universal Precautions Toolkit[17]	A set of 21 tools to increase patient understanding of health information and enhance support for patients of all health literacy levels.
AHRQ Pharmacy Health Literacy Center[104]	A Web site that contains medication-related health literacy tools, including evidence-based prescription medicine instructions.
AHRQ's Making Informed Consent an Informed Choice: Training for Health Care Leaders and Professionals[72]	Two interactive training modules that teach health-literacy-informed strategies that health care organizations and clinical teams can use to ensure that people understand their choices.
Always Use Teach-back![105]	Interactive training to help health care providers learn to use teach-back, every time it is indicated, to support patients and families throughout the care continuum.
American Academy of Pediatrics Resources (Health Literacy and Pediatrics)[106]	A list of resources compiled by the American Academy of Pediatrics, including a Pedialink Continuing Medical Education Course, a webinar, and conference materials.
Building Health Literate Organizations: A Guidebook to Achieving Organizational Change[107]	A resource that helps health care organizations of any size engage in organizational change to become health literate.
Clear Communication Index (CCI)[108]	An assessment tool that provides a set of research-based criteria to develop and assess public communication products.
The Health Literacy Environment of Hospitals and Health Centers[109]	A guide to analyzing literacy-related barriers to health care access and navigation and using the results to create an action plan.
Health Literacy Maintenance of Certification (MOC) Modules	Pediatricians and family physicians taking the Health Literacy Knowledge Self-Assessment Module (MOC Part 2) or Improve Health Literacy Performance Improvement Modules (MOC Part 4) through the American Board of Pediatrics or the American Academy of Family Physicians can earn credit for recertification.
Health Literacy Online[110]	A guide to writing and designing easy-to-use health Web sites.
HELPix Medication Sheets[111]	Plain language, pictogram-based medication instruction sheets to support medication counseling for parents with low literacy and limited English proficiency.
How-to Guide: Improving Transitions from the Hospital to Community Settings to Reduce Avoidable Rehospitalizations[9]	A guide to support inpatient teams and community partners in collaborating in the design and implementation of processes to ensure optimal transitions of care after hospital discharge.
IDEAL Discharge Planning from the Guide to Patient and Family Engagement in Hospital Quality and Safety[23]	Summary of key components for ideal discharge planning and how to implement them.

(*continued on next page*)

Table 3 (*continued*)	
Patient Education and Materials Assessment Tool (PEMAT)[33]	A systematic method to evaluate and compare the understandability and actionability of print and audiovisual patient education materials.
Plain Language Pediatrics: Health Literacy Strategies and Communication Resources for Common Pediatric Topics[32]	A guide for using plain language communication strategies, including 25 bilingual (English/Spanish) patient education handouts.
Re-Engineered (RED) Discharge Toolkit[112]	A set of tools to help hospitals re-design the discharge process, particularly hospitals that serve diverse populations, to reduce readmissions and post-hospital emergency department visits.
The SHARE Approach[25]	A train-the-trainer curriculum that supports the training of health care professionals on how to engage patients in their health care decision making.
Taking Care of Myself: A Guide for When I Leave the Hospital[24]	A fillable PDF that allows patients to record information they need to remember about appointments and medicines and how to care for themselves when they get home.
Ten Attributes of Health Literate Health Care Organizations[3]	A set of 10 attributes that health-literate health care organizations can adopt and invest in to help everyone benefit fully from the nation's health care systems.
Toolkit for Clear and Effective Written Materials[39]	A resource that provides a detailed and comprehensive set of tools to help make written materials easier for people to read, understand, and use.

- Hospital policy requires teach-back of benefits, harms, risks, and other information about tests, procedures, and medicines as part of obtaining informed consent.
- Patients are not discharged until successful teach-back of discharge instructions is documented in the medical record.

For hospitals to adopt health literacy universal precautions, champions are needed at every level of the organization, from executive sponsors to frontline staff, to lead the required quality improvement efforts. It also means allocating resources to create supports, such as easy-to-understand patient education and informed consent materials. Hospitals that aim to become health literate go even further.[3] They integrate health literacy into planning, evaluation measures, patient safety, and quality improvement. They include the populations they serve in the design, implementation, and evaluation of health information and services. They provide easy access to health information and services and navigation assistance. They systematically hardwire the hospital to make it easy for people to navigate, understand, and use information and services to take care of their health. The resources listed in **Table 3** can help hospitals along their health literacy improvement journey.

SUMMARY

Health literacy has implications for patients and families in the events leading up to hospitalization, during the hospital stay, and post-discharge. Hospitals and providers should use a universal precautions approach and routinely incorporate health-literacy-informed strategies in communicating with all patients and families to ensure that they can understand health information, follow medical instructions, participate actively in their own/their child's care, and successfully navigate the health care system. Interventions that go beyond the individual provider level are essential to keep patients safe from harm. Addressing the problem of health literacy necessitates health care systems matching the demands they place on individuals with those individuals' skills and abilities. Future work should focus on studying the effects of limited health literacy in pediatric inpatients and their parents as much of the work in this field has come from the adult literature. Additional strategies to provide education to providers and trainees about health literacy should be developed and implemented.

REFERENCES

1. Agency for Healthcare Research and Quality. HCUPnet, healthcare cost and utilization project 2018. Available at: https://hcupnet.ahrq.gov/. Accessed April 20, 2018.
2. Ratzan S, Parker R. Introduction. In: Selden C, Zorn M, Ratzan S, et al, editors. National Library of Medicine current bibliographies in medicine: health literacy. Bethesda (MD): National Institutes of Health, U.S. Department of Health and Human Services; 2000. p. v–vii.
3. Brach C, Keller D, Hernandez LM, et al. Ten attributes of health literate health care organizations. Washington, DC: National Academy of Medicine; 2012.
4. Karsenty C, Landau M, Ferguson R. Assessment of medical resident's attention to the health literacy level of newly admitted patients. J Community Hosp Intern Med Perspect 2013;3(3–4):23071.
5. Ahmed AM. Deficiencies of history taking among medical students. Saudi Med J 2002;23(8):991–4.
6. Vashi A, Rhodes KV. "Sign right here and you're good to go": a content analysis of audiotaped emergency department discharge instructions. Ann Emerg Med 2011;57:315–22.e1.
7. Yin HS, Dreyer BP, van Schaick L, et al. Randomized controlled trial of a pictogram-based intervention to reduce liquid medication dosing errors and improve adherence among caregivers of young children. Arch Pediatr Adolesc Med 2008;162(9):814–22.
8. Glick A, Farkas J, Tomopoulos, S, et al. Role of discharge plan complexity and health literacy in parent understanding and execution of discharge instructions. In: Pediatric Academic Societies Meeting. San Francisco, May 7, 2017.
9. Wiens MO, Kumbakumba E, Larson CP, et al. Scheduled follow-up referrals and simple prevention kits including counseling to improve post-discharge outcomes among children in Uganda: a proof-of-concept study. Glob Health Sci Pract 2016;4:422–34.
10. Wu S, Tyler A, Logsdon T, et al. A quality improvement collaborative to improve the discharge process for hospitalized children. Pediatrics 2016;138(2):e20143604.
11. Kutner M, Greenberg E, Jin Y, et al. The health literacy of America's adults: results from the 2003 national assessment of adult literacy. Washington, DC: National Center for Educational Statistics; 2006. https://doi.org/10.1592/phco.22.5.282.33191.

12. U.S. Department of Health and Human Services. America's health literacy: why we need accessible health information 2008. Available at: https://health.gov/communication/literacy/issuebrief/. Accessed May 26, 2018.
13. Yin HS, Johnson M, Mendelsohn AL, et al. The health literacy of parents in the United States: a nationally representative study. Pediatrics 2009;124:S289–98.
14. OECD. Time for the U.S. To reskill?: What the survey of adult skills says. Paris: OECD Publishing; 2013. https://doi.org/10.1787/9789264204904-en.
15. van Bruinessen IR, van Weel EM, Gouw H, et al. Barriers and facilitators to effective communication experienced by patients with malignant lymphoma at all stages after diagnosis. Psychooncology 2013;22(12):2807–14.
16. Chappuy H, Taupin P, Dimet J, et al. Do parents understand the medical information provided in paediatric emergency departments? A prospective multicenter study. Acta Paediatr 2012;101(10):1089–94.
17. Brega A, Barnard J, Mabachi N, et al. AHRQ health literacy universal precautions Toolkit. Second Edition 2015. Available at: https://www.ahrq.gov/professionals/quality-patient-safety/quality-resources/tools/literacy-toolkit/index.html.
18. Baker DW, Williams MV, Parker RM, et al. Development of a brief test to measure functional health literacy. Patient Educ Couns 1999;38(1):33–42. http://www.ncbi.nlm.nih.gov/pubmed/14528569.
19. Weiss B, Mays M, Martz W. Quick assessment of literacy in primary care: the newest vital sign. Ann Fam Med 2005;3:514–22.
20. Kumar D, Sanders L, Perrin EM, et al. Parental understanding of infant health information: health literacy, numeracy, and the parental health literacy activities test (PHLAT). Acad Pediatr 2010;10(5):309–17.
21. Morris NS, Maclean CD, Chew LD, et al. The single item literacy screener: evaluation of a brief instrument to identify limited reading ability. BMC Fam Pract 2006;7(21). https://doi.org/10.1186/1471-2296-7-21.
22. Fagerlin A, Zikmund-Fisher BJ, Ubel PA, et al. Measuring numeracy without a math test: development of the subjective numeracy scale. Med Decis Making 2007;27(5):672–80.
23. Health literacy tool shed. Available at: https://healthliteracy.bu.edu/. Accessed May 26, 2018.
24. The Joint Commission. A crosswalk of the national standards for culturally and linguistically appropriate services (CLAS) in health and health care to the Joint Commission Hospital Accreditation Standards 2014. Available at: https://www.jointcommission.org/assets/1/6/Crosswalk-_CLAS_-20140718.pdf. Accessed May 26, 2018.
25. National Quality Forum (NQF). Safe practices for better healthcare–2010 update: a consensus report. Washington, DC: National Quality Forum; 2010.
26. Agency for Healthcare Research and Quality. Making health care safer: a critical analysis of patient safety practices. Rockville (MD): Agency for Healthcare Research and Quality; 2001.
27. Rutherford P, Nielsen G, Taylor J, et al. How-to guide: improving transitions from the hospital to community settings to reduce avoidable rehospitalizations. Cambridge (MA): Institute for Healthcare Improvement; 2012.
28. Griffey RT, Shin N, Jones S, et al. The impact of teach-back on comprehension of discharge instructions and satisfaction among emergency patients with limited health literacy: a randomized, controlled study. J Commun Healthc 2015;8(1):10–21.

29. Kornburger C, Gibson C, Sadowski S, et al. Using “teach-back” to promote a safe transition from hospital to home: an evidence-based approach to improving the discharge process. J Pediatr Nurs 2013;28:282–91.
30. Davis TC, Wolf MS, Bass PF, et al. Literacy and misunderstanding prescription drug labels. Ann Intern Med 2006;145(12):887–94.
31. Wilson EAH, Wolf MS. Working memory and the design of health materials: a cognitive factors perspective. Patient Educ Couns 2009;74:318–22.
32. Abrams MA, Dreyer BP. Plain language pediatrics: health literacy strategies and communication resources for common pediatric topics. Elk Grove Village (IL): American Academy of Pediatrics; 2008.
33. Shoemaker S, Wolf M, Brach C. The patient education materials assessment tool and user's guide. Rockville (MD): Agency for Healthcare Research and Quality; 2013.
34. Auger KA, Simon TD, Cooperberg D, et al. Summary of STARNet: seamless transitions and (Re)admissions Network. Pediatrics 2015;135(1):164–75.
35. Use health education material effectively: tool #12. Available at: http://www.ahrq.gov/professionals/quality-patient-safety/quality-resources/tools/literacy-toolkit/healthlittoolkit2-tool12.htm. Accessed May 17, 2018.
36. Turner T, Cull WL, Bayldon B, et al. Pediatricians and health literacy: descriptive results from a national survey. Pediatrics 2009;124(Suppl 3):S299–305.
37. Katz MG, Kripalani S, Weiss BD. Use of pictorial aids in medication instructions: a review of the literature. Am J Health Syst Pharm 2006;63:2391–7.
38. Houts PS, Doak CC, Doak LG, et al. The role of pictures in improving health communication: a review of research on attention, comprehension, recall, and adherence. Patient Educ Couns 2006;61:173–90.
39. U.S. Department of Health and Human Services Centers for Medicare and Medicaid. Toolkit for making written material clear and effective. Baltimore (MD): U.S. Department of Health and Human Services Centers for Medicare and Medicaid; 2011.
40. Harrington KF, Zhang B, Magruder T, et al. The impact of parent's health literacy on pediatric asthma outcomes. Pediatr Allergy Immunol Pulmonol 2015;28(1):20–6.
41. Macy ML, Davis MM, Clark SJ, et al. Parental health literacy and asthma education delivery during a visit to a community-based pediatric emergency department: a pilot study. Pediatr Emerg Care 2011;27(6):469–74.
42. Janisse HC, Naar-King S, Ellis D. Brief report: parent's health literacy among high-risk adolescents with insulin dependent diabetes. J Pediatr Psychol 2010;35(4):436–40.
43. Pulgarón ER, Sanders LM, Patiño-Fernandez AM, et al. Glycemic control in young children with diabetes: the role of parental health literacy. Patient Educ Couns 2014;94(1):67–70.
44. Rosas-Salazar C, Ramratnam SK, Brehm JM, et al. Parental numeracy and asthma exacerbations in Puerto Rican children. Chest 2013;144(1):92–8.
45. DeWalt DA, Dilling MH, Rosenthal MS, et al. Low parental literacy Is associated with worse asthma care measures in children. Ambul Pediatr 2007;7(1):25–31.
46. Morrison AK, Schapira MM, Gorelick MH, et al. Caregiver low health literacy and nonurgent use of the pediatric emergency department for febrile illness. Acad Pediatr 2014;14(5):505–9. http://ovidsp.ovid.com/ovidweb.cgi?T=JS&PAGE=reference&D=emed12&NEWS=N&AN=2014571011.

47. Williams MV, Baker DW, Parker RM, et al. Relationship of functional health literacy to patients' knowledge of heir chronic disease. Arch Intern Med 1998;158:166–72.
48. Teo KGW, Tacey M, Holbeach E. Understanding of diagnosis and medications among non-English-speaking older patients. Aust J Ageing 2018. https://doi.org/10.1111/ajag.12503.
49. Aitken J, Bain C, Ward M, et al. How accurate is self-reported family history of colorectal cancer? Am J Epidemiol 1995;141(9):863–71.
50. Ivanovich J, Babb S, Goodfellow P, et al. Evaluation of the family history collection process and the accuracy of cancer reporting among a series of women with endometrial cancer. Clin Cancer Res 2002;8:1849–56.
51. Bryant MD, Schoenberg ED, Johnson TV, et al. Multimedia version of a standard medical questionnaire improves patient understanding across all literacy levels. J Urol 2009;182(3):1120–5.
52. Yin HS, Gupta RS, Mendelsohn AL, et al. Use of a low-literacy written action plan to improve parent understanding of pediatric asthma management: a randomized controlled study. J Asthma 2017;54(9):919–29.
53. Bickley LS, Szilagyi PG, Hoffman RM. Bates' guide to physical examination and history taking. 12th edition. Philadelphia: Wolters Kluwer; 2017.
54. Grover G, Berkowitz CD, Lewis RJ. Parental recall after a visit to the emergency department. Clin Pediatr (Phila) 1994;33:194–201.
55. Musso MW, Perret JN, Sanders T, et al. Patients' comprehension of their emergency department encounter: a pilot study using physician observers. Ann Emerg Med 2015;65(2):151–1550.e4.
56. Bourquin C, Stiefel F, Mast MS, et al. Well, you have hepatic metastases: use of technical language by medical students in simulated patient interviews. Patient Educ Couns 2015;98(3):323–30.
57. Schillinger D, Bindman A, Wang F, et al. Functional health literacy and the quality of physician-patient communication among diabetes patients. Patient Educ Couns 2004;52(3):315–23.
58. Khan A, Baird J, Rogers JE, et al. Parent and provider experience and shared understanding after a family-centered nighttime communication intervention. Acad Pediatr 2017;17(4):389–402.
59. Béranger A, Pierron C, de Saint Blanquat L, et al. Provided information and parents' comprehension at the time of admission of their child in pediatric intensive care unit. Eur J Pediatr 2018;177(3):395–402.
60. O'Leary KJ, Kulkarni N, Landler MP, et al. Hospitalized patients' understanding of their plan of care. Mayo Clin Proc 2010;85(1):47–52.
61. Khan A, Rogers JE, Forster CS, et al. Communication and shared understanding between parents and resident-physicians at night. Hosp Pediatr 2016;6:319–29.
62. Tait AR, Voepel-Lewis T, Snyder RM, et al. Parents' understanding of information regarding their child's postoperative pain management. Clin J Pain 2008;24(7):572–7.
63. Menendez ME, van Hoorn BT, Mackert M, et al. Patients with limited health literacy ask fewer questions during office visits with hand surgeons. Clin Orthop Relat Res 2017;475(5):1291–7.
64. Khan A, Furtak SL, Melvin P, et al. Parent-provider miscommunications in hospitalized children. Hosp Pediatr 2017;7(9):505–15.
65. Kripalani S, Jacobson TA, Mugalla IC, et al. Health literacy and the quality of physician-patient communication during hospitalization. J Hosp Med 2010;5(5):269–75.

66. Jubbal K, Chun S, Chang J, et al. Parental and youth understanding of the informed consent process for pediatric endoscopy. J Pediatr Gastroenterol Nutr 2015;60(6):769–75.
67. Pianosi K, Gorodzinsky AY, Chorney JM, et al. Informed consent in pediatric otolaryngology: what risks and benefits do parents recall? Otolaryngol Head Neck Surg 2016;155(2):332–9.
68. Tait AR, Voepel-Lewis T, Gauger V. Parental recall of anesthesia information: informing the practice of informed consent. Anesth Analg 2011;112(4):918–23.
69. Tan M, Hooper Evans K, Braddock CH, et al. Patient whiteboards to improve patient-centered care in the hospital. Postgrad Med J 2013;89(1056):604–9.
70. Lin R, Gallagher R, Spinaze M, et al. Effect of a patient-directed discharge letter on patient understanding of their hospitalisation. Intern Med J 2014;44(9):851–7.
71. Schenker Y, Fernandez A, Sudore R, et al. Interventions to improve patient comprehension in informed consent for medical and surgical procedures: a systematic review. Med Decis Making 2011;31(1):151–73.
72. Agency for Healthcare Research and Quality (AHRQ). Making informed consent an informed choice: training for health care leaders audio script 2017. Available at: https://www.ahrq.gov/professionals/systems/hospital/informedchoice/audio-script-leaders.html#slide13. Accessed May 17, 2018.
73. Subramony A, Hametz PA, Balmer D. Family-centered rounds in theory and practice: an ethnographic case study. Acad Pediatr 2014;14(2):200–6.
74. Subramony A, Schwartz T, Hametz P. Family-centered rounds and communication about discharge between families and inpatient medical teams. Clin Pediatr (Phila) 2012;51(8):730–8.
75. Lion KC, Mangione-Smith R, Martyn M, et al. Comprehension on family-centered rounds for limited English proficient families. Acad Pediatr 2013;13(3):236–42.
76. Khan A, Spector ND, Baird JD, for the Patient and Family Centered I-PASS Study Group. Patient safety after implementation of a coproduced family centered communication programme: multicenter before and after intervention study. BMJ 2018;363:k4764.
77. Glick AF, Farkas JS, Nicholson J, et al. Parental management of discharge instructions: a systematic review. Pediatrics 2017;140(2):e20164165.
78. Howard LM, Tique JA, Gaveta S, et al. Health literacy predicts pediatric dosing accuracy for liquid zidovudine. AIDS 2014;28(7):1041–8.
79. Al-Harthy N, Sudersanadas KM, Al-Mutairi MM, et al. Efficacy of patient discharge instructions: a pointer toward caregiver friendly communication methods from pediatric emergency personnel. J Family Community Med 2016;23:155–60.
80. McPhail GL, Ednick MD, Fenchel MC, et al. Improving follow-up in hospitalised children. Qual Saf Health Care 2010;19(5):e35.
81. Isaacman DJ, Purvis K, Gyuro J, et al. Standardized instructions: do they improve communication of discharge information from the emergency department? Pediatrics 1992;89:1204–8.
82. Hwang V, Trickey AW, Lormel C, et al. Are pediatric concussion patients compliant with discharge instructions? J Trauma Acute Care Surg 2014;77:117–22.
83. Kun S, Warburton D. Telephone assessment of parents' knowledge of homecare treatments and readmission outcomes for high-risk infants and toddlers. Am J Dis Child 1987;141:888–92.
84. Bhansali P, Washofsky A, Romrell E, et al. Parental understanding of hospital course and discharge plan. Hosp Pediatr 2016;6(8):449–55.

85. Berry JG, Ziniel SI, Freeman L, et al. Hospital readmission and parent perceptions of their child's hospital discharge. Int J Qual Health Care 2013;25:573–81.
86. Cox SR, Liebl MG, McComb MN, et al. Association between health literacy and 30-day healthcare use after hospital discharge in the heart failure population. Res Social Adm Pharm 2017;13(4):754–8.
87. Bailey SC, Fang G, Annis IE, et al. Health literacy and 30-day hospital readmission after acute myocardial infarction. BMJ Open 2015;5(6). https://doi.org/10.1136/bmjopen-2014-006975.
88. Mitchell SE, Sadikova E, Jack BW, et al. Health literacy and 30-day postdischarge hospital utilization. J Health Commun 2012;17(SUPPL. 3):325–38.
89. Sterling MR, Safford MM, Goggins K, et al. Numeracy, health literacy, cognition, and 30-day readmissions among patients with heart failure. J Hosp Med 2018;13(3):145–51.
90. Copeland LA, Zeber JE, Thibodeaux LV, et al. Postdischarge correlates of health literacy among Medicaid inpatients. Popul Health Manag 2018. https://doi.org/10.1089/pop.2017.0095.
91. Waisman Y, Siegal N, Chemo M, et al. Do parents understand emergency department discharge instructions? A survey analysis. Isr Med Assoc J 2003;5:567–70.
92. Wright JP, Edwards GC, Goggins K, et al. Association of health literacy with postoperative outcomes in patients undergoing major abdominal surgery. JAMA Surg 2018;153(2):137–42.
93. Wallace AS, Perkhounkova Y, Bohr NL, et al. Readiness for hospital discharge, health literacy, and social living status. Clin Nurs Res 2016;25(5):494–511.
94. Unaka NI, Statile A, Haney J, et al. Assessment of readability, understandability, and completeness of pediatric hospital medicine discharge instructions. J Hosp Med 2017;12(2):98–101.
95. Yin HS, Gupta RS, Tomopoulos S, et al. Readability, suitability, and characteristics of asthma action plans: examination of factors that may impair understanding. Pediatrics 2013;131(1):e116–26.
96. Davis TC, Wolf MS, Bass PF, et al. Low literacy impairs comprehension of prescription drug warning labels. J Gen Intern Med 2006;21:847–51.
97. Ismail S, McIntosh M, Kalynych C, et al. Impact of video discharge instructions for pediatric fever and closed head injury from the emergency department. J Emerg Med 2016;50(3):e177–83.
98. Jack BW, Chetty VK, Anthony D, et al. A reengineered hospital discharge program to decrease rehospitalization: a randomized trial. Ann Intern Med 2009;150:178–87.
99. Mallory LA, Osorio SN, Prato BS, et al. Project IMPACT pilot report: feasibility of implementing a hospital-to-home transition bundle. Pediatrics 2017;139(3):e20154626.
100. Agency for Healthcare Research and Quality (AHRQ). Guide to patient and family engagement in hospital quality and safety 2017. Available at: https://www.ahrq.gov/professionals/systems/hospital/engagingfamilies/index.html. Accessed May 27, 2018.
101. Agency for Healthcare Research and Quality (AHRQ). Taking care of myself: a guide for when I leave the hospital 2010. Available at: https://www.ahrq.gov/sites/default/files/publications/files/goinghomeguide.pdf. Accessed May 17, 2018.

102. Agency for Healthcare Research and Quality (AHRQ). The SHARE approach. 2017. Available at: https://www.ahrq.gov/professionals/education/curriculum-tools/shareddecisionmaking/index.html. Accessed May 17, 2018.
103. Brach C. The journey to become a health literate organization: a snapshot of health system improvement. In: Logan R, Siegel E, editors. Health literacy: new directions in research, theory, and practice. Amsterdam: IOS Press; 2017. p. 203–37.
104. Agency for Healthcare Research and Quality (AHRQ). AHRQ pharmacy health literacy center 2017. Available at: http://www.ahrq.gov/professionals/quality-patient-safety/pharmhealthlit/index.html. Accessed May 30, 2018.
105. Always use teach-back!. Available at: http://www.teachbacktraining.org/. Accessed May 17, 2018.
106. American Academy of Pediatrics. Health literacy and pediatrics 2018. Available at: https://www.aap.org/en-us/professional-resources/Research/research-resources/pages/Health-Literacy-and-Pediatrics.aspx. Accessed May 31, 2018.
107. Abrams M, Kurtz-Rossi S, Riffenburgh A, et al. Building health literate organizations: a guidebook to achieving organizational change 2018. Available at: http://www.healthliterateorganization.org. Accessed June 1, 2018.
108. Baur C, Prue C. The CDC clear communication index is a new evidence-based tool to prepare and review health information. Health Promot Pract 2014;15(5):629–37.
109. Rudd RE, Anderson JE. The health literacy environment of hospitals and health centers. Partners for action: making your healthcare facility literacy-friendly 2006. Available at: https://cdn1.sph.harvard.edu/wp-content/uploads/sites/135/2012/09/healthliteracyenvironment.pdf. Accessed May 17, 2018.
110. U.S. Department of Health and Human Services, Office of Disease Prevention and Health Promotion. Health literacy online: a guide to writing and designing easy to use health websites 2010. Available at: http://www.health.gov/healthliteracyonline/interactive.htm. Accessed May 17, 2018.
111. The HELPix Intervention. Available at: https://med.nyu.edu/helpix/helpix-intervention. Accessed May 30, 2018.
112. Jack B, Paasche-Orlow M, Mitchell S, et al. Re-engineered discharge (RED) Toolkit. AHRQ Publ No 12(13)-0084. Rockville (MD): Agency for Healthcare Research and Quality; 2013.

Family-Centered Rounds

Past, Present, and Future

Lauren A. Destino, MD[a,*], Samir S. Shah, MD, MSCE[b],
Brian Good, MB BCh, BAO[c]

KEYWORDS

• Family-centered rounds • Patient centeredness • Education of trainees
• Hospitalist medicine

KEY POINTS

- Hospital medicine and family-centered rounds have evolved concurrently.
- Family-centered rounds is an in-patient vehicle that accomplishes both the Institute of Medicine's and the American Academy of Pediatrics goal of patient-centered care.
- Participant perspectives of family-centered rounds are generally positive but there is still opportunity for improvement.
- Integrating different perspectives into rounds could improve patient safety and educational opportunities for a broad range of learners.

FROM BEDSIDE ROUNDS TO FAMILY-CENTERED ROUNDS

The current model of family-centered rounds has evolved alongside advances in medicine and technology, the growth of hospitalist medicine and patient-centered care. Traditionally, when a person's illness became too severe to be managed safely at home, their outpatient medical provider often fluidly assumed responsibility for that patient's in-patient medical care.[1] In the hospital, the provider would complete "rounds" by visiting and examining their patient, and discussing the medical management with the patient in a natural extension of the outpatient relationship. Medicine was less complex and diagnoses and therapeutic interventions were limited. In teaching settings, physicians would additionally use this in-patient experience to further education. Sir William Osler used bedside rounds as the cornerstone of his education

Disclosure: Dr S.S Shah holds equity in the I-PASS Patient Safety Institute. The I-PASS Patient Safety Institute is a company that seeks to train institutions in best handoff practices and aid in their implementation.

[a] Stanford University, Lucile Packard Children's Hospital, 300 Pasteur MC 5776, Palo Alto, CA 94034, USA; [b] Cincinnati Children's Hospital Medical Center, University of Cincinnati College of Medicine, 3333 Burnet Avenue ML 9016, Cincinnati, OH 45229, USA; [c] University of Utah, Primary Children's Hospital, 100 North Mario Capecchi Drive, Salt Lake City, UT 84113, USA
* Corresponding author.
E-mail address: ldestino@stanford.edu

Pediatr Clin N Am 66 (2019) 827–837
https://doi.org/10.1016/j.pcl.2019.03.008
pediatric.theclinics.com

and gradual promotion of learners.[2] His emphasis on having learners experience illness through the words and the physical examination of their patients is well documented.[3]

Bedside rounding continued to be used as a clinical and educational tool well into the last century. Studies during this period not only illustrate its prevalence and benefits, but also started to describe some challenges, which persist today. A study published in 1964 looked at teaching in 10 medical centers and documented that attending physicians taught learners at the bedside for nearly 75% of the team's patients.[4] This simultaneous presence on rounds allowed the learners to articulate their thought process while more senior members of the team could engage in valuable role modeling and bedside teaching, using the patients' stories and examination findings as learning material. However, this same study characterized difficulties of bedside teaching and noted that it can come across as "mediocre and haphazard" without preparation.[4] Another study questioned the benefit of involving patients in health-related decisions.[5] It is clear that, although bedside rounding was valued for teaching, opportunities to incorporate shared decision making and patient centeredness remained.

In the decades to follow, changing practitioner work flows further affected the bedside rounding environment (**Fig. 1**). Information gleaned from discussions with and examination of the patient were superseded by the easy availability and abundance of vital sign, laboratory, and imaging data. The entry point to this data, the electronic medical record (EMR), drew teams from patient rooms to hallways and conference rooms for rounds. With improvements in EMR technology, there has been continued concern that this mass of electronic patient data, or the "ipatient," is being prioritized over actual patient interaction.[14] This worry is reinforced and

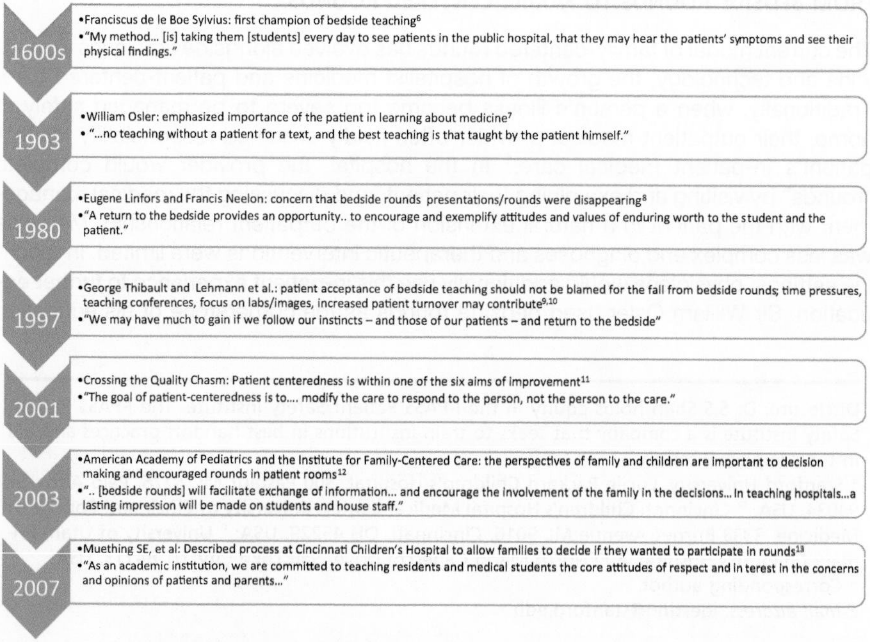
1600s
•Franciscus de le Boe Sylvius: first champion of bedside teaching6
•"My method... [is] taking them [students] every day to see patients in the public hospital, that they may hear the patients' symptoms and see their physical findings."
1903
•William Osler: emphasized importance of the patient in learning about medicine7
• "...no teaching without a patient for a text, and the best teaching is that taught by the patient himself."
1980
•Eugene Linfors and Francis Neelon: concern that bedside rounds presentations/rounds were disappearing8
•"A return to the bedside provides an opportunity.. to encourage and exemplify attitudes and values of enduring worth to the student and the patient."
1997
•George Thibault and Lehmann et al.: patient acceptance of bedside teaching should not be blamed for the fall from bedside rounds; time pressures, teaching conferences, focus on labs/images, increased patient turnover may contribute9,10
•"We may have much to gain if we follow our instincts – and those of our patients – and return to the bedside"
2001
•Crossing the Quality Chasm: Patient centeredness is within one of the six aims of improvement11
•"The goal of patient-centeredness is to.... modify the care to respond to the person, not the person to the care."
2003
•American Academy of Pediatrics and the Institute for Family-Centered Care: the perspectives of family and children are important to decision making and encouraged rounds in patient rooms12
•".. [bedside rounds] will facilitate exchange of information... and encourage the involvement of the family in the decisions... In teaching hospitals...a lasting impression will be made on students and house staff."
2007
•Muething SE, et al: Described process at Cincinnati Children's Hospital to allow families to decide if they wanted to participate in rounds13
•"As an academic institution, we are committed to teaching residents and medical students the core attitudes of respect and in terest in the concerns and opinions of patients and parents..."

Fig. 1. A brief history of rounds at the bedside moving from a focus on teaching to a focus on teaching and patient centeredness.[6–13]

supported by time-motion studies in both internal medicine and pediatric, demonstrating that trainees spent less than 8 minutes per hour on direct patient care.[15,16] The distance from the bedside allows for more private structured mini-lectures from a senior team member, which often encourages more passive learning.[8,17] The conference room teaching and rounding environment has also been often viewed comfortably in comparison with bedside rounding, which demands integration of all people present and requires adaptation to learners and to the introduction of unanticipated topics.[8] Duty hour limitations for learners and frequent interruption of team members (eg, returning pages, subspecialty interactions, reading charts, and entering documentation) have further decreased the ability of the full team complement to be at each bedside together and, as a consequence, total bedside time has decreased.[16,18–20] One survey found that most discussions regarding medical decision making, teaching, and feedback occurred away from the bedside.[21] As a newer generation of physicians spend less time rounding at the bedside, there is concern that they will be less comfortable teaching at the bedside, thus propagating the deficit.[8]

Concurrent with the movement of medical care and education away from the bedside, multiple governing bodies, including the American Academy of Pediatrics (AAP) and the Institute for Patient- and Family-Centered Care, began to focus on the importance of patient centeredness.[12,22] Of the 6 aims emphasized by the Institute of Medicine (IOM) to improve the quality of US health care, 2 relate directly to communication and patient empowerment.[11] In this report, the IOM states "an informed patient is a safe patient" and recommends full clinical transparency. They also highlight the importance of "patient-centered care," asking caregivers to share all information necessary to engage patients and families into the decision-making process. Further, this information needs to be provided in a manner that is culturally and intellectually at the level of the patients and their families.[11] In 2003, and again in 2012, the AAP took this 1 step further and directly suggested that family-centered rounds (FCR) in the in-patient setting was a vehicle to accomplish these IOM aims.[11,22] This emphasis once again called physicians and trainees back to the patient bedside for rounding and learning.

Pediatric hospitalist medicine has blossomed and matured in the past decade.[23] Not only have fellowships proliferated but, in 2016, the American Board of Medical Specialties officially recognized Pediatric Hospital Medicine as an official pediatric subspecialty. Currently, approximately 98% of hospitals with academic Pediatric departments employ hospitalists.[24] Because of their clinical emphasis of improving the in-patient care of children, their focus on systems improvement and their consistent presence directly in hospitals, pediatric hospitalists are uniquely situated and trained to integrate the aims of the IOM and AAP into the in-patient setting. As such, they have been instrumental in bringing teaching and rounds back to the bedside. Wide-ranging implementation of family-centered rounding has been a means to achieve relationship building, patient centeredness, shared decision making, and continuing the education of learners.

THE CURRENT STATE OF FAMILY-CENTERED ROUNDS

Family-centered rounding is formally defined as "multidisciplinary bedside rounds whereby both the patient and family are able to participate in medical decision making."[25] Many institutions have instituted FCR and have studied their experiences or enhancements to the rounding process. Despite this, many of these publications focus on stakeholder perspectives of FCR, rather than what actually occurs during rounds and how content may vary within and between institutions. Thus, it is difficult to know what content elements are required for successful implementation of FCR incorporating patient centeredness, shared decision making, and education. Muething and colleagues[13] provide one of the few descriptions of a specific framework for FCR. This framework indicates that the team should start with introductions and welcoming the family to participate, then discuss the current status of the patient and treatment options. Further the framework emphasizes that, in academic institutions, the supervisory level physicians (senior residents, fellows, attendings) are present to observe, model, and teach in the presence of the patient and family. The authors of this framework state the model was well received and provide limited data on rounding time, discharge time, and percentage of families requesting to be involved in rounds.[13] One single-site study evaluated the use of a checklist that encompassed many elements included in Muething's framework (introductions, assessment, and plan). In this study, the checklist did not improve the use of these specific elements. Both before and after the checklist, summarization of the plan was done frequently, whereas providing an assessment and introducing the team was only done about 40% of the time.[26]

Beyond content, individuals participating in rounds and the effect of interventions on the duration of rounds need to be considered. By definition a member of the patient's family must be present, but the question of who composes the "medical team" is often raised.[17] In addition to physician attendance, the importance of nursing presence is most often emphasized.[13,25,27] Although nursing presence is often thought to be essential, improvement projects aimed at increasing nurse presence on FCR would indicate that this ideal is not always achieved.[28,29] In addition to nursing and physician providers, the medical team also often includes case managers, social workers, pharmacists, respiratory therapists, occupational and physical therapists, dieticians, consulting subspecialist providers, and others. When patients have limited English proficiency, the presence of an interpreter (either in person or using iPad) is preferred.[30,31] Depending on the needs of the individual patient and the institution's resources and processes, FCR may include a variety of these providers.[32] Because of the widespread concern that FCR prolongs rounds, studies often include rounding time as an outcome measure. There is no clear answer as to whether FCR actually lengthens rounds, but studies have documented that FCR varies from 3 to 23 minutes, averaging about 10 minutes per patient.[28,33-35] This time invested on rounds is often thought to improve communication and create a better shared mental model with both nurses and families resulting in decreased questions and clarifications later in the day.[13]

The variation in content, length, and composition on FCR suggests that there may be competing priorities from rounds participants. Perspectives of families, attendings, and learners on FCR demonstrate some existing tensions on rounds. Families have a high desire to participate and are largely satisfied with FCR. They understand the need for teaching at academic centers, are often reassured by that teaching, and feel that they, themselves, can serve as teachers.[36] Barriers for families on FCR include the use of medical jargon, not always being welcomed to participate, and variation in how teams might collaborate.[37]

Pediatric trainees recognize FCR as a time for patient/family involvement, patient care, and clinical education, as well as a place of evaluation.[38] However, tensions have arisen. There is some evidence that time spent teaching has decreased, and trainees often feel the need to appear competent on rounds and perceive that there are missed opportunities for feedback.[38,39] Interestingly, as families seem to recognize the learning process and have a positive view of the trainees,[36] the learner's perceptions about needing to appear competent are potentially unfounded. Trainees appreciate the ability to be autonomous during FCR. There were early concerns that hospitalists may decrease resident autonomy,[40,41] but there is limited evidence that this has happened. In fact, 1 qualitative analysis suggested that hospitalists often promote resident autonomy.[42]

Attending perceptions on how to promote autonomy aligns with resident perceptions,[42] but despite this appreciation of autonomy, 1 study demonstrated that attending physicians speak most.[34] Relative to attendings in internal medicine, pediatric attending physicians emphasize patient/family communication and increasing rapport with patients.[39] This difference may be driven by FCR.

Nursing perceptions of rounds have also been assessed. Consistent with other participants they recognize the importance of teaching, introductions, and focus on the family. They may not always perceive that their own presence at FCR is important,[28] and in 1 study were noted to speak the least.[34] Based on the opinions of some family members, lack of consistent nursing presence and their active participation may be a lost opportunity.[27] Nurses are the primary caregiver at the bedside throughout the day, must carry out the intended plan, and have situational awareness about their patient's expected disease course and potential complications. It stands to reason then that having the nurse actively engaged in FCR is beneficial to patient care.

Moving beyond the literature focused on participant perspectives, several institutions and studies have built on the initial framework of FCR through adjunctive tools, structure, and interventions. These tools are often targeted at enhancing family and nurse engagement, patient and nursing education, and ensuring completion of tasks. The patient- and family-centered I-PASS intervention uses multiple techniques to enhance a shared mental model among the care team. Techniques include: (1) have the family begin with their concerns and perception of their child's illness severity; (2) use skills in health literacy to present the child's current assessment and plan by problems; (3) emphasize actions for that hospital day; (4) ensure teach back at the end of FCR by the family; and (5) use written communication through use of a rounds report or the room white board. The intervention was implemented in 7 centers across the United States and Canada and was associated with increased nursing and family engagement and improved patient safety—a decrease in harmful medical errors by 38%.[43] Of note, training of all members was also emphasized in the patient- and family-centered I-PASS intervention with modules and tools for medical students, residents, attendings, nurses, and family members. A qualitative study of rounding stakeholders suggested the use of scheduled rounds and more training for all members participating in FCR to improve family engagement.[44] Mobile devices have been explored with the goal of increasing access to patient care information and educational materials.[35] The authors found improved perceptions around trainees feeling prepared for rounds and teaching. Another institution embedded a clinical librarian on FCR with the goal of increasing the number of clinical questions asked and application of evidence-based medicine.[45] As FCR is a complex task, checklists have been applied with improvement in task performance as well as family engagement and perceptions of the safety climate[26] and trainee's perceptions of clear guidelines for FCR presentations.[46] In summary, although there are many challenges to conducting FCR effectively, various countermeasures have been explored with some success at individual institutions. Pairing the countermeasures with objective outcome measures could help describe the success or lack thereof and highlight which countermeasure might be appropriate for wider implementation (**Table 1**).

Table 1
Challenges of family-centered rounds, potential countermeasures, and outcomes measures

Challenge	Potential Countermeasure(s)	Outcome Measure(s)
Varying content	Structured Communication Checklists	Work-based assessment of content Concordance between providers and family
Physical space	Schedule rounds Unit-based teams Adapt team size	Number of teams rounding on unit at same time Family preference for round location met
Nursing (or other necessary provider) presence and participation	Schedule rounds Ensuring active role Adjusting provider work outside of rounds	Attendance by key providers Active participation by providers and family Family and provider perception of appropriate team member presence
Concerns about less teaching for trainees	Focus learning on topics that benefit families and learners Use mobile devices Include clinical librarian Prepare participants before rounds Debrief following rounds	Time-motion studies Work-based assessment: quantity and quality of teaching on rounds Learner perceptions
Tendency to use medical jargon	Training in health literacy principles Use check back to ensure understanding	Work-based assessment of language used Concordance between providers and family
Assessment of quality	Regular observations with feedback Use check back to ensure understanding	Concordance between providers and family Family perceptions of miscommunication Family engagement Safety events

POTENTIAL FUTURE DIRECTIONS FOR FAMILY-CENTERED ROUNDS

What then might be the next steps to build on the current state of FCR? Rounding is the critical interface between the care team and patients and their families. When done effectively, all parties are fully engaged, informed, and share a similar understanding of the patient's illness and the subsequent care plan. Creating this shared mental model requires that the medical teams communicate effectively and at a family-appropriate level. True "family-centered rounding" takes energy, coordination, resources, and training to function well. Objective measures are necessary to ensure this personal and institutional investment is producing the anticipated outcomes. One study attempted to describe the actual quality of communication on rounds. As simultaneous surveys of physician teams and families identified a low degree of concordant understanding of the medical plan,[47] further investigations of the efficacy of the communication process during FCR is necessary.

Formally assessing nursing, family, and physician concordance might help establish whether a shared understanding actually develops as a result of FCR. As there is more evidence to suggest that an engaged family can also detect more errors than traditional medical teams alone,[48] further studies objectively measuring family engagement and patient safety outcomes in the context of FCR are also necessary. At

Table 2
Published strategies for improving teaching on rounds[a]

Author	Article Name and Brief Summary	Model Tenets
Fitzgerald,[52] 1993	"Bedside teaching" Earlier paper describing barriers and solutions to improve bedside teaching	• Pre-rounds: prepare patient and teacher, reassure learners • Bedside: appropriate demeanor, illness correlation, seek patient interaction • Debrief: following interaction debrief and suggestions for improvement
Ramani,[51] 2003	"12 tips to improve bedside teaching" The paper lists and describes 12 high yield ideas to improve the ability of bedside teaching	• Pre-rounds: preparation, planning, orientation • Rounds: introduction, interaction, observation, instruction, summarization • Post-rounds: debriefing, feedback, reflection, preparation
Reilly,[54] 2007	"Inconvenient truths about effective clinical teaching" The author shares experience of 8 traits of exemplary teachers, formed into a mnemonic, TALK WALK	• Think out loud • Activate the learner • Listen smart • Keep it simple • Wear gloves • Adapt • Link learning to caring • Kindness
Williams et al,[53] 2008	"Improving bedside teaching" Authors share data from 6 student and resident focus groups on the barriers and solutions to improve bedside rounding	• Orient and include the patient • Address time constraints through flexibility, selectivity, and integration • Provide learners with reassurance, reinforce autonomy, and incorporate them • Develop faculty attitudes, knowledge, and skill for bedside teaching
Chi et al,[56] 2016	"5-min moment" A brief structured model of teaching physical examination findings	• Start with narrative or relevant clinical vignette • Demonstrate the examination finding • Interpretation variations of examination findings • Caveats and errors: have learners attempt maneuver and provide feedback
Lichstein & Atkinson,[55] 2018	"Patient-centered bedside rounds and the clinical examination" Authors delve further into Fitzgerald's 1993 work and describe additional opportunities and steps to improve bedside teaching	• Before bedside: prepare team and patient, set expectations • At the bedside: introduce team, limit jargon, engage all learners, limit teaching points • After the bedside: check back with patient, learner debrief, and feedback

[a] PubMed search criteria: "bedside teaching," with further source identification through each article's reference list.

present, only 1 study has shown that an FCR model that focuses on health literacy principles to increase family engagement and understanding has led to decreased errors and improved patient safety.[43] As rounds can be a large time commitment for all present, processes and outcomes should be followed to track efficiency and common barriers to implementation of an effective model. One challenge is recognizing that the optimal composition of services necessary for round depends on each child's illness, complexity, and psychosocial factors, and often varies daily. Once identified, further coordination effort is required to ensure the presence of the individuals who make up that composition of services during rounds. Many families, nurses, and providers agree that a process to identify and publish when rounds will take place would be beneficial. Institutions have focused on the area of creating a "rounding scheduler." Although evidence is lacking, the expenditure could be validated by increased rounding presence of multiple teams, earlier discharges, and safer care. Studies that focus on quality of communication and appropriate resource use are beneficial to a more diffuse endorsement of FCR.

As Osler believed that the bedside is an ideal place for learning, effective teachers should be able to use the simultaneous presence and cumulative knowledge and experience of patients, families, nurses, learners, and attending physicians to create a uniquely rich learning environment. However, as the model for FCR adapts to local institutional pressures, many barriers to bedside teaching have been identified. In addition to the time constraints and draw of "conference room teaching" mentioned previously, there are team misperceptions about family attitudes toward honest bedside conversation. The belief that teaching will increase family anxiety or will undermine the learners' intelligence and importance on the team is unfounded and not supported by evidence.[17,49,50] Perhaps then, additional effort needs to be focused on changing learner's perceptions of bedside teaching, which in reality provides many benefits relative to what can be learned within the confining walls of a classroom. Many strategies to achieve effective bedside teaching have been described (**Table 2**).[19,51–56] Certain elements of bedside learning are obvious, such as emphasizing an element of a patient's history or elucidating a pertinent physical examination finding. There are many other elements that are equally valuable, but less overt, such as the way an attending creates a comfortable environment before a difficult conversation, or fosters autonomy by encouraging the learner to be the primary communicator. Further, when the attending either explains his or her thought process to a family or encourages the trainee to do the same, all participants learn about clinical reasoning. As is true of subtle communication, such as feedback, labeling the specific conversation or learning point as "bedside teaching" (either within the room or outside of it) could help emphasize the occurrence of education on rounds. Appropriate faculty development, pre-round preparation, and certain teacher characteristics have been shown to improve education on rounds.[19,51–55] Successful teachers are adaptable, recognize time constraints, and create a positive learning environment in the setting of FCR. They can also promote autonomy by allowing residents to "step up"[57] using such techniques as senior resident empowering actions, while also adapting to the learner and the clinical scenario.[58]

SUMMARY

Bedside rounds have always been at the forefront of medical care and even more so for the teaching of medicine. FCR has taken bedside rounds 1 step further, incorporating principles of family centeredness in its ideal state. Although the use of FCR has grown in the pediatric in-patient setting, there remain continued opportunities to ensure the goals of all participants are achieved.

REFERENCES

1. Weil E. PCP vs hospitalist. Boston (MA): Forum CRICO/RMF; 2009. p. 8.
2. John Hopkins Medicine Website. The four founding fathers. Available at: https://www.hopkinsmedicine.org/about/history/history5.html. Accessed May 15, 2018.
3. Stone MJ. Historical review: William Osler's legacy and his contribution to haematology. Br J Haematol 2013;123:3–18.
4. Reichsman F, Browning FE, Hinshaw JR. Observations of undergraduate teaching in action. J Med Educ 1964;39:147–63.
5. Hurst JW. The art and science of presenting a patient's problems (as an extension of the Weed system). Arch Intern Med 1971;126:463–5.
6. Sylvius F. Epistola apolegetica. In: Opera medica. Amsterdam: Elsevir and Wolfgang; 1679. p. 907.
7. Osler W. On the need of a radical reform in our methods of teaching senior students. Med News 1903;82:49–53.
8. Linfors EW, Neelon FA. The case for bedside rounds. N Engl J Med 1980;303:1230–3.
9. Thibault GE. Bedside rounds revisited. N Engl J Med 1997;336:1174–5.
10. Lehmann LS, Brancati FL, Chen MC, et al. The effect of bedside case presentations on patients' perceptions of their medical care. N Engl J Med 1997;336:1150–5.
11. Institute of Medicine. Crossing the quality chasm. A new health care system for the 21st century. Washington, DC: National Academy Press; 2001.
12. Committee on Hospital Care. Family-centered care and the pediatrician's role. Pediatrics 2003;112:691–6.
13. Muething SE, Kotagal UR, Schoettker PJ, et al. Family-centered bedside rounds: a new approach to patient care and teaching. Pediatrics 2007;119:829–32.
14. Verghese A. Culture shock-patient as icon, icon as patient. N Engl J Med 2008;359:2748–51.
15. Destino LA, Valentine M, Sheikhi FH, et al. Inpatient hospital factors and resident time with patients and families. Pediatrics 2017;139 [pii:e20163011].
16. Block L, Habicht R, Wu AW, et al. In the wake of the 2003 and 2011 duty hours regulations, how do internal medicine interns spend their time? J Gen Intern Med 2018;28:1042–7.
17. Peters M, Ten Cate O. Bedside teaching in medical education: a literature review. Perspect Med Educ 2014;3:76–88.
18. Miller M, Johnson B, Greene HL, et al. An observational study of attending rounds. J Gen Intern Med 1992;7:646–8.
19. Gonzalo JD, Heist BS, Duffy BL, et al. Identifying and overcoming the barriers to bedside rounds: a multicenter qualitative study. Acad Med 2014;89:326–34.
20. Crumlish CM, Yialamas MA, McMahon GT. Quantification of bedside teaching by an academic hospitalist group. J Hosp Med 2009;4:304–7.
21. Stickrath C, Noble M, Prochazka A, et al. Attending rounds in the current era. What is and is not happening. JAMA Intern Med 2013;173:1084–9.
22. American Academy of Pediatrics Committee on Hospital Care and Institute for Patient- and Family- Centered Care. Patient- and family-centered care and the pediatrician's role. Pediatrics 2012;129:394–404.
23. Wachter RM, Goldman L. Zero to 50,000 – the 20th anniversary of the hospitalist. N Engl J Med 2016;15:1009–11.
24. Barrett DJ, McGuinness GA, Cunha CA, et al. Pediatric Hospital Medicine: a proposed new subspecialty. Pediatrics 2017;139 [pii:e20161823].

25. Sisterhen LL, Blaszak RT, Woods MB, et al. Defining family-centered rounds. Teach Learn Med 2007;19:319–22.
26. Cox ED, Jacobsohn GC, Rajamanickam VP, et al. A family-centered rounds checklist, family engagement, and patient safety: a randomized trial. Pediatrics 2017;139 [pii:e20161688].
27. Gleason M, Gleason A. A family's perspective on family-centered rounds: progress and frustrations. Hosp Pediatr 2016;6:437–8.
28. Aragona E, Ponce-Rios J, Garg P, et al. A quality improvement project to increase nurse attendance on pediatric family centered rounds. J Pediatr Nurs 2016;31: e3–9.
29. Sharma A, Norton L, Gage S, et al. A quality improvement initiative to achieve high nursing presence during patient- and family-centered rounds. Hosp Pediatr 2014;4:1–5.
30. Anttila A, Rappaport DI, Tijerino J, et al. Interpretation modalities used on family-centered rounds: perspectives of Spanish-speaking families. Hosp Pediatr 2017; 7:492–8.
31. O'Toole JK, Alvarado-Little W, Ledford CJW. Communication with diverse patients: addressing culture and language. Pediatr Clin N Am 2019. in press.
32. Mittal V, Sigrest T, Ottolini M, et al. Family-centered rounds on pediatric wards: a PRIS network survey of US and Canadian hospitalists. Pediatrics 2010;126(1): 37–43.
33. Levin AB, Fisher KR, Cato KD, et al. An evaluation of family-centered rounds in the PICU: room for improvement suggested by families and providers. Pediatr Crit Care Med 2015;16:801–7.
34. Pickel S, Shen MW, Hovinga C. Look who's talking: comparing perceptions versus direct observations in family-centered rounds. Hosp Pediatr 2016;6: 387–93.
35. Byrd AS, McMahon PM, Vath RJ, et al. Integration of mobile devices to facilitate patient care and teaching during family-centered rounds. Hosp Pediatr 2018;81: 44–8.
36. Beck J, Meyer R, Kind T, et al. The importance of situational awareness: a qualitative study of family members' and nurses' perspectives on teaching during family-centered rounds. Acad Med 2015;90:1401–7.
37. Rea KE, Rao P, Hill E, et al. Families' experiences with pediatric family-centered rounds: a systemic review. Pediatrics 2018;141. https://doi.org/10.1542/peds.2017-1883.
38. Rabinowitz R, Farnan J, Hulland O, et al. Rounds today: a qualitative study of internal medicine and pediatrics resident perceptions. J Grad Med Educ 2016;8: 523–31.
39. Hulland O, Farnan J, Rabinowitz R, et al. What's the purpose of rounds? A qualitative study examining the perceptions of faculty and students. J Hosp Med 2017;12:892–7.
40. Landrigan CP, Muret-Wagstaff S, Chiang VW, et al. Effect of a pediatric hospitalist system on housestaff education and experience. Arch Pediatr Adolesc Med 2002;156:877–83.
41. Kemper AR, Freed GL. Hospitalists and residency medical education: measured improvement. Arch Pediatr Adolesc Med 2002;156:858–9.
42. Beck J, Kind T, Meyer R, et al. Promoting resident autonomy during family-centered rounds: a qualitative study of resident, hospitalist, and subspecialty physicians. J Grad Med Educ 2016;8:731–8.

43. Khan A, Spector ND, Baird JD, for the Patient and Family Centered I-PASS Study Group. Patient safety after implementation of a coproduced family centered communication programme: multicenter before and after intervention study. BMJ 2018;363:k4764.
44. Kelly MM, Xie A, Carayon P, et al. Strategies for improving family engagement during family-centered rounds. J Hosp Med 2013;8:201–7.
45. Hermann LE, Winer JC, Kern J, et al. Integrating a clinical librarian to increase trainee application of evidence-based medicine on patient family-centered rounds. Acad Pediatr 2017;17:339–41.
46. Austin J, Bumsted T, Brands C. Teaching and evaluating oral presentations on family-centered rounds using the FREE TIPS tool. MedEdPORTAL 2013;9:9553.
47. Khan A, Rogers JE, Forster CS, et al. Communication and shared understanding between parents and resident-physicians at night. Hosp Pediatr 2016;6:319–29.
48. Khan A, Coffey M, Litterer KP, et al. Families as partners in hospital error and adverse event surveillance. JAMA Pediatr 2017;171:372–81.
49. LaCombe MA. On bedside teaching. Ann Intern Med 1997;126(3):217–20.
50. Nair BR, Coughlan JL, Hensley MJ. Student and patient perspectives on bedside teaching. Med Educ 1997;31:341–6.
51. Ramani S. Twelve tips to improve bedside teaching. Med Teach 2003;25:112–5.
52. Fitzgerald FT. Bedside teaching. West J Med 1993;158:418–20.
53. Williams KN, Ramani S, Fraser B, et al. Improving bedside teaching: findings from a focus group study of learners. Acad Med 2008;83:257–64.
54. Reilly BM. Inconvenient truths about effective clinical teaching. Lancet 2007;370:705–11.
55. Lichstein PR, Atkinson HH. Patient-centered bedside rounds and the clinical examination. Med Clin North Am 2018;102:509–19.
56. Chi J, Artandi M, Kugler J, et al. The five-minute moment. Am J Med 2016;129:792–5.
57. Balmer DF, Giardino AP, Richards BF. The dance between attending physicians and senior residents as teachers and supervisors. Pediatrics 2012;129:910–5.
58. Weisberger M, Toth H, Brewer C, et al. The instructor's guide for the SREA-21 (senior resident empowerment action-21) item checklist and the SOS-REACH (suspected observable senior resident empowerment action checklist); tools for evaluating senior resident empowerment during family-centered rounds. MedEdPORTAL 2011;7:8547.

Section 3: Education in the Inpatient Setting

The Clinical Learning Environment and Workplace-Based Assessment

Frameworks, Strategies, and Implementation

Duncan Henry, MD[a,*], Daniel C. West, MD[b]

KEYWORDS

- Clinical learning environment • Competency-based medical education
- Entrustable professional activities • Mastery learning • Self-regulated learning
- Assessment for learning

KEY POINTS

- Assessments should drive learning by providing a framework for and information to inform trainee goal setting and inquiry.
- A competency-based assessment framework is a key component in transitioning from a normative-based assessment strategy to a criterion-based assessment strategy.
- Entrustable professional activities translate abstract competency domains and milestones into observable activities that are intuitive to trainees and supervisors.
- Programs of assessment should foster self-regulated learning behaviors including goal setting, self-monitoring, and feedback seeking to support the development of intrinsic motivation.
- Supporting learners through advising and coaching for clinical skill and professional development is an essential component of a program of assessment.

THE CLINICAL LEARNING ENVIRONMENT

The clinical learning environment (CLE) can be defined as the "social, cultural, and material context" in which trainees learn while helping to care for patients in the clinical

Conflicts of Interest: Dr D. Henry has no conflicts of interest to report. Dr D.C. West holds equity in and has consulted with the I-PASS Patient Safety Institute. The I-PASS Patient Safety Institute is a company that seeks to train institutions in best handoff practices and aid in their implementation. Dr West has additionally received monetary awards, honoraria, and travel reimbursement from multiple academic and professional organizations for teaching and consulting on physician performance and handoffs. The authors report no external funding for this article.
[a] Department of Pediatrics, University of California San Francisco, 550 16th Street, 5th floor, Box 0110, San Francisco, CA 94143-0110, USA; [b] Department of Pediatrics, University of California San Francisco, 550 16th Street, 4th floor, Box 0110, San Francisco, CA 94143-0110, USA
* Corresponding author.
E-mail address: duncan.henry@ucsf.edu

Pediatr Clin N Am 66 (2019) 839–854
https://doi.org/10.1016/j.pcl.2019.03.010 pediatric.theclinics.com

workplace.[1] Social theories of learning, particularly those by Lave and Wenger,[2,3] suggest that the environment, and the learner's interaction with that environment, are critical aspects of learning. When the CLE is functioning well it supports trainees in acquiring knowledge and skill while leading to improved outcomes for patients.[4] However, in the context of growing demands from patients and payers for more cost-effective and higher-quality care and from health systems for increased clinical productivity, the CLE often is not optimized for learning.[5]

Understanding how trainees learn in the CLE is one essential step toward optimizing the CLE for learning. There is evidence that most of the learning in the CLE occurs through workplace-based activities (eg, conducting rounds, making patient care decisions, interacting with consultants).[6] In other words, the day-to-day activities of caring for patients in the CLE drive acquisition of knowledge and skills as residents interpret (eg, read the situation, use consultant input, and make reasoned clinical decisions) and construct meaning out of these experiences. A key element of this process is when trainees reflect on these experiences to compare their performance with their own expectations and those of others. This process helps drive additional learning by informing how trainees might need to adjust specific techniques or strategies and/or seek out additional or new experiences to further improve their performance.[6] Considering that learning in this environment is such a complex entity with many variables that can influence the process, it is not surprising that there are significant challenges in optimizing learning in the CLE.

One group of investigators used a process called Group Concept Mapping to develop a consensus opinion on what are the most important elements for improving learning for residents in the CLE.[7] Their work identified 10 essential elements of the CLE and identified the barriers that can inhibit learning each of them. **Table 1** summarizes those elements and the barriers they create along with some potential solutions. Among the elements that were rated highest in importance were those that centered on establishing and nurturing connection between residents and senior clinicians and facilitating feedback through those interactions. "Organization and conditions of work" was identified as another important element, which highlights how very busy clinical work environments that focus on efficiency and high throughput can interfere with trainees' ability to reflect on their experiences, assess their own performance, and consolidate knowledge. Other elements of high importance included resident support, time to learn with senior doctors, and interaction and feedback in clinical teams. Aspects of the CLE thought to be easier to modify included clinical experience content, assessment methods and process, faculty supervisor skill and support, and continuity of training experiences.[7]

In summary, the CLE is both a rich and challenging place for learners to acquire knowledge and skills. Competing pressures of productivity and patient care are often in conflict with elements essential to facilitating resident learning, especially time for reflection and interactions with supervising senior clinicians. Understanding how learners use the CLE, and the barriers and facilitators of learning in that environment, can help in the design programs of training and assessment that meet the needs of learners, and foster these critical elements of learning in the workplace and still achieve the goals of efficient, cost-effective, and high-quality patient care. The remainder of this article focuses on using assessment frameworks and strategies to support learning in the CLE.

COMPETENCY FRAMEWORKS: EVOLUTION AND EXAMPLE

History of Competency-Based Medical Education

Medical education is increasingly shifting from a time-based and process-based training system, in which competency was inferred from completing a defined set of

Table 1
Key elements of clinical learning environments

Element	Challenge	Potential Solutions
Organization and conditions of work	Tension between providing clinical service and time for learning, reflection, and knowledge consolidation	• Optimize the number and types of patients trainees cover • Provide scheduled, protected time for reflection
Learning from clinical supervisors	Time and productivity pressures limit interactions with senior clinical supervisors	• Optimize the number and types of patients trainees cover • Set focused, realistic, and transparent goals for teaching and learning in clinical workplace
Management and facilities	Physical space and workflows often prioritize health care system and delivery needs over training and education	• Create and maintain physical space for learning activities
Workplace culture	Trainees, clinical teachers, and learning need to be valued in the clinical workplace	• In addition to clinical productivity, incentivize and reward clinical supervisors for high-quality teaching
Development of clinical supervisors	Clinical supervisors need the skills to teach and give feedback in busy clinical workplace	• Time-efficient faculty development programs • Realistic adaptation of teaching and feedback methods to clinical workplace • Use trained observers in multiple clinical contexts
Supervision, autonomy, and feedback for trainees on clinical teams	Balancing patient safety, quality, and efficiency with allowing trainees to practice, make decisions, reflect, and gradually gain more independence	• Develop clinical supervisor skills in supervision, teaching, and feedback • Develop trainee skills in seeking and processing feedback • Develop and communicate shared mental model about learning goals in each clinical workplace
Content, assessment, and continuity of training	Clinical training activities in a particular clinical workplace need to match goals of assessment, and supervisors need to apply assessments and draw conclusions appropriately	• Match assessments to clinical workplace and supervisor skills • Train supervisors in appropriate use of assessment tools • Provide supervisors with ongoing feedback about how they are applying assessments
Motivation and morale	Stress, burnout, and overwork can lead to fatigue and undermine working and learning in the clinical environment	• Optimize the number and types of patients trainees cover • Provide backup systems to offload excessive workload • Wellness programs to support trainees, supervisors, and interprofessional team members

(*continued on next page*)

Table 1
(*continued*)

Element	Challenge	Potential Solutions
Trainee treatment and support in the clinical workplace	Creating a welcoming and respectful environment for trainees who lack knowledge, experience, and relationships with senior clinicians and interprofessional team members who work regularly in the clinical workplace	• Provide effective orientation to the clinical workplace • Develop shared mental model among trainees, supervisors, and interprofessional team members about trainee responsibility and roles • Engage interprofessional team members in the training process
The role of patients in the clinical learning environment	Balancing patients' expectations of care with their willingness to support trainee learning	• Provide patients with effective orientation learning and supervision in the clinical workplace • Provide opportunities for patients/families to provide guided feedback to trainees

Adapted from Kilty C, Wiese A, Bergin C, et al. A national stakeholder consensus study of challenges and priorities for clinical learning environments in postgraduate medical education. BMC Med Educ 2017;17(1). https://doi.org/10.1186/s12909-017-1065-2.

clinical experiences over a fixed duration of time, to a competency-based framework that provides explicit sets of skills and behaviors that trainees must demonstrate that they can perform well enough to care for patients independently. Competency frameworks play an essential role in providing a shared understanding, or mental model, between faculty supervisors and trainees about the goals and objectives of training. They also provide the basis for designing curricula (eg, training experiences) and assessment strategies, and a structure for both formative feedback and summative decision making. Beginning in the 1990s with the development of Tomorrow's Doctors in the UK, there has been widespread adoption of competency frameworks internationally for both undergraduate and graduate medical education. Examples include CanMEDS,[8] Scottish Doctor,[9] Accreditation Council for Graduate Medication Education (ACGME) Outcomes Project,[10] and the Australian Curriculum Framework for Junior Doctors[11,12] Although each of these frameworks are different, they all provide an educational and cultural perspective on the qualities and behaviors that are important for being an effective physician. For the purposes of this article, the focus here is on the development and evolution of competency-based medical education (CBME) frameworks for graduate medical education (GME) training in the United States.

Evolution of Competency-Based Medical Education in the United States

In the United States, the ACGME and the American Board of Medical Specialties worked together to develop the Outcomes Project in 1999. In the Outcomes Project, physician competencies were organized into 6 domains: Patient Care, Medical Knowledge, Practice-based Learning and Improvement, Interpersonal and Communication Skills, Professionalism, and Systems-based Practice. In 2009, in an effort to further define these broad competency domains, the Milestones Project began as each specialty developed a set of specialty-specific competencies within each domain and accompanying developmental levels for each competency that defined 4 to 5 levels of performance as residents progress through training.[13] Twice each academic year, all ACGME accredited training programs are required to use a Clinical Competency Committee (CCC) to determine the level at which milestone level each trainee in their program is currently performing for a subset of competencies and report those ratings to the ACGME. In Pediatrics there are a total of 21 reporting milestones or competencies representing the 6 domains of competence. For example, in the Patient Care domain, one reported competency (PC4) is to "make informed diagnostic and therapeutic interventions."[10,14,15] Theoretically this competency framework with its developmental structure can be used for formative feedback to guide further development toward competence. However, the ACGME Milestones have been criticized as being so detailed and reductionist that they miss the big picture and are not intuitive for faculty supervisors and trainees.[16,17]

Example of an Evolving Competency Framework: Pediatric Entrustable Professional Activities

Entrustable professional activities (EPAs) are a competency framework that synthesizes and provides clinical context for ACGME Competencies and Milestones. EPAs provide a simplified, more holistic view of a trainee's progress in learning to perform the common tasks of a particular specialty and allow for more intuitively useful assessment strategies.[18] First proposed in 2005 by ten Cate[19] with further elucidation by ten Cate and Scheele,[20] EPAs incorporate competencies into a framework centered around large-scale, observable clinical care and other activities that a physician routinely performs in the CLE. Thus EPAs can be thought of as defining a profession, because they describe the critical activities that a physician practicing a particular specialty or subspecialty must be able to perform without supervision in order to practice independently. Central to the application of EPAs in a training environment is the concept of "trust"—the idea that a trainee is working toward earning the trust of supervisors to perform a given EPA independently, without supervision.

EPAs and competencies are inter-related because to perform an EPA, a trainee must be able to effectively perform multiple competencies. Using this logic, multiple domains of competence (ie, patient care, medical knowledge, professionalism) and individual competencies can be "mapped" to EPAs. In this way, EPAs provide a conceptual model that links the abstract qualities and characteristics of physicians described in the ACGME Milestone Competencies with observable, patient-care–related activities that are recognizable to supervising clinicians and trainees.[21] One additional advantage of the EPA model is the shift from a normative (eg, how does a trainee do compared with peers or a supervisor's expectations) to a criterion-based (eg, how much supervision does a trainee require or can a supervisor "trust" them to perform an EPA unsupervised) standard.[22] The concept of "trust" or "level of supervision" provides a criterion standard that is intuitive for supervisors and trainees.

Increasingly, the EPA competency model has been embraced in both undergraduate and GME throughout the world. In the United States, this has resulted in the development of EPAs for multiple specialties and some subspecialties. In 2013 the American Board of Pediatrics worked with stakeholders to develop 17 EPAs that "define" the practice of a general pediatrician and could plausibly be assessed to determine when a trainee is ready to practice independently and graduate from residency training. Each EPA carries a description of the key elements of the activity and is parsimoniously mapped to critical ACGME competency domains and individual competencies. For example, EPA 3 (Care for the Well Newborn) incorporated specific competencies related to medical knowledge, patient care, and communication.

Linking Competency Frameworks to Assessment Strategies

Assessment can be viewed through the lens of Miller's Pyramid with the bottom level of "Knows," followed by "Knows How," then "Shows," and finally the highest level of "Does."[23] Assessment strategies for lower levels are relatively straightforward and common. For example, multiple-choice questions can be effective in assessing whether a trainee "knows" something, but assessment of complex tasks that require integration of knowledge, skills, and attitudes, such as those required to care for patients, means focusing on the top 2 levels of Miller's Pyramid. Competency frameworks, such as the ACGME Milestone Competencies or EPAs, provide a shared mental model of the skills, behaviors, and abilities that trainees are trying to learn and supervisors are trying to assess. Miller's Pyramid can help us identify how we should look for it. However, it is important to remember that no single assessment method or tool will be valid for assessing trainee performance in the complex tasks of caring for patients, regardless of competency framework. Effectively determining whether a trainee is ready to practice their intended specialty of medicine independently requires a program of assessment (eg, multiple assessment tools, appropriate sampling strategy) that measures the full range of competencies necessary to practice that discipline. However, the authors consider it equally important that a program of assessment be designed in such a way that it provides useful feedback for trainees such that they can effectively use it to guide their learning.

PROGRAM OF ASSESSMENT FOR LEARNING: A VIEW THROUGH THE LENS OF MOTIVATIONAL THEORIES

Before discussing the specifics of a program of assessment to support CBME, it is worthwhile to discuss the concept of assessment in general, competing purposes of assessment, and underlying educational theories that can be used to help design a program of assessment. In the context of CBME, assessment is commonly thought of as an important component of a summative process in which competence is determined by assessment of what a trainee has learned (ie, assessment *of* learning). Often this process is heavily informed by high-stakes assessments and comparisons of a trainee's performance to a normative standard.[24] More recently, there has been a movement to develop a strategy whereby assessment can be used to provide feedback to learners to inform development of learning goals (ie, assessment *for* learning). The core principles in this process should emphasize the low-stakes nature of any given assessment, ensure that every assessment provides meaningful feedback to learners to use in their own development, and provide support and coaching for trainees in the context of a safe and trusting relationship with an advisor.[25–27]

Among the more negative effects of high-stakes, normative-based assessment is that it can reinforce a "performance" or "entity" rather than a "mastery" or "incremental" mindset. Goal Orientation Theory, first elucidated by Carol Dweck,[28] describes 2 broad orientations, or mindsets, to learning. In a "performance" orientation, learners focus on looking better than others or avoiding the perception of being unintelligent. These learners can be characterized as having an "entity mindset" whereby there is a belief that intelligence and ability are fixed, innate characteristics that cannot change over time. In contrast, learners with an "incremental" mindset focus on the intrinsic value of learning (ie, acquisition of new knowledge or skills). This concept is paired with a belief that intelligence and ability can increase with training.[29] Perhaps most applicable to this discussion is that an incremental mindset can be taught, and that randomized controlled trials have shown that learners, when taught about the malleability of the brain and an incredible capacity for learning, will take on more difficult tasks and persevere even when faced with occasional failures.[28,29]

Assessment strategies should work to reinforce opportunities for incremental improvement *and* promote and sustain a "mastery" orientation. The concept of mastery learning emphasizes deliberate practice with reflection and coaching within a set of defined and well-articulated learning goals.[30–32] This can be achieved through the development of a program of assessment *for* learning, which has been defined as "an approach in which routine information about the learner's competence and progress is continually collected, analyzed and, where needed, complemented with purposively collected additional assessment information, with the intent to both maximally inform the learner and their mentor and allow for high-stakes decisions at the end of a training phase."[26,33] In brief, the concept involves developing targeted assessments that are optimized to the CLE and occur at spaced intervals that allow for the development of a holistic view of the learner. A core principle in this approach is that any single assessment forces a compromise between utility and its quality and that there is no single "silver bullet" for learner assessment.[34] A critical additional element to this type of assessment program is support in the form of mentorship and coaching designed to allow learners the opportunity for critical reflection, goal setting, and defining opportunities to seek additional clinical experience and practice to inform iterative improvement toward achieving competence.

Although there are many theories that inform the program of assessment literature, it is useful to consider 2 in more detail: Self-Determination Theory and Self-Regulated Learning. Self-Determination Theory posits that to encourage intrinsic motivation (defined as free engagement in an activity out of interest or inherent satisfaction and the most desirable form of motivation as compared with amotivation or extrinsic motivation), learning environments should promote 3 characteristics: autonomy, competency, and relatedness.[35–38] Autonomy refers to the ability of the individual to choose what they consider a useful course of action and is supported by creating an environment in which learners are empowered to set their own goals and direct their learning. Competency is embodied in the desire to feel effective in action and performance. Relatedness refers to a sense of interconnectedness, belonging, and engagement in reciprocal caring relationships, for example, incorporation of the learner into the larger professional or clinical group.[39] Self-Regulation Theory, originally developed by Zimmerman, characterized self-regulated learning in individuals as an internal desire to achieve mastery through metacognitive, motivational, and behavioral strategies. Such behaviors are highly valued in medicine. One key characteristic of self-regulated learning is intrinsic motivation, whereby learners use strategies to set goals and monitor progress as well as seek activities to enhance progress toward those learning goals. The key behaviors of self-regulated learning are goal setting, feedback seeking, and monitoring of one's self and abilities to promote intrinsic motivation aimed at performance improvement.[40–42]

Using the lenses of Self-Determination Theory and Self-Regulation Theory helps illustrate several key points about programmatic assessment. Learners need to demonstrate autonomy by being fully engaged in the process and feel that they have an ability to direct the content and nature of feedback. In addition, learners need to set goals and monitor their own performance relative to those goals and then seek out additional feedback to validate their feelings of growing competence. Finally, learners need to establish relatedness to a trusted individual who can coach them as they regularly review their assessment data and work to revise their learning plans as they progress to competence. In other words assessment should drive feedback, which in turn drives learning by helping trainees identify, create, and monitor progress toward achieving learning and professional goals and, ultimately, competence.

Table 2 outlines several key elements that are necessary for successful implementation of a program of assessment that supports learning.[26,27] For example, there are structural elements such as an overarching roadmap that incorporates learning environments and targeted assessments, in essence defining who does what, where, and with whom. Additional structural pieces include a physical means of capturing assessment data, a way to display aggregate data, and a place to record reflection and critique. This involves systems designed to be easily useable and ideally nimble enough to capture feedback and observations (ie, mobile applications) as well as systems designed to aggregate and display these data in user-friendly formats (eg, dashboards, e-portfolios).[43] In addition to the structural elements, there are also processes that need to be in place to adequately support reflection and goal setting beyond a physical/electronic system. These processes include ways to facilitate review and

Table 2
Elements of program assessment

Structural Elements	Processes and Procedures	Faculty/Trainee Development
Overarching assessment plan • Roadmap of learning environments and targeted assessments matched to competency framework • Clearly identify who does what, where, and with whom Assessment data • Outline method to collect, summarize, and display assessment data • Collect written feedback comments to inform learning • Make assessments mobile, easy to use, efficient Dashboard and learning plans • Display aggregate data in user-friendly format • Collect and organize learner reflections and coach comments • Create a place to write learning goals, share with advisor, and track progress Faculty advisors/coaches • Develop a cohort of faculty advisors/coaches to guide trainees in processing feedback and creating learning plans	Reflection activities • Provide protected times for learners to participate in guided reflection experiences, feedback review, and generation of learning plans Intermediate summative assessment • Perform periodic summative assessments to assess trainee progress toward high-stakes competency decision • Identify trainees who may need additional support/ remediation Quality assurance program • Create a system to monitor number, timeliness, and quality of assessments • Measure key elements of clinical learning environment to identify areas for continued improvement • Implement a program to assess quality/utility of assessment tools/dashboard and revise as required to optimize effectiveness • Provide regular assessment and review of learning plans, advisor/trainee interactions to identify areas for improvement	Mentorship/Advising/ Coaching • Build shared understanding of overarching goals for program of assessment • Enhance understanding of competency framework • Develop skills for trainees to aid processing of feedback and creation of actionable learning goals Clinical supervisor feedback • Build skills of clinical supervisors in giving effective feedback • Build skills in applying appropriate supervision • Build skills in appropriate use of assessment tools Trainee feedback seeking • Enhance trainee skills in initiating or seeking out assessments and helping direct supervisor feedback to align with learning goals • Build trainee skills in processing feedback and converting it into actionable learning goals

reflection. In addition, it is important to have planned intermediate "certification points" that validate that learners are making adequate progress and to help identify when trainees are struggling or might need remediation. Finally there are human aspects of the program that may require additional faculty and learner development, such as delivering feedback and teaching faculty how to be effective mentors and coach learners in contextualizing feedback and building skills in feedback seeking.[44,45] Although these factors provide list of key elements for a program of assessment for learning, ultimately individual training programs need to mobilize local resources or modify existing structures to adapt these elements for implementation in their systems and CLE.

COMMON ASSESSMENT STRATEGIES

In designing a program of assessment for learning it can be useful to consider the Hindu parable of the blind men and an elephant, in which the perspective of feeling only a smaller part of the elephant (eg, feeling the tusk, the trunk, the leg) may not necessarily allow each individual to identify what they are feeling as an elephant.[46] In a similar way, considering only the perspective of a single assessment tool or single assessment encounter is imperfect and unlikely to provide a full picture of how a trainee is progressing toward competency. Fortunately, there is a large and ever-growing toolbox of quality assessment tools that when combined in a thoughtful and planned manner can provide a robust and holistic view of the learner to inform self-regulated, mastery learning for the trainee. The same assessment data, when considered together, can be used by CCCs and training program leadership to make high-stakes competency and advancement decisions. The key to this latter process is to consider the body of low-stakes assessments in its totality and avoid the temptation to place too much weight on a few individual assessments. **Table 3** lists types of workplace-based assessment tools that can be used or adapted for use in a broad range of CLEs. **Table 3** also provides a brief summary of the tools and pros and cons of each, and provides several essential references.

IMPLEMENTATION AND SUSTAINMENT CHALLENGES FOR A PROGRAM OF WORKPLACE-BASED ASSESSMENT FOR LEARNING

Despite the significant improvements that can be gained from conversion to competency-based frameworks, workplace-based assessments, and incorporating a program of assessment for learning, there are significant challenges in implementing and sustaining such a program. These challenges can be grouped into 3 categories: (1) logistical; (2) instrument (or assessment tool) related; and (3) faculty and trainee development.[27]

In the logistics category there are several simple but key elements that must be addressed. For example, should the program of assessment use a single data management system to collect and collate information, or will users be required to access and manage multiple systems? Ensuring up-to-date enrollment in the system (not a trivial task in complex CLEs) so that trainees and faculty can engage in meaningful assessment and capture that data for later review is also essential. Issues of data management must also be addressed including answering questions such as who inputs data, who manages data, and who has access to what? Finally, it is imperative to provide easy visualization of such large amounts of assessment data in a way that can be understood by trainees, mentors/coaches, and faculty supervisors. Learners and mentor/coaches can and will be quickly overwhelmed by trying to sort through and make sense of an unorganized mound of assessments, regardless of the quality.

Table 3
Examples of workplace-based assessment tools

Tool	Description	Advantages	Limitations	References
Global assessment	• Based on big picture impressions of trainee performance rather than direct observation of discrete patient encounter • Often constructed from elements that directly map to competency framework	• Usually understandable to clinical supervisors • Can be delivered to and collected from assessors electronically on a large scale • Often use numbered rating scales that can be summarized efficiently • Can support mastery orientation, depending on design	• Rating scales often lack value and utility for learners • Context and rater variability can affect reliability, especially if number of assessments is small • If used as summative assessment at end of clinical training experience, it will promote performance, rather than mastery, orientation	51–54
Multisource assessment	• Provides assessments from individuals with different perspectives (eg, peers, patients, families, nurses, other clinical team members, etc) • Can include self-assessment • Assessment can be global or discrete patient encounters • Can be in the form of checklists with rating scales or free-text comments	• Provides information about aspects of behavior and skills not generally seen by faculty • Provides information about impacts of behaviors that may not be apparent to trainee • Can support mastery orientation, depending on design	• Logistical and technical challenges of collecting assessments from diverse group of assessors • Requires cooperation and training of multiple assessors with variable investment in the process • Trainees often express discomfort in assessing peers	23,55–57
Structured clinical observation	• Structured assessment of a discrete or series/sequence of discrete patient encounters • Assessment process usually requires observer or rater to assess a structured list of specific behaviors or skills	• Some assessments have substantial evidence supporting their validity (eg, mini-CEX) • Can be designed to assess a focused activity in a particular clinical environment • Can be designed to capture multisource assessment • Can support mastery orientation, depending on design	• Requires significant investment of time and resources (ie, faculty development and observation) with direct conflict in revenue-generating priorities • Checklist-oriented design may not provide the type of feedback that a trainee desires (ie, may not support self-determination and self-regulated learning)	23,58,59

Direct observation of procedural skills	• Observation and assessment of trainee performing a procedure • Can be done in clinical workplace or simulated procedure • Usually asks observer to assess trainee on a structured list of specific behaviors, skills, or steps related to a procedure • Often rated on a yes/no response scale	• Several of these tools have significant validity evidence to support their use • Particularly effective if determining that a trainee can perform the steps to a procedure • Depending on what decisions will be made based on the assessment, can support mastery orientation	• Depending on design, often not as effective in assessing the quality of how well the trainee performed the procedure • Checklist-oriented design may not provide the type of feedback that a trainee desires (ie, may not support self-determination and self-regulated learning)	60
Chart-stimulated recall	• Interview, or oral examination, of trainee based on reviewing a specific case in the medical record (chosen by trainee or assessor) • Similar to a "talk aloud" assessment where trainee explains their approach and decision making in a specific case • Also allows for assessment of trainee's written documentation in the chart	• Several validated forms exist in a variety of specialties • Case can be chosen to align with trainee learning goals, thus supporting self-determination and self-regulated learning • Can be used to target action plans for improvement around clinical decision making or other specific aspects of competency framework	• Time intensive for assessor and trainee • Requires significant training of assessors • Several threats to validity including inadequate number of cases, bias of assessor, focus of encounter • Usually is a high-stakes assessment, thus tends to foster performance, rather than mastery, orientation	61,62

In terms of assessment instruments or tools, there should be acknowledgment that many of the tools likely to be used in a workplace-based assessment are inherently subjective, because the complex competencies (regardless of the competency framework) that one is attempting to measure *are* subjective. For example, one system that uses EPA-based assessments uses a supervision-anchored scale whereby faculty supervisors are asked to rate how much supervision they think the trainee they are assessing requires.[47,48] However, faculty ratings of need for supervision are situated in clinical context, the degree to which a relationship has been fostered between trainee and assessor that promotes trust, time spent in observation, and a faculty supervisor's own expectations, experiences, and bias. In a program of assessment for learning, this type of variability from assessment to assessment is perfectly acceptable because any individual assessment is low-stakes. From an assessment psychometric perspective, this variability evens out by viewing the assessment data not as individual components each with their own validity, but in aggregate with a large number of assessments from many different clinical contexts and different supervisors. Taking this approach, it is possible to make highly valid and reliable decisions about level of competence and advancement through the training program.

Finally, a key area to consider is faculty and trainee development focusing on such topics as: (1) the changing nature of assessment and the idea of workplace-based assessment using criterion-based referents[49]; (2) the roles, responsibilities, and skills necessary for feedback seeking and feedback delivery situated in a competency-based framework[44]; (3) developing self-regulated learning skills such as goal setting and self monitoring[50]; (4) enhancing skills in mentorship/coaching/advising. In short, attention should be paid to not only the framework and content of assessments but also the supporting infrastructure of electronic and human resources that such a program of assessment requires.

SUMMARY

This article has reviewed the concepts of the CLE, the rationale for and examples of CBME frameworks, and the learning theories that support this transition to a new focus of assessment. In addition, it describes how a program of assessment can provide information to the learner to guide intrinsically motivated, self-regulated mastery learning and can be used to inform high-stakes competency and advancement decisions. The key elements to successful workplace-based assessment and the promotion of assessment for learning are:

- Assessments should drive new learning by providing a framework for and information to inform trainee goal setting and inquiry, rather than focusing on testing previously learned material
- A competency-based assessment framework is essential in transitioning from a normative-based assessment strategy (eg, how do I compare with my peers, a gold standard) to a criterion-based assessment strategy (eg, am I ready for independent/unsupervised practice)
- EPAs have the potential to translate abstract competency domains and milestones into observable activities, even at the level of the individual faculty supervisor
- Programs of assessment should foster self-regulated learning behaviors including goal setting, self-monitoring, and feedback seeking to support the development of intrinsic motivation
- No single assessment tool is sufficient to provide a holistic, unbiased view of the learner. Instead multiple, varied, and planned assessments are required to provide a complete picture of a trainee

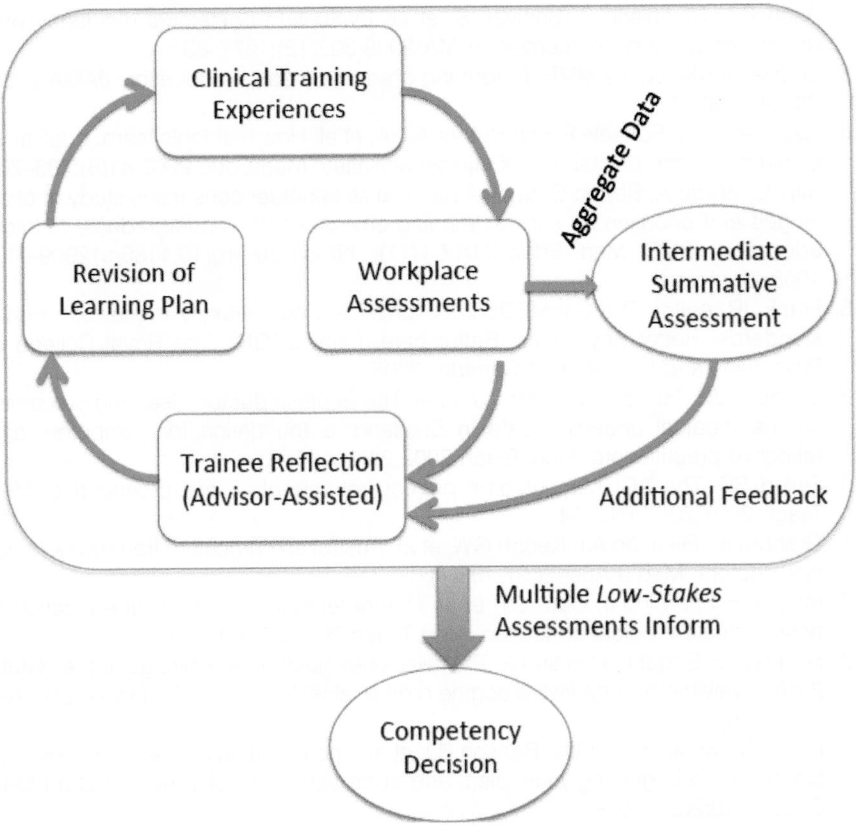

Fig. 1. Program of assessment for learning in the clinical learning environment.

- Supporting the learner through advising and coaching for clinical skill and professional development is an essential component of any program of assessment
- In addition to the structure of assessment (how they happen, when and with whom), attention to the systems and people that support them including development of both learners and faculty in this process is vital

In summary, how a program of assessment might work in an iterative cycle of continuous self-improvement is described (**Fig. 1**). Through structured assessments and the feedback inherently contained within them, facilitated reflection with trusted advisors, and support and development in goal setting and feedback seeking, learners will not only engage in, but also find reinforcement of their behavior in becoming an intrinsically motivated, self-regulated mastery learner for the rest of their career.

REFERENCES

1. Dornan T, editor. Medical education: theory and practice. Edinburgh (Scotland): Elsevier; 2011.
2. Lave J, Wenger E. Situated learning: legitimate peripheral participation. New York: Cambridge University Press; 1991.
3. Wenger E. Communities of practice: learning, meaning, and identity. Cambridge (England): Cambridge Univ. Press; 2008.

4. Asch DA, Nicholson S, Srinivas S, et al. Evaluating obstetrical residency programs using patient outcomes. JAMA 2009;302(12):1277–83.
5. Ludmerer KM, Johns MME. Reforming graduate medical education. JAMA 2005; 294(9):1083–7.
6. Teunissen PW, Scheele F, Scherpbier AJJA, et al. How residents learn: qualitative evidence for the pivotal role of clinical activities. Med Educ 2007;41(8):763–70.
7. Kilty C, Wiese A, Bergin C, et al. A national stakeholder consensus study of challenges and priorities for clinical learning environments in postgraduate medical education. BMC Med Educ 2017;17(1). https://doi.org/10.1186/s12909-017-1065-2.
8. Frank JR, editor. The CanMEDS 2005 physician competency framework. Better standards. Better physicians. Better care. Ottawa (ON): The Royal College of Physicians and Surgeons of Canada; 2005.
9. Simpson JG, Furnace J, Crosby J, et al. The Scottish doctor—learning outcomes for the medical undergraduate in Scotland: a foundation for competent and reflective practitioners. Med Teach 2002;24(2):136–43.
10. Swing SR. The ACGME outcome project: retrospective and prospective. Med Teach 2007;29(7):648–54.
11. Graham IS, Gleason AJ, Keogh GW, et al. Australian curriculum framework for junior doctors. Med J Aust 2007;186(7):6.
12. Iobst WF, Sherbino J, Cate OT, et al. Competency-based medical education in postgraduate medical education. Med Teach 2010;32(8):651–6.
13. Holmboe E, Edgar L, Hamstra S. The milestones guidebook. Chicago (IL): ACGME; 2016. Available at: http://www.acgme.org/Portals/0/MilestonesGuidebook.pdf. Accessed April 4, 2019.
14. Hicks PJ, Schumacher DJ, Benson BJ, et al. The pediatrics milestones: conceptual framework, guiding principles, and approach to development. J Grad Med Educ 2010;2(3):410–8.
15. Schumacher DJ, Lewis KO, Burke AE, et al. The pediatrics milestones: initial evidence for their use as learning road maps for residents. Acad Pediatr 2013; 13(1):40–7.
16. Brooks MA. Medical education and the tyranny of competency. Perspect Biol Med 2008;52(1):90–102.
17. Touchie C, ten Cate O. The promise, perils, problems and progress of competency-based medical education. Med Educ 2016;50(1):93–100.
18. Carraccio C, Englander R, Gilhooly J, et al. Building a framework of entrustable professional activities, supported by competencies and milestones, to bridge the educational continuum. Acad Med 2017;92(3):324–30.
19. Ten Cate O. Entrustability of professional activities and competency-based training. Med Educ 2005;39(12):1176–7.
20. ten Cate O, Scheele F. Viewpoint: competency-based postgraduate training: can we bridge the gap between theory and clinical practice? Acad Med 2007;82(6): 542–7.
21. Carraccio C, Englander R, Holmboe ES, et al. Driving care quality: aligning trainee assessment and supervision through practical application of entrustable professional activities, competencies, and milestones. Acad Med 2016;91(2): 199–203.
22. Pereira AG, Woods M, Olson APJ, et al. Criterion-based assessment in a norm-based world: how can we move past grades? Acad Med 2017. https://doi.org/10.1097/ACM.0000000000001939.
23. Norcini JJ. Peer assessment of competence. Med Educ 2003;37(6):539–43.

24. Shepard LA. The role of assessment in a learning culture. Educ Res 2000;29(7): 4–14.
25. van der Vleuten CPM, Schuwirth LWT. Assessing professional competence: from methods to programmes. Med Educ 2005;39(3):309–17.
26. van der Vleuten CPM, Schuwirth LWT, Driessen EW, et al. A model for programmatic assessment fit for purpose. Med Teach 2012;34(3):205–14.
27. Van Der Vleuten CPM, Schuwirth LWT, Driessen EW, et al. Twelve tips for programmatic assessment. Med Teach 2015;37(7):641–6.
28. Dweck CS. Self-theories: their role in motivation, personality, and development. Philadelphia: Psychology Press; 2000.
29. Cook DA, Artino AR. Motivation to learn: an overview of contemporary theories. Med Educ 2016;50(10):997–1014.
30. Lineberry M, Soo Park Y, Cook DA, et al. Making the case for mastery learning assessments: key issues in validation and justification. Acad Med 2015;90(11): 1445–50.
31. McGaghie WC. Mastery learning: it is time for medical education to join the 21st century. Acad Med 2015;90(11):1438–41.
32. Eppich WJ, Hunt EA, Duval-Arnould JM, et al. Structuring feedback and debriefing to achieve mastery learning goals. Acad Med 2015;90(11):1501–8.
33. Schuwirth L, van der Vleuten C, Durning SJ. What programmatic assessment in medical education can learn from healthcare. Perspect Med Educ 2017;6(4): 211–5.
34. Schuwirth LWT, van der Vleuten CPM. Programmatic assessment and Kane's validity perspective: programmatic assessment and Kane's validity perspective. Med Educ 2012;46(1):38–48.
35. Deci EL, Vallerand RJ, Pelletier LG, et al. Motivation and education: the self-determination perspective. Educ Psychol 1991;26(3–4):325–46.
36. Ryan RM, Deci EL. Intrinsic and extrinsic motivations: classic definitions and new directions. Contemp Educ Psychol 2000;25(1):54–67.
37. Deci EL, Ryan RM. The "what" and "why" of goal pursuits: human needs and the self-determination of behavior. Psychol Inq 2000;11(4):227–68.
38. Ryan RM, Deci EL. Self-determination theory and the facilitation of intrinsic motivation, social development, and well-being. Am Psychol 2000;55(1):68.
39. ten Cate OTJ, Kusurkar RA, Williams GC. How self-determination theory can assist our understanding of the teaching and learning processes in medical education. AMEE Guide No. 59. Med Teach 2011;33(12):961–73.
40. Zimmerm B. Self-regulated learning and academic achievement - an overview. Educ Psychol 1990;25(1):3–17.
41. Schunk DH, Greene JA. Handbook of self-regulation of learning and performance 2018. Available at: http://search.ebscohost.com/login.aspx?direct=true&scope=site&db=nlebk&db=nlabk&AN=1554356. Accessed September 16, 2018.
42. Sandars J, Cleary TJ. Self-regulation theory: applications to medical education: AMEE guide no. 58. Med Teach 2011;33(11):875–86.
43. Bok HG, Teunissen PW, Favier RP, et al. Programmatic assessment of competency-based workplace learning: when theory meets practice. BMC Med Educ 2013;13(1):123.
44. Ramani S, Könings KD, Ginsburg S, et al. Twelve tips to promote a feedback culture with a growth mind-set: swinging the feedback pendulum from recipes to relationships. Med Teach 2018;1–7. https://doi.org/10.1080/0142159X.2018.1432850.

45. Bing-You R, Hayes V, Palka T, et al. The art (and artifice) of seeking feedback: clerkship students' approaches to asking for feedback. Acad Med 2018;93(8): 1218–26.
46. Goldstein EB, editor. Encyclopedia of perception. Los Angeles (CA): SAGE; 2010.
47. Henry D. Developing an assessment program to support self-regulated learning: the UCSF pediatric residency experience. Oral Platform Presentation presented at the 2018 World Summit on Competency-based Medical Education, Basel, Switzerland, August 25, 2018.
48. Chen HC, van den Broek WES, ten Cate O. The case for use of entrustable professional activities in undergraduate medical education. Acad Med 2015;90(4): 431–6.
49. Boulet JR, Durning SJ. What we measure … and what we should measure in medical education. Med Educ 2018. https://doi.org/10.1111/medu.13652.
50. Leggett H, Sandars J, Roberts T. Twelve tips on how to provide self-regulated learning (SRL) enhanced feedback on clinical performance. Med Teach 2017;1–5. https://doi.org/10.1080/0142159X.2017.1407868.
51. Lurie SJ, Mooney CJ, Lyness JM. Measurement of the general competencies of the accreditation council for graduate medical education: a systematic review. Acad Med 2009;84(3):301–9.
52. Williams RG, Dunnington GL, Mellinger JD, et al. Placing constraints on the use of the ACGME milestones: a commentary on the limitations of global performance ratings. Acad Med 2015;90(4):404–7.
53. Hicks PJ, Margolis M, Poynter SE, et al. The pediatrics milestones assessment pilot: development of workplace-based assessment content, instruments, and processes. Acad Med 2016;91(5):701–9.
54. Turner TL, Bhavaraju VL, Luciw-Dubas UA, et al. Validity evidence from ratings of pediatric interns and subinterns on a subset of pediatric milestones. Acad Med 2017;92(6):809–19.
55. Wood L, Hassell A, Whitehouse A, et al. A literature review of multi-source feedback systems within and without health services, leading to 10 tips for their successful design. Med Teach 2006;28(7):e185–91.
56. Whitehouse A, Hassell A, Bullock A, et al. 360 degree assessment (multisource feedback) of UK trainee doctors: field testing of team assessment of behaviours (TAB). Med Teach 2007;29(2–3):171–6.
57. Archer JC, Norcini J, Davies HA. Use of SPRAT for peer review of paediatricians in training. BMJ 2005;330(7502):1251–3.
58. Norcini JJ. The Mini-CEX (clinical evaluation exercise): a preliminary investigation. Ann Intern Med 1995;123(10):795.
59. Kogan JR, Holmboe ES, Hauer KE. Tools for direct observation and assessment of clinical skills of medical trainees: a systematic review. JAMA 2009;302(12): 1316.
60. Holmboe ES, Hawkins RE, Huot SJ. Effects of training in direct observation of medical residents' clinical competence: a randomized trial. Ann Intern Med 2004;140(11):874.
61. Reddy ST, Endo J, Gupta S, et al. A case for caution: chart-stimulated recall. J Grad Med Educ 2015;7(4):531–5.
62. Sinnott C, Kelly MA, Bradley CP. A scoping review of the potential for chart stimulated recall as a clinical research method. BMC Health Serv Res 2017;17(1). https://doi.org/10.1186/s12913-017-2539-y.

Simulation in Medical Education for the Hospitalist

Moving Beyond the Mock Code

Jennifer H. Hepps, MD[a], Clifton E. Yu, MD[a],
Sharon Calaman, MD[b,*]

KEYWORDS

• Simulation • Debriefing • Interprofessional education • Procedural training
• Clinical reasoning • Patient safety • Just-in-time training • Role plays

KEY POINTS

- The need for simulation in inpatient education has intensified within the last decade because of decreased patient care exposure and increased health care system complexities.
- Simulation uses 4 main modalities: human patient simulators, task trainers, standardized patients, and virtual reality, to provide structured clinical experiences without endangering patients.
- As an educational strategy, simulation should fill a curriculum gap. Goals and objectives must be developed, and the simulation modality, location, and case flow chosen accordingly.
- The prebrief, brief, and debrief are phases that surround the actual simulation exercise and help to create a respectful and collaborative learning environment.
- Best practices for inpatient simulation can be found in the areas of communication skills, interprofessional education, clinical reasoning, procedural training, and patient safety surveillance.

SIMULATION OVERVIEW

Background and Definitions

Background

The widespread need for simulation in medical education, particularly in the inpatient setting, reflects the recognition that there is decreased time for training as well as

Disclosure Statement: Dr S. Calaman holds stock options and has done consulting work for the I-PASS Patient Safety Institute. The I-PASS Patient Safety Institute is a company that seeks to train institutions in best handoff practices and aid in their implementation.

[a] Department of Pediatrics, Walter Reed National Military Medical Center, Uniformed Services University of the Health Sciences, 8901 Wisconsin Avenue, Bethesda, MD 20889, USA; [b] St. Christopher's Hospital for Children, Drexel College of Medicine, 160 East Erie Avenue, Philadelphia, PA 19134, USA
* Corresponding author.
E-mail address: Sc493@drexel.edu

Pediatr Clin N Am 66 (2019) 855–866
https://doi.org/10.1016/j.pcl.2019.03.014
0031-3955/19/

decreased length of hospital stay, both of which lead to less exposure to clinical situations. In addition, there is increasing complexity in the health care system, with constantly evolving new technologies, which requires advanced training. Finally, the patient safety movement has highlighted that learners need more hands-on clinical skills practice and assessment, not just lectures and tests, to ensure professional competence.[1–4] Simulation allows exposure to different clinical scenarios in a structured fashion, without a patient at risk, to bridge some of these gaps.[4]

Modern day medical simulation began in the 1960s when Asmund S. Laerdal, a toy manufacturer, and Dr Peter Safar, a leader in the concept of cardiopulmonary resuscitation (CPR), developed the Resusci-Anne manikin to facilitate training in CPR.[1,5,6] During this time period, Dr Steven Abrahamson and his team developed the SimOne simulator, with simulated heart tones, pulse, and physiologic responses.[1,5] However, the technology was not well accepted until the 1980s, when several groups began to reexamine the concept of human patient simulators. At Stanford University, Dr David Gaba developed the Comprehensive Anesthesia Simulation Environment, and at the University of Florida, Drs Michael Good and J.S. Gravenstein developed the Gainesville anesthesia simulator. These products were commercialized and helped initiate the widespread use of human patient simulators.[1,5]

Simulation modalities

There are 4 main types of simulation modalities: human patient, task trainers, standardized patients (SPs), and virtual reality (**Table 1**).[2,4,7–9] Human patient simulators are whole body simulators with physiologic features, such as lung and heart sounds, chest rise, and seizure activity, which can be manipulated by computer. They have been referred to as both high technology and high fidelity; however, the former terminology is most appropriate. Task trainers, such as intubation heads or intravenous (IV) arms, are less costly than these high-technology simulators and allow repeated practice of a specific procedure until proficiency is attained. SPs are actors who have been trained to simulate actual patients and are used for teaching history and physical examination skills as well as communication skills.[4,8] Finally, virtual reality simulators are computer-based modules that create an immersive 3-dimensional environment, often using haptic devices, which provide tactile feedback to the user, such as the sensation of cutting tissue.[4,8] Hybrid simulation refers to applying 2 or more of these modalities, for example, simulating IV placement using a simulated patient and a task trainer IV arm.[8] All of these modalities exist on a spectrum from low fidelity to high fidelity. Fidelity reflects how closely the simulation replicates the actual event and includes physical fidelity (how the simulator replicates the body), environmental fidelity (how the

Table 1
Simulation modalities and uses

Modality	Possible Use in Inpatient Setting
Human patient simulator	Team training for a medical emergency like cardiac arrest
Task trainer	Demonstrating competency before performing an actual procedure, such as lumbar puncture
Simulated patient	Practicing difficult conversation skills like delivering bad news
Virtual reality simulator	Practicing pediatric resuscitation algorithms in a computer-based setting
Hybrid simulation	Practicing bag valve mask skills for apnea while talking to a simulated parent about what is happening to their infant

simulation environment mimics the clinical setting), and psychological fidelity (how the simulation evokes the same behaviors as the actual situation).[2,4,7–9]

Building a Simulation Exercise from Start to Finish

Educators often fall into the trap of being distracted by the technology that simulation has to offer, instead of focusing on how simulation can enhance the educational content. To be effective, simulation needs to be considered as an educational strategy within a larger curriculum.[2–4,10] In this section, the authors focus on how to develop the simulation exercise from identifying educational gaps (ie, performing a needs assessment), to articulating goals and objectives based on that assessment, to choosing a simulation modality that best addresses the goals and objectives, to designing the exercise itself, and finally to implementing the exercise and evaluating its effectiveness.

Considerations for goals and objectives

The first step in building a simulation exercise is to identify a gap in the broader curriculum, which can best be addressed by simulation. This gap could be in knowledge, skills, or attitudes; some examples of gaps and possible simulation applications are listed in **Table 2**. Once a gap is identified, the next step is to develop clear goals and objectives for the simulation exercise itself.[4,10]

Goals and objectives guide content development by ensuring that the exercise addresses the gap identified in the needs assessment as well as by guiding the choice of simulation modality. Too often this step is skipped or not recorded, which can lead to problems in simulation design and sustainability.[4,10] Goals provide the overarching vision for the exercise, and objectives are the means to achieve that goal, representing discretely measurable items. For example, a goal might be for interns to understand the management of a patient with apnea, whereas objectives could be to recognize apnea in a pediatric patient, to demonstrate bag-mask ventilation using the E-C technique, and to activate team members by calling for help. There are several considerations when developing simulation goals and objectives. First, the number of objectives has to be achievable within the timeframe of the exercise. Second, it is important to consider the balance of cognitive versus communication objectives. If the goal is to improve teamwork, the clinical complexity of the case may need to be minimized to best address the communication objectives. Finally, the objectives will vary according to the needs of the learner. For example, in managing a patient with apnea, the expectation for fellows may be to demonstrate the ability to intubate, whereas for the intern or medical student, it may be to recognize the apneic patient. This consideration is particularly relevant to interprofessional simulation, which is discussed later.

Table 2
Example of curricular gaps that simulation might address

Gap	Simulation Exercise
Recognizing clinical signs of possible complications of meningitis, such as increased intracranial pressure	Human patient simulator with a case of an infant with concern for meningitis who has vital sign changes and seizures
Managing the airway in a seizure patient	Human patient simulator case with an active seizure and vital sign changes
Appreciating the importance of the 2-challenge rule in preventing error	Simulated participant case or a role play of a medical error

Design considerations

There are several templates available to help structure the design of a simulation experience.[9,11–13] The 3 most critical elements reflected in simulation templates are knowing "who will be trained, what they must learn, and how it will be learned."[12] In this section, the authors discuss considerations for "how it will be learned," to include determining the simulation modality, establishing the simulation environment, and scripting the evolution of the clinical scenario.

Once goals and objectives are established, the most appropriate simulation modality must be chosen. For example, if in the apnea case an important objective is to communicate the change in status to the parent, then a simulated parent will be more important than a high-technology simulator. On the other hand, if the main objective is to recognize the progression of vital signs toward apnea and to demonstrate intubation, then a high-technology simulator might be critical. In addition to simulation modality, the location of the exercise must be chosen based on the objectives. If one of the objectives is to identify whether the right equipment is available in a unit, then an in situ simulation is essential. On the other hand, if the focus is on technical skills, an off-site location may be more appropriate.

The next design step is to think through the flow of the simulated exercise by determining the initial clinical state of the patient as well as the circumstances that bring the participants to the scenario (eg, an alarm sounding, a routine admission, a nurse calling for help). Then, one must determine how the patient will improve or deteriorate as a result of learner actions. The learning objectives will dictate the desired actions that result in a positive change in the simulator (eg, initiating bag mask ventilation in an apneic patient). There are also potentially unexpected actions that will result in a negative change in the simulator (eg, applying oxygen to the apneic patient without ventilation). An important element of scenario design is determining how to redirect learners when something unexpected happens. These strategies are referred to as scenario "lifesavers"[14] and include changing vital signs or having a simulated participant offer suggestions.[11,14] Both expected and unexpected actions represent learning opportunities to be explored during the postexercise debrief.

Implementation: stages of a scenario, facilitation, and debriefing strategies

A simulation exercise is often divided into 4 parts: the prebrief, the brief, the exercise, and the debrief.[8,10] In each part, the facilitator is responsible for creating a respectful and collaborative environment, which promotes the experiential learning essential for simulation. In this section, the authors discuss each stage of the simulation exercise.

Prebrief and brief The prebrief establishes a "safe container" for exploring together, where learners are able to "practice at the edge of their ability" and take risks without feeling embarrassed.[4,15] An effective prebrief will include the following steps: (1) An orientation to the environment, the simulator, and the logistics of the day; (2) The expectations of learners, including confidentiality, as well as the type of evaluation (ie, formative or summative); and (3) The establishment of the fiction contract, that is, asking learners to behave as if it is a real environment to maximize learning.[15,16] The prebrief emphasizes what has been referred to as the "the basic assumption," the idea that all participants are well trained, well educated, and motivated to do their best and learn from mistakes.[15,17]

Although the prebrief outlines the overarching goals and objectives of the simulation experience, the brief addresses the specific details of the simulated case. The brief introduces learners to the patient background and initial state, through verbal instruction from the facilitator or visual aids like the patient chart.[8]

Simulation exercise After the brief, the simulation exercise begins. The facilitator observes the actions of the participants, identifying areas for exploration during the debrief.[9] The facilitator also monitors the case flow, noting when the case is diverting from its intended objectives and providing scenario "lifesavers."[14] As previously discussed, "lifesavers" may be embedded into the scenario as vital sign changes or a simulated participant verbalization, or they may need to be developed spontaneously. The former strategy is more effective, because it promotes the fiction contract (eg, having a simulated nurse say "I don't think the baby is breathing," rather than the facilitator simply describing the patient state).

Debrief The final stage, the debrief, is generally identified as the most valuable component of the exercise.[10,11,18–21] It allows learners to reflect on what has happened and to make sense of the experience, independently and as a group.[4,9,17,18,22] This opportunity for both self-analysis and group discussion is a unique strength of simulation as an educational strategy.[4,9] Debriefing challenges the instructor to facilitate a conversation focused on the intended learning objectives as well as unexpected learning opportunities that may have arisen.[9,11,17,18] There are multiple published frameworks and techniques for debriefing.[9,19,21,23–25] These frameworks generally include 3 or more phases, with some overlap in the literature.[20] The authors focus on 4 phases of debriefing: (1) Reactions, (2) Description with a brief summary of facts, (3) Analysis, and (4) Summary.[10,17,19–21]

The reactions phase is a chance for participants to air their emotional responses to the case. It is also a chance for the debriefer to use these emotional reactions to guide further discussion (eg, Are the learners angry? Are they satisfied or dissatisfied about a performance and why?). It is important for the debriefer to be flexible, because the planned agenda may not contain the most valuable lessons. Not allowing participants to express their initial feelings can serve as a barrier to subsequent phases. Recall that critical to an effective debrief is an environment where participants are comfortable sharing their reflections; without a reactions phase, emotions may be too intense for this to occur.[17,18,21,26]

The next phase is a brief summary of the facts of the case, generated by the participants with the support of the debriefer. This few-sentence summary is essential, because it ensures a shared understanding before progressing to the analysis phase.[9,20,21,26] Without a shared mental model, the analysis may be derailed by lingering questions or misunderstanding about the medical details of the case.

The analysis phase is generally the longest portion, where the debriefer explores the actions observed during the simulation. There are many different methods for conducting this phase, and the choice depends on factors such as time, debriefer expertise, and types of observations made.[9,10,21,23,25,26] "Advocacy and inquiry" is a questioning technique that is part of the "debriefing with good judgment" framework. It involves sharing an observation (eg, I noticed that you did compressions at a rate of 15:2), explaining what the debriefer is concerned about (eg, I am concerned because the guidelines say for a single rescuer you should do compressions at 30:2), and inquiring about the learners' frames (eg, Tell me about that?).[19,21,26,27] The "advocacy and inquiry" technique is useful when one is truly not sure why a learner did what was observed (eg, Did they not know the ratio? Did they think someone else was helping?).[19,26] An alternate technique is "plus delta," or learner-facilitated discussion. The debriefer asks the learner what they thought went well and then asks what they would have changed. The "plus delta" technique can be helpful in a more time-limited situation and requires less training.[10,21,26]

The final stage of the debrief is the summary phase, whereby learners are encouraged to express take-away points. It is important to check for final questions and understanding to allow the debrief to conclude after the summary phase.[9,21,26]

BEST PRACTICES FOR IMPLEMENTATION

In the next section, the authors discuss the application of simulation to the following curricular needs for the inpatient hospitalist: communication skills, interprofessional education (IPE), clinical reasoning, procedural training, and patient safety.

Communication Skills

Simulation techniques to teach communication skills

Simulation is a highly effective strategy to teach communication skills through the use of simulated patients, role plays, and trigger videos. SPs are lay people trained to realistically portray a patient in order to teach and evaluate learners.[28] Performance may be standardized for the purposes of assessment, for example, in Observed Structured Clinical Exams, or may be more improvisational, where the actor receives a basic description of the case instead of a script. SPs are a valuable educational resource, but require substantial resources in recruiting and training.

In contrast, role plays are less costly than SPs and in some studies have been found to be just as effective.[29,30] Role plays promote skill acquisition by allowing learners to experience a situation from a different viewpoint and to demonstrate expertise.[31,32] Role plays need to be carefully scripted so that participants are oriented to their roles and expectations. Similarly, the facilitator must craft a learning environment where participants feel comfortable and where there is sufficient time for debriefing afterward.[31,32]

Trigger videos are another technique for teaching communication skills, in addition to professionalism, diagnostic decision making, and ethics.[33–36] Trigger videos are brief vignettes based on a simple case, intended to provoke discussion. The facilitator must orient the learners to the case and then facilitate the discussion using the debriefing techniques described earlier.[33]

In the authors' experience, they used both role plays and trigger videos to teach handoff skills in the I-PASS study.[37,38] They used trigger videos to stimulate discussion about ideal versus nonideal handoff practices as well as team communication techniques, and then the learners practiced these skills through a series of role plays. In addition, the authors developed trigger videos to train faculty on handoff assessment using a validated observation tool, a skill they later practiced during the role plays and translated to actual handoff observations on their inpatient units.[39]

Interprofessional Education

Utility and definitions

As opposed to the traditional educational model whereby practitioners learn primarily within their disciplines, IPE allows different types of professionals to learn together in teams and to effectively collaborate, much as they are expected to do in real-life clinical situations.[40–42] In Jennifer Baird and colleagues' article, "Interprofessional Teams: Current Trends and Future Directions," in this issue, a variety of evidence-based models were introduced to conduct IPE. Here, the authors focus on simulation a way to re-create a team-based environment for the purposes of IPE.

Educators are often unclear as to what defines an IPE exercise. Hammick and colleagues[41] define IPE as "those occasions when members (or students) of two or more professions learn with, from and about one another to improve collaboration and the quality of care." Critical to this definition is the concept that professions are learning actively from each other, as opposed to a multiprofessional exercise where participants from multiple professions are learning side by side.[42] For example, an exercise designed for residents, in which a nurse is invited to play the nurse role, is not interprofessional unless he or she is also expected to achieve specific goals and objectives.

Key design and facilitation strategies

Like any simulation exercise, the first design step requires identifying the key stakeholders and understanding how the exercise fits into the broader curriculum.[40,41] Ideally, content experts from each of the clinical areas should be actively involved in developing learning objectives relevant for each provider.[40] Authenticity is critical in an IPE simulation.[41] Numbers and types of participants should reflect the actual clinical environment, but should also allow for balance (eg, no specialty or provider group should have priority in case design; no provider should only be in an observer role). To achieve both aims, the scenario may need to be adjusted for complexity or length to allow *all* participants to perform in their roles. For example, if 1 goal is to highlight the role of the respiratory therapist within a rapid response team, then the scenario must include airway issues for the team to address.

IPE simulations use more resources than a traditional simulation, so they should be used for topics best learned interactively with other professions.[40] For example, an exercise focused on the skill of bag mask ventilation for apnea would not necessarily need to be done as an IPE. However, if the objectives are to demonstrate teamwork in responding to a patient with apnea (eg, managing resources, delegating roles, and communicating with the team), an IPE may be highly appropriate.

Benefits and challenges of implementing interprofessional education in the inpatient setting

Jennifer Baird and colleagues' article, "Interprofessional Teams: Current Trends and Future Directions," in this issue discusses the challenges of IPE, such as trying to accommodate scheduling issues, ever-changing team compositions, and the tendency to default to multiprofessional, rather than interprofessional, teams. In addition, for interprofessional simulations specifically, facilitating and debriefing can be more challenging because of both real and perceived hierarchical relationships among team members, which make it harder to achieve the "safe container."[4,15,40] One approach to minimizing this problem is to have co-debriefers representing the different types of providers.

Despite the logistical challenges of IPE simulations, studies are beginning to demonstrate the positive impact on outcomes when teams train together. In obstetrics, for example, IPE interventions have increased Apgar scores and decreased the incidence of hypoxic ischemic encephalopathy.[43] In trauma, IPE simulation exercises have impacted times to task completion and mortality.[44,45] Finally, in pediatrics, a small study suggested that team training with mock codes potentially decreased mortality.[46] These studies support the benefits of implementing IPE training in the inpatient setting to improve communication and patient care.

Clinical Reasoning Skills

Simulation can also be a powerful tool for teaching clinical reasoning skills essential to the inpatient setting. For example, programs have been developed to improve recognition of the deteriorating patient in multiple disciplines and among multiple learner levels.[47–51] In addition, simulation has been used to teach clinical reasoning in the "first 5 minutes" of a code, encompassing multiple scenarios ranging from respiratory distress to full cardiac arrest.[52]

Although these curricula have been effective, they can be time intensive for a hospitalist educator to integrate into the daily flow of an inpatient unit. Alternative models that may be more educationally feasible include just-in-time mock codes. One model uses 1 to 2 mock codes per month conducted by chief residents, drawing from a real patient case and integrating the patient's nurse plus the full code team.[53] Similar curricula have focused on the recognition of the deteriorating patient and the implementation of contingency plans, which have been folded into monthly exercises for the inpatient team based on their real patients.[54]

Procedural Training: Beyond See One Do One Teach One

Simulation plays an important role in preparing inpatient providers to perform procedures, moving beyond the paradigm of "see one, do one, teach one." Task trainers allow deliberate practice of a procedure coupled with focused feedback until the skill is done successfully.[4,55] Like any simulation exercise, procedural training requires clear learning objectives that are measurable. A meta-analysis by McGaghie and colleagues,[55] although limited by a small number of articles, showed that deliberate practice with simulation was more effective at teaching procedures than traditional medical education techniques. As an extension of deliberate practice, *mastery learning* progresses from a baseline assessment, to standardized instruction and deliberate practice with coaching, to demonstrated independent practice using an assessment tool.[4,55,56]

Just-in-time and just-in-place training have also been used to allow real-time refresher training for procedural skills, such as central venous catheter care, CPR, and pediatric lumbar puncture.[57–59] For pediatric lumbar puncture, Kessler and colleagues[57] developed a program using mastery learning for initial training, followed by just-in-time refreshers before a procedure. Although this program did not impact overall success, it resulted in better trainee adherence to the procedural steps and fewer required lumbar puncture attempts.[57] In the Emergency Department, Thomas and colleagues[60] developed a just-in-time procedure training room for sutures, lumbar puncture, and splinting with 24-hour access. Trainee and supervisor confidence was increased for these procedures, with less need for intervention reported by supervisors. Such a resource could be readily adapted for use in the inpatient setting as well.

The Role of Simulation in Identifying Latent Safety Threats

Simulation can be used not only for educational purposes but also as a way to identify latent safety threats, similar to crash testing. Simulation for patient safety is typically conducted in situ, because although an offsite exercise may identify knowledge gaps or issues in team performance, it may not reveal vulnerabilities in the system itself.[61] With this concept in mind, in situ simulation has been used as a way to evaluate new hospital spaces, where multiple latent safety threats, from lack of crash carts and defibrillators to inadequate oxygen flow, code alarms, and phone locations, have been found.[62–65]

In addition to evaluating new clinical spaces, in situ simulations have been used during the actual work day.[61,66] Threats, such as missing equipment, medications not being available, and lack of clear labeling of equipment, were revealed.[61,66] In situ, real-time simulations have the benefit of using the actual care team in their environment to identify systems issues and latent safety threats. However, these simulations can often be logistically challenging to implement, because staff are balancing clinical responsibilities and may have limited time to participate. Working with the leadership of units is crucial to generate buy-in and to plan productive sessions.

SUMMARY

The use of simulation in inpatient medical education has grown over the last few decades based on an evolution in health care and training, which has led to decreased learner exposure to clinical situations, increased medical and technological complexity, and enhanced focus on patient safety vulnerabilities. As a result of these trends, educators have been tasked to build learner knowledge, skills, and attitudes through experiential learning with the goal of improving patient care.

Using simulation in the inpatient unit requires first considering the broader goals and objectives of the curriculum and determining if simulation best meets these educational needs. If so, the simulation exercise can be designed with thoughtful selection of the simulation modality (ie, human patient simulators, task trainers, SPs, or virtual reality simulators), location, and case flow, to include "lifesavers" if learners need redirection. Once the "script" is written, the exercise is primed for implementation, which includes the 4 phases of prebrief, brief, exercise, and debrief. The authors emphasized that the debrief, which also generally includes 4 phases (reactions, summary of facts, analysis, and summary), is where the learning happens, as long as there is opportunity for both self and group reflection.

Given the imperative to provide learners with realistic clinical training without jeopardizing patient safety, hospitalists have developed novel applications of simulation to meet inpatient learning requirements. The use of simulation in teaching communication skills, interprofessional team dynamics, clinical reasoning, and procedural competencies, as well as for identifying latent patient safety threats, has been discussed. For many of these applications, there are multiple training options: for example, longitudinal or "just-in-time," intradisciplinary or interprofessional, deliberate practice or mastery learning, and off-site or in situ. As the complexity of inpatient care continues to increase, and processes to improve patient safety become more urgent, simulation needs to be considered an essential element of the inpatient educator's toolbox.

REFERENCES

1. Bradley P. The history of simulation in medical education and possible future directions. Med Educ 2006;40:254–62.
2. Clerihew L, Rowney D, Ker J. Simulation in paediatric training. Arch Dis Child Educ Pract Ed 2016;101(1):8–14.
3. Issenberg SB, McGaghie WC, Petrusa ER, et al. Features and uses of high-fidelity medical simulations that lead to effective learning: a BEME systematic review. Med Teach 2005;27(1):10–28.
4. Lopreiato JO, Sawyer T. Simulation-based medical education in pediatrics. Acad Pediatr 2015;15(2):134–42.
5. Cooper JB, Taqueti VR. A brief history of the development of mannequin simulators for clinical education and training. Qual Saf Health Care 2004;13:i11–8.
6. Tjomsland N, Baskett P. The resuscitation greats: Asmund S. Laerdal. Resuscitation 2002;53:115–9.
7. Dieckmann P, Gaba D, Rall M. Deepening the theoretical foundations of patient simulation as social practice. Simul Healthc 2007;2(3):183–93.
8. In: Lopreiato JOE, Downing D, Gammon W, and the Terminology & Concepts Working Group, et al, editors. Healthcare simulation dictionary. In. Available at: http://www.ssih.org/dictionary.2016. Accessed June 10, 2018.
9. Rall M, Gaba DM, Dieckmann P, et al. Patient simulation. In: Miller RD, Eriksson LI, Fleisher LA, et al, editors. Miller's anesthesia. 8th edition. Philadelphia: Elsevier/Saunders; 2015. p. 167–209.

10. Motola I, Devine LA, Chung HS, et al. Simulation in healthcare education: a best evidence practical guide. AMEE Guide No. 82. Med Teach 2013;35(10): e1511–30.
11. Alinier G. Developing high-fidelity health care simulation scenarios: a guide for educators and professionals. Simul Gaming 2010;42(1):9–26.
12. Benishek LE, Lazarra EH, Gaught WL, et al. The template of events for applied and critical healthcare simulation (TEACH Sim) a tool for systematic simulation scenario design. Simul Healthc 2015;10:21–30.
13. Seropian MA. General concepts in full scale simulation: getting started. Anesth Analg 2003;97(6):1695–705.
14. Dieckmann P, Lippert A, Glavin R, et al. When things do not go as expected: scenario life savers. Simul Healthc 2010;5:219–25.
15. Rudolph JW, Raemer DB, Simon R. Establishing a safe container for learning in simulation: the role of the presimulation briefing. Simul Healthc 2014;9(6):339–49.
16. Simon R, RD, Rudolph J. Debriefing assessment for simulation in healthcare (DASH) Rater's handbook 2009. Available at: https://harvardmedsim.org/wp-content/uploads/2017/01/DASH.handbook.2010.Final.Rev.2.pdf. Accessed March 14, 2018.
17. Gardner R. Introduction to debriefing. Semin Perinatol 2013;37(3):166–74.
18. Fanning RG, Gaba DM. The role of debriefing in simulation-based learning. Simul Healthc 2007;2(2):115–25.
19. Rudolph JS, Simon R, Dufresne RL, et al. There's no such thing as "nonjudgmental" debriefing: a theory and method for debriefing with good judgment. Simul Healthc 2006;1:49–55.
20. Sawyer T, Eppich W, Brett-Fleegler M, et al. More than one way to debrief: a critical review of healthcare simulation debriefing methods. Simul Healthc 2016; 11(3):209–17.
21. Eppich W, Cheng A. Promoting excellence and reflective learning in simulation (PEARLS): development and rationale for a blended approach to health care simulation debriefing. Simul Healthc 2015;10(2):106–15.
22. Savoldelli GL, Naik VN, Park J, et al. Value of debriefing during simulated crisis management. Anesthesiology 2006;105:279–85.
23. Zigmont JJ, Kappus LJ, Sudikoff SN. The 3D model of debriefing: defusing, discovering, and deepening. Semin Perinatol 2011;35(2):52–8.
24. Jaye P, Thomas L, Reedy G. 'The Diamond': a structure for simulation debrief. Clin Teach 2015;12(3):171–5.
25. Phrampus P, O'Donnell J. Debriefing using a structured and supported approach. In: Levine A, DeMaria S, Schwartz A, et al, editors. The comprehensive textbook of healthcare simulation. New York: Springer; 2013. p. 73–84.
26. Cheng A, Grant V, Robinson T, et al. The promoting excellence and reflective learning in simulation (PEARLS) approach to health care debriefing: a faculty development guide. Clinical Simulation in Nursing 2016;12(10):419–28.
27. Rudolph JW, Simon R, Rivard P, et al. Debriefing with good judgment: combining rigorous feedback with genuine inquiry. Anesthesiol Clin 2007;25(2):361–76.
28. Cleland JA, Abe K, Rethans JJ. The use of simulated patients in medical education: AMEE Guide No 42. Med Teach 2009;31(6):477–86.
29. Bosse HM, Nickel M, Huwendiek S, et al. Peer role-play and standardised patients in communication training: a comparative study on the student perspective on acceptability, realism, and perceived effect. BMC Med Educ 2010;10:27.
30. Nestel D, Tierney T. Role-play for medical students learning about communication: guidelines for maximising benefits. BMC Med Educ 2007;7:3.

31. Joyner B, Young L. Teaching medical students using role play: twelve tips for successful role plays. Med Teach 2006;28(3):225–9.
32. Steihert Y. Twelve tips for using role-plays in clinical teaching. Med Teach 1993; 15(4):1993.
33. Ber R, Alroy G. Twenty years of experience using trigger films as a teaching tool. Acad Med 2001;76:656–8.
34. Ber R, Alroy G. Teaching professionalism with the aid of trigger films. Med Teach 2002;24(5):528–31.
35. Alroy G, Ber R. Doctor-patient relationship and the medical student - the use of trigger films. J Med Educ 1982;57:334–6.
36. Losh DP, Mauksch LB, Arnold RW, et al. Teaching inpatient communication skills to medical students: an innovative strategy. Acad Med 2005;80:118–24.
37. Spector N, Starner A, Allen A, et al. I-PASS handoff curriculum: core resident workshop. MedEdPORTAL 2013;9:9311.
38. Calaman S, Hepps J, Spector N, et al. I-PASS handoff curriculum: handoff simulation exercises. MedEdPORTAL 2013;9:9402.
39. Starmer AJ, O'Toole JK, Rosenbluth G, et al. Development, implementation, and dissemination of the I-PASS handoff curriculum: a multisite educational intervention to improve patient handoffs. Acad Med 2014;89(6):876–84.
40. Boet S, Bould MD, Layat Burn C, et al. Twelve tips for a successful interprofessional team-based high-fidelity simulation education session. Med Teach 2014; 36(10):853–7.
41. Hammick M, Freeth D, Koppel I, et al. A best evidence systematic review of interprofessional education: BEME Guide no. 9. Med Teach 2007;29(8):735–51.
42. Hammick M, Olckers L, Campion-Smith C. Learning in interprofessional teams: AMEE Guide no 38. Med Teach 2009;31(1):1–12.
43. Draycott T, Sibanda T, Owen L, et al. Does training in obstetric emergencies improve neonatal outcome? BJOG 2006;113(2):177–82.
44. Capella J, Smith S, Philp A, et al. Teamwork training improves the clinical care of trauma patients. J Surg Educ 2010;67(6):439–43.
45. Steinemann S, Berg B, Skinner A, et al. In situ, multidisciplinary, simulation-based teamwork training improves early trauma care. J Surg Educ 2011;68(6):472–7.
46. Andreatta P, Saxton E, Thompson M, et al. Simulation-based mock codes significantly correlate with improved pediatric patient cardiopulmonary arrest survival rates. Pediatr Crit Care Med 2011;12(1):33–8.
47. Theilen U, Leonard P, Jones P, et al. Regular in situ simulation training of paediatric medical emergency team improves hospital response to deteriorating patients. Resuscitation 2013;84(2):218–22.
48. Odell M. Detection and management of the deteriorating ward patient: an evaluation of nursing practice. J Clin Nurs 2015;24(1–2):173–82.
49. Hogg G, Miller D. The effects of an enhanced simulation programme on medical students' confidence responding to clinical deterioration. BMC Med Educ 2016; 16:161.
50. Connell CJ, Endacott R, Jackman JA, et al. The effectiveness of education in the recognition and management of deteriorating patients: a systematic review. Nurse Educ Today 2016;44:133–45.
51. O'Leary J, Nash R, Lewis P. Standard instruction versus simulation: educating registered nurses in the early recognition of patient deterioration in paediatric critical care. Nurse Educ Today 2016;36:287–92.

52. Hunt EA, Walker AR, Shaffner DH, et al. Simulation of in-hospital pediatric medical emergencies and cardiopulmonary arrests: highlighting the importance of the first 5 minutes. Pediatrics 2008;121(1):e34–43.
53. Sam J, Pierse M, Al-Qahtani A, et al. Implementation and evaluation of a simulation curriculum for paediatric residency programs including just-in-time in situ mock codes. Paediatr Child Health 2012;17(2):e16–20.
54. Wheaton T, Topiol E, Dickinson B, et al. Implementation of a just-in-time simulation curriculum aimed at improving care of "watchers". Crit Care Med 2016;44(12):182.
55. McGaghie WC, Issenberg SB, Cohen ER, et al. Does simulation-based medical education with deliberate practice yield better results than traditional clinical education? A meta-analytic comparative review of the evidence. Acad Med 2011;86(6):706–11.
56. McGaghie WC, Issenberg SB, Barsuk JH, et al. A critical review of simulation-based mastery learning with translational outcomes. Med Educ 2014;48(4):375–85.
57. Kessler D, Pusic M, Chang TP, et al. Impact of just-in-time and just-in-place simulation on intern success with infant lumbar puncture. Pediatrics 2015;135(5):e1237–46.
58. Lengetti E, Monachino AM, Scholtz A. A simulation-based "just in time" and "just in place" central venous catheter education program. J Nurses Staff Dev 2011;27(6):290–3.
59. Niles D, Sutton RM, Donoghue A, et al. "Rolling Refreshers": a novel approach to maintain CPR psychomotor skill competence. Resuscitation 2009;80(8):909–12.
60. Thomas AA, Uspal NG, Oron AP, et al. Perceptions on the impact of a just-in-time room on trainees and supervising physicians in a pediatric emergency department. J Grad Med Educ 2016;8(5):754–8.
61. Knight P, MacGloin H, Lane M, et al. Mitigating latent threats identified through an embedded in situ simulation program and their comparison to patient safety incidents: a retrospective review. Front Pediatr 2017;5:281.
62. Geis GL, Pio B, Pendergrass TL, et al. Simulation to assess the safety of new healthcare teams and new facilities. Simul Healthc 2011;6(3):125–33.
63. Villamaria FJ, Pliego JF, Wehbe-Janek H, et al. Using simulation to orient code blue teams to a new hospital facility. Simul Healthc 2008;3(4):209–16.
64. Kobayashi L, Shapiro MJ, Sucov A, et al. Portable advanced medical simulation for new emergency department testing and orientation. Acad Emerg Med 2006;13(6):691–5.
65. Adler MA, Mobley BL, Eppich WJ, et al. Use of simulation to test systems and prepare staff for a new hospital transition. J Patient Saf 2018;14(3):143–7.
66. Patterson MD, Blike GT, Nadkarni VM. Advances in patient safety in situ simulation: challenges and results. In: Henriksen K, Battles JB, Keyes MA, et al, editors. Advances in patient safety: new directions and alternative approaches, vol. 3. Rockville (MD): Agency for Healthcare Research and Quality (US); 2008. Performance and Tools. p. 1–18.

A Focus on Feedback

Improving Learner Engagement and Faculty Delivery of Feedback in Hospital Medicine

Kheyandra D. Lewis, MD[a,*,1,2], Aarti Patel, MD, MEd[b,1,2], Joseph O. Lopreiato, MD, MPH, CHSE[c]

KEYWORDS

• Feedback • Medical education • Hospital medicine • Teacher • Learner • Performance improvement • Direct observation • Self-assessment

KEY POINTS

- Feedback is a crucial aspect of medical education that involves communication between a teacher and a learner to improve performance.
- The inpatient setting allows hospitalists to directly observe learner performance during and outside of family-centered rounds.
- Various feedback models can be used to communicate learner strengths and areas of improvement, depending on what works best for each situation.
- Important characteristics for any feedback encounter include self-assessment, specificity, timeliness, privacy, bidirectional communication, and learner centeredness.
- Feedback should end with a learner-initiated plan of action for performance improvement.

INTRODUCTION

Feedback is the dynamic delivery of communication to a learner to improve or modify previous performance.[1,2] It is an integral aspect of medical education, providing insight for a learner's acquisition of clinical skills and knowledge.[1] Defining and providing feedback is met with several challenges, particularly in a demanding clinical environment such as hospital medicine. However, when embraced by both the learner

Disclosures: The authors have no conflicts of interest to disclose.
[a] Section of Hospital Medicine, St. Christopher's Hospital for Children, Drexel University College of Medicine, 160 East Erie Avenue, Philadelphia, PA 19134, USA; [b] Division of Pediatric Hospital Medicine, Rady Children's Hospital, University of California San Diego, 3020 Children's Way, MC 5064, San Diego, CA 92123, USA; [c] Medicine and Nursing, Uniformed Services University of the Health Sciences, 4301 Jones Bridge Road, Bethesda, MD 20814, USA
[1] Drs K.D. Lewis and A. Patel contributed equally to this article.
[2] Co-first authors.
* Corresponding author.
E-mail address: kdl62@drexel.edu

Pediatr Clin N Am 66 (2019) 867–880
https://doi.org/10.1016/j.pcl.2019.03.011

and teacher, and viewed as a teaching tool—not simply commentary, its influence can be greatly impactful in developing mastery of clinical practice. In hospital medicine, the longitudinal nature of teacher and learner interaction offers ample opportunity to provide feedback on several observable daily tasks and procedures, as well as patient, interprofessional, and peer interactions.

IMPORTANCE OF FEEDBACK AND IMPROVING LEARNER ENGAGEMENT

What Can Go Wrong If It Is Not Done or Done Badly?

Without feedback, an emphasis on ideal performance is not nurtured, and suboptimal performance is not rectified.[3] The omission of feedback may not equate to good performance. When teachers fail to give feedback, the guidance toward improvement is lost.[2] Learners may seek input from unreliable sources, or worse yet, falsely assume they are performing well.[3] The literature has previously shown that physician learners often hold inaccurate self-assessments and frequently overestimate their own capabilities.[4] Withholding feedback is a disservice to the learner as well as the patients they care for.

Feedback, when delivered, should be revisited on more than one occasion (**Table 1**). Once an action plan to improve performance has been established, teachers must ensure they reobserve the behavior to help navigate the learner to proficiency.

Barriers to Giving Feedback

Teachers miss opportunities to provide feedback to learners owing to time and place constraints, as well as competing patient care priorities. However, more frequently, teachers avoid giving feedback because they may lack formal training or feel uncomfortable, particularly if the feedback is negative.[1] If negative feedback is delivered without concrete examples of a learner's performance, it can be perceived as a judgmental critique. The careless delivery of negative feedback could discourage a learner or cause a deterioration of their performance.[3,5] In addition, teachers often fear fracturing the educational relationship.[3,6]

Building a Teacher–Learner Alliance

It is important for learners to feel equipped to receive and respond to feedback.[6] This foundation begins with trust, much like the trust built between an athlete and a coach, and is designed from the beginning to help the learner to improve their performance. The team dynamic inherent to hospital medicine lends itself well to establishing a safe learning environment where teachers and learners can work as allies. This team connection promotes and builds dialogue where feedback can be reciprocated between teacher and learner. When a teacher role models welcomed receipt of feedback

Table 1
Characteristics of feedback

Effective Feedback	Ineffective Feedback
Specific	Not based on first-hand data
Learner centered	Judgmental
Private	Public
Timely and periodic	Given once
Goal oriented	Punitive

from their learner, rapport between this partnership increases.[3] This modeling exemplifies to the learner that the attending physician is also a lifelong learner and continually working on self-improvement. Alternatively, learners who fail to identify receipt of feedback or dismiss feedback have more often received feedback from a teacher with whom they lack a connection.[6]

Ensuring Feedback Is Meaningful and Timely

Teachers should aim to help learners recognize that the feedback focus is on the action that can be improved or changed.[6] The incorporation of active reflection provides an avenue for personal growth, whereas feedback alone promotes proficiency.[7] Furthermore, the timing of feedback is critical, because it has independent influence over the efficacy of feedback.[5]

DEFINITIONS

Feedback versus Evaluation

It is important to clearly distinguish feedback from evaluation, because they provide different information to a learner, although they often overlap in content.[7] Evaluation is a method of summative assessment that measures the achievement or competence of an individual either through formal knowledge-based testing or observation of skills demonstration (Please see Duncan Henry and Daniel C. West's article, "The Clinical Learning Environment and Workplace-based Assessment: Frameworks, Strategies, and Implementation," in this issue for further information of assessment). Feedback searches for the learner's understanding of the problem, provides strategies to remedy it, and is followed by an action plan.[5,7] Evaluation is then used to assess if a learner was able to correct the issue.

Facilitative versus Directive Feedback

Directive feedback simply instructs the learner on actions to be corrected.[5] The teacher does not seek out the learner's perspective or interpretation.[8] Facilitative feedback provides suggestions to help the learner in their own revision through the exploration of what went well and what performance areas need improvement.[5]

Just-in-Time Feedback

Also known as "on-the-job" or "brief" feedback, just-in-time feedback is specific to a certain behavior followed by a plan for improvement in the future.[3] It can be used when demonstrating the correct way to perform a physical examination, procedural skill, or reporting on a patient. The impact of just-in-time feedback is that it forces the teacher to develop meaningful and concrete suggestions in the moment and not delay feedback until a later time and place.[7] A strategic way to ensure a learner is aware that just-in-time feedback is occurring is to preface the suggestion with, "Let me give you some quick feedback."[7]

Formative versus Summative Assessment

The terms formative and summative assessment are often confused and happen contemporaneously in medical education. Formative assessment or feedback is designed to observe and comment on performance, with the goal of helping the learner to improve. It is not meant as a final judgment or grade. Summative assessment is a judgment about performance after a period of observations that usually occurs at the end of a learning experience (please see Duncan Henry and Daniel C. West's article, "The Clinical Learning Environment and Workplace-based Assessment: Frameworks, Strategies, and Implementation," in this issue for more information regarding workplace-based assessment). Further, when feedback is obtained from multiple sources, it can help to give the learner a holistic summation of their observed performance; multisource feedback from interdisciplinary team members can share perspectives not typically realized. Formative assessment can occur at any time, but summative assessment is set with a distinct time and place agreed upon by both the teacher and the learner.[5,7] Often, formative assessment and summative assessment are delivered at the same time or at a later date, and this strategy does not allow the learner interval time to demonstrate their ability to improve. Ideally, there have been several instances of formative assessment (feedback) before a summative assessment is rendered. This process requires the teacher to set the expectation that, in the clinical environment, frequent feedback will be given, and that the learner will have the opportunity to self-reflect and improve before the summative assessment. Feedback should be interactive and initiated with the learner's self-reflection: "How did that case go for you?"[7]

THEORETIC FRAMEWORK FOR FEEDBACK

To understand feedback, there are 3 main learning theories that are relevant and used in medical education (**Fig. 1**). Feedback is a key feature in self-regulated learning theory. This theory posits that learning occurs when learners set goals, choose learning strategies, monitor their progress, and adjust their goals and strategies.[9] Feedback in a self-regulated learner is designed to assist in the process of learner goal setting, choosing learning strategies, and monitoring. Effective feedback should promote learning and serve as a catalyst for self-regulated learning activities.[10] Self-regulated learning theory also predicts that learners use feedback to compare their performances with their internal learning goals. Students benefit most when they understand the standard for which to aim, the difference between their performance and the ideal, and how to bridge the divide.[10] External feedback from teachers and peers influences how learners feel about themselves and what they can learn.[11] Cultivating learners who possess feedback-seeking behavior increases likelihood of success for the desired learning goal.[12]

Feedback in education is also a feature of the social constructivism view of learning. In this theory, learning is an active process by which the learner brings their own prior knowledge and experience to a learning situation. Feedback to learners from teachers, peers, examinations, and patient experiences (the social aspect) are integrated by learners to

Self-regulated Theory	Social Constructivist Theory	Cognitive Theory
• Learning occurs when learners set their own goals, choose strategies, monitor their progress, and adjust based on feedback • Helps them to understand the difference between their performance and the expected standard	• Feedback from various sources, including teachers, peers, examinations, and experiences, are integrated by the learner to make connections and construct knowledge • Learn by doing rather than observing	• Reframing prior knowledge with guidance from teachers on incorporation of new knowledge allows for learners to improve their performance • Feedback can occur through facilitation by teachers in identifying learning goals and coaching learner self-assessment

Fig. 1. Theory basis of feedback.

construct meaning and make connections.[10] This new knowledge can influence future behavior and decisions. A lack of feedback will only reinforce previous behaviors.

The importance of reframing knowledge is central to the cognitive theory of feedback, where guidance from teachers can help to understand new information, adjust performance, and be more engaged in learning in the future.[3] The key is performing ongoing feedback to regular intervals to improve clinical performance. This can be done through facilitation of learner self-reflection, coaching, and assistance in identification of educational goals.[13] Through these informed self-assessments, the student can then work toward behavior modification.

SETTING THE STAGE WITH STRATEGIES THAT WORK IN HOSPITAL MEDICINE

Ongoing Nature

Improvement is not limited to a fixed endpoint; the continuous development of expertise makes feedback valuable in nearly all situations.[2] The continuum of learning in hospital medicine provides ample opportunity for teachers and learners to reaffirm performance and modify plans for improvement on a daily, weekly, and monthly basis. To maintain the integrity and momentum of feedback, it should be performed as a progressive process.[5]

Daily Observation on Family-Centered Rounds

Observation is essential and critical to providing meaningful feedback. Without direct observation, feedback is simply judgment. Family-centered rounds are a vital component of hospital medicine and an ideal aspect of patient care that allows direct observation. When providing feedback based on observation that occurred during family-centered rounds, a key introductory phrase such as "I noticed" helps the learner to recognize feedback is being delivered.[3]

Setting Expectations from the Beginning

When feedback is viewed as an everyday aspect of clinical education, it increases the likelihood that it will be performed and received. To establish a culture of feedback among learners, teachers should provide expectations on the first clinical day to all learners on the service. Additionally, trainees should be empowered to set goals that are meaningful and learning oriented.[5] This discussion should be followed by a statement that frequent and timely feedback linked to these goals and expectations will be given. Feedback is designed to reinforce good performances and to point out where performances could be improved to make the learner successful.

Identifying Learning Gaps at the Start of a Clinical Rotation

Although the promotion of self-directed learning and reflection is an integral aspect of adult learning, insight into a learner's deficits may be lacking. It is also important that the teacher clearly outline the expectations for what signifies good performance. This step eliminates the need for the learner to identify the gap between actual and desired performance.[3]

Preparation for Feedback Delivery

Given how vital feedback is to a learner's progression toward clinical excellence, care must be taken to prepare for feedback delivery, not just with timing but also location. Taking notes during clinical interactions, such as on family-centered rounds, can be used by a teacher to more accurately reference details of a given encounter during the discussion. Particularly when the feedback is negative, it is crucial that it occurs in a private setting, such as a conference room or office; learners may be less likely to seek feedback in front of their peers.[12] Other brief and less critical feedback may occur in the hallway between patient rooms.[7]

Ensuring Feedback Is Meaningful and Timely

For feedback to be effective, it should be a priority for both the teacher and learner, and learners should feel empowered to ask for it.[6] It should be given at the time of an event or shortly after.[3] Conducting feedback closer to the observed behavior allows for more detailed assessment and for the guidance to be more relevant to the receiver.[14] It should be reflective of a limited number of observations at a given time to allow the learner to focus on 1 to 2 items.[6] Avoid general performance remarks, like "good job," without providing specific comments on what went well, which can guide future performance.[3]

The timing of feedback is also important to consider. Conducting feedback partway through a clinical rotation allows the student time to show improvement, compared with when this discussion occurs on the last day. Although having immediate feedback is important, especially with a high-stakes situation, there is also benefit to delaying feedback if the recipient is not in the right mental state to receive it, such as after breaking bad news or in the event of a medical error.[15] Allowing the learner time to process the experience may help them to be in a better mental state to participate in self-assessment and goal setting. Being mindful of the needs of the learner in terms of context, timing, and location can help to make the feedback interaction more conducive to clinical improvement.

GUIDELINES FOR GIVING FEEDBACK

Ende's Guidelines for Giving Feedback

Considered to be the grandfather of feedback in clinical medicine, Jack Ende published about guiding principles for giving feedback to learners as early as 1983 (**Box 1**).[1]

Feedback Models

There are a variety of models that have been developed since Ende's guideline. Several models can be used in hospital medicine, and each has unique strengths

Box 1
Ende's guidelines for giving feedback

- Feedback should be undertaken with the teacher and trainee working as allies, with common goals.
- Feedback should be well-timed and expected.
- Feedback should be based on first-hand data.
- Feedback should be regulated in quantity and limited to behaviors that are remediable.
- Feedback should be phrased in descriptive, nonevaluative language.
- Feedback should deal with specific performances, not generalizations.
- Feedback should offer subjective data, labeled as such.
- Feedback should deal with decisions and actions, rather than assumed intentions or interpretations.

Data from Ende J. Feedback in clinical medical education. JAMA 1983;250(6):777–81.

and challenges. Ultimately, the selection of one model over the other should be assessed based on the teacher and learner's needs (**Fig. 2**).

Feedback Sandwich

Although there is not one correct model, there have been some feedback strategies that have fallen by the wayside, one of those being the infamous "feedback sandwich." With the feedback sandwich, a teacher begins with a positive or reinforcing statement, followed by a negative or corrective statement, and ends with another positive or reinforcing statement.[3] Commonly the teacher will use the word "but" before the corrective statement, which often leads learners to ignore the initial positive statements. Additionally, in an effort to maintain self-esteem, the teacher may focus too much effort on the final positive statements, causing the learner to leave with a falsely positive assessment.[8] Although the perception of the learner may change, their performance does not.[16] At its core, the feedback sandwich is flawed, because all the power is in the hands of the teacher; communication is only occurring in 1 direction.[3] Although it is not an ideal method, it is easy to remember and may be used in situations where there is limited time for feedback or a lack of familiarity with other feedback models.

Learner Self-Assessment

The vital component missing from the feedback sandwich is self-assessment by the learner. A central tenet of andragogy is that adult learners should be able to cultivate self-directed learning based on their specific needs in their individual environment.[17] Having an awareness of their knowledge and skills gaps helps the learner to understand areas of needed improvement. Unfortunately, this method relies on adult

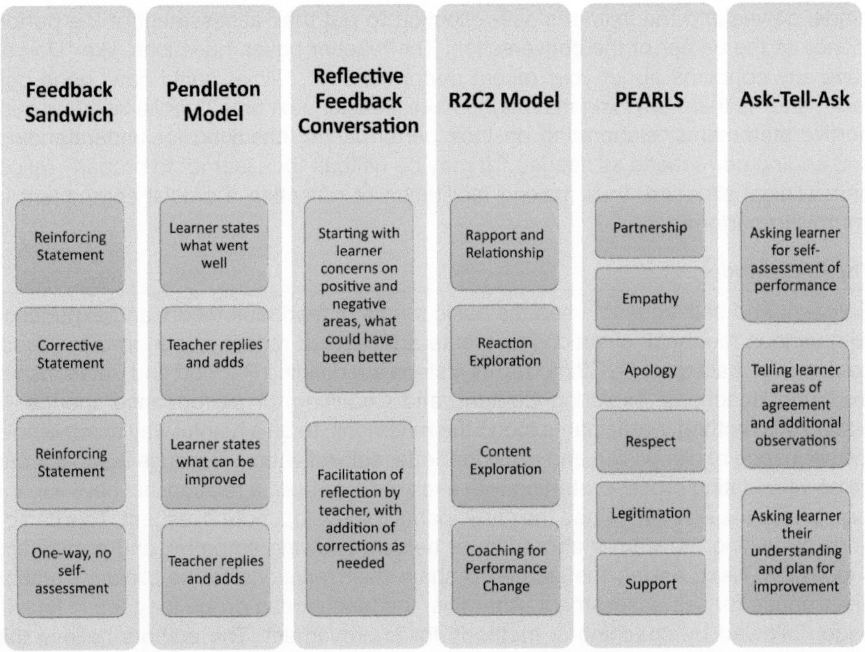

Fig. 2. Major feedback models.

learners having insight into their shortcomings, and humans naturally gravitate toward experiences that they enjoy or skills at which they excel.

There are multiple reasons for why learners may not be able to self-assess. They may have "information neglect" or "memory biases" that lead them to unconsciously ignore or selectively remember their performance.[17] Adapting to a more optimistic viewpoint of themselves may also be a reason for not identifying their weaknesses. Last, they may have never received negative feedback and, therefore, have an inaccurate assessment of their abilities.[17] However, even with this condition, instructing learners to reflect on their behavior may help to begin the feedback conversation.

Reflection is an integral part of self-assessment; however, external feedback also aids the learner in better self-monitoring of their abilities in certain situations.[5] Metacognition, which is thinking about one's own thoughts, is an important skill for self-assessment, but likely one that has to develop over time to be truly self-critical.[4] Therefore, novice learners have to rely on adequate feedback from their teachers to better understand their abilities and their limitations, and teachers need training in delivering feedback effectively.

The Pendleton Model

The Pendleton model attempts to build on the feedback sandwich to include learner observations.[3] It begins with the learner sharing what they did well, followed by the teacher replying with areas of agreement and adding additional reinforcing comments; then, the learner shares what could have been better about their performance, and the teacher supplementing with what they think could be improved in the future. This style of feedback caters better to sit-down discussion, rather than brief feedback while on the wards, because it involves more detailed assessment of performance.

The Reflective Feedback Conversation

Taking the Pendleton model one step further, the reflective feedback conversation model delves into the learner's self-reflection to put their assessment of the performance at the center of the conversation. The teacher poses questions, like "Do you have any concerns about your recent performance?", "What could have gone better?", and "Is there anything that might make it easier next time?" while inserting supportive statements, elaborating on their performance, checking for understanding, and adding corrections as needed.[3] It may be difficult for a learner to properly reflect on a clinical situation, thus making facilitation of reflection a crucial component of improving performance.[7]

The R2C2 Model

Sargeant and colleagues[13] used the basic tenets of feedback theory and experience with various feedback situations to create a facilitated reflective performance feedback model, called the R2C2 model. Its 4 steps are building Rapport and Relationship, exploring Reactions, exploring Content, and Coaching for performance change. In testing this method, participants found the mnemonic to be a helpful way to remember the sequence of discussion and allow for better self-reflection. Because feedback can be an intimidating process, starting with a reminder to build a relationship between the learner and the teacher helped the participants to develop mutual respect. This can be done by asking the learner about him or herself, showing empathy, and applauding successes. Next, asking the learner to share their reactions to the clinical situation gives space for self-assessment. After this, the teacher can probe for gaps in knowledge, followed by coaching in methods for improvement. The authors believe this model allows the learner to take ownership of their performance.[13] In a subsequent study, Sargeant and colleagues[18] further tested their model with residents in internal medicine and pediatrics and found that it helped the learners to have more meaningful feedback interactions with their teachers, with an emphasis on the helpfulness of the coaching phase. This model works well with reflective learners.

PEARLS Model

Another feedback model that takes advantage of the utility of mnemonics is the PEARLS model. Milan and colleagues[19] first presented this technique at a conference in 2003 and later published their method in 2006. PEARLS, or Partnership Empathy Apology Respect Legitimation and Support, centers on helping a learner to be receptive to change in their behavior in a supportive environment. The teacher begins by partnering with the learner in sharing the understanding of a problem, apologizing for barriers to success, having respect for a learner's choices, legitimizing feelings, and supporting their efforts to improve.[19] The learner's response to the feedback may vary depending on their readiness to change. By diagnosing the learner, the teacher can make targeted interventions to help them understand where their performance lies compared with the expected standard. Because this model is more teacher directed, it may be useful with learners who have more difficulty with reflection or the identification of errors.

Ask–Tell–Ask

As feedback models become more elaborate, they can be difficult to remember on a busy clinical day. French and others have adopted a simple method from patient care to use for reflective feedback. To promote better doctor–patient communication, Clark and colleagues[20] published an easy-to-remember framework called Ask–Tell–Ask in 1998. In this 3-function model, the clinician would probe the patient for information or concerns (ask), use an emphatic statement to acknowledge any emotions (tell), and ask another question to assist the patient in making future plans (ask). Barnett[21] proposed that this framework be used by hospitalists to improve rapport with patients. French and colleagues[22] at the Cleveland Clinic then published their adaption of the Ask–Tell–Ask framework for feedback; in this context, teachers giving feedback to learners would first ask for the learner's self-assessment of their performance, followed by the teacher acknowledging the learners' assessment and stating their own observations (tell), and then asking the learner for their understanding of the feedback and their plan for improvement (ask). The benefit of this method is that it allows the learner to first reflect on their performance before the teacher gives their opinion. This model is especially useful when their perspectives are discordant, because it instructs the teacher on the learner's self-assessment and where to begin the discussion to reach common ground.

No matter the feedback method used, the incorporation of certain phrases can help to make the conversation less intimidating and more conducive to reflection and self-improvement (**Box 2**).[23,24]

HELPING LEARNERS REACT TO AND RECOGNIZE FEEDBACK

Being a Credible Source

For feedback to be accepted, it must come from a source that the learner considers to be credible. Being proficient in feedback delivery and being a good role model improves the likelihood of success. One study from Johns Hopkins found that 6 behaviors correlated with better feedback delivery: (1) discussing the learner's emotional reaction, (2) asking about the learner's goals, (3) documenting personal professional

Box 2
Helpful phrasing when giving feedback

- Ask questions of the learner's self-assessment, before telling him or her how he or she did: "How do you think that went?" or "Tell me what you thought about your performance."
- Avoid nonspecific positive statements, because they may relate more to self-image than particular behaviors: Consider "Your documentation was very thorough, especially your assessment in the daily progress note," rather than "You are an excellent trainee."
- Use "I" statements to emphasize that this is how the actions were perceived, rather than assuming intentions: "I noticed that you did not finish your notes until 10 PM. Tell me about that."
- Focus more on the action or observed event, rather than the person: "I saw that you tried once for the lumbar puncture and then the senior resident took over for the second try."
- Acknowledge their feelings if a learner becomes emotional, and ask them to elaborate on the situation, thus giving them space to debrief: "I can see that seemed very frustrating."
- Check for understanding: "Does this make sense?" or "Does this seem reasonable?"
- Help the learner to develop a plan: "How would you handle a similar situation in the future?" with "Okay, so we have agreed that next time, you will try to..."

Data from Ende J, Fosnocht KM. Clinical examination: still a tool for our times? Trans Am Clin Climatol Assoc. 2002;113:137–150; Thomas JD, Arnold RM. Giving feedback. J Palliat Med 2011;14(2):233–9.

goals in the past year, (4) working with learners on mutually agreed upon goals, (5) permitting learners to do their own problem solving, and (6) using conflict resolution techniques.[17] Building a relationship with the learner and cultivating trust allows the receiver to see the feedback as valid. Making the feedback feel relevant by setting expectations and shared goals increases its relevance.[5] Demonstrating inattentiveness or a low level of knowledge or experience can undermine the message.[14] In contrast, having high enthusiasm for learning, experience, knowledge, and communication skills can help the learner to aspire to emulate this role model behavior and request guidance to do so.[7] The benefit of working in the inpatient setting is that these qualities can be demonstrated on a daily basis through family-centered rounds and allow for multiple opportunities to build rapport. Johnson and colleagues[25] conducted a comprehensive literature review and determined 25 behaviors that demonstrate high-quality feedback in clinical practice, including many of the characteristics discussed herein regarding observation, specificity, timeliness, sharing differences between the learner's performance and the standard, and helping the learner to create an action plan for future improvement.

Learner Perceptions of Feedback

A major barrier that leads to ineffective feedback results when learners do not perceive feedback was delivered. This can be due to the feedback not being labeled as such, but too often this can occur because feedback is not given.[7] In the absence of specific directed feedback, learners may misconstrue other cues as criticism of their performance when they may be unrelated to the teacher's assessment of their behavior.[1] Making feedback explicit and an expected part of the clinical rotation may help to lessen these misperceptions. Because of difficulties in assessing learner perceptions of feedback, Bing-You and colleagues[26] performed a review of the literature to find validated instruments that targeted this issue. They were able to test 2 feedback instruments with teachers and learners, one on culture and another on provider traits. They found that these instruments facilitated delivery of feedback in the clinical environment. The Feedback Culture instrument asked learners 16 Likert scale questions, including rating of frequency of feedback, whether they self-assess or reflect, if they were given specific details or suggestions for improvement, and if it helped to improve their performance.[26] The 13-item Feedback Provider instrument asked about the learner's perception of their teacher, including comfort, respect, knowledge and skills, if they have worked with the learner long enough to assess them, and if it was a 2-way conversation. Whether a teacher uses a feedback instrument or verbal discussion, the valuable lesson is that feedback with learners may need to be more explicitly labeled and structured so that all who take part are aware that it is occurring.

Psychology of Attitude and Ability to Change

Because we are all human and adult learners, it can be difficult to accept constructive feedback and change a behavior that may be long standing. There are countless theories that examine the psychology of attitudes, attitude change, and behavior.[27] An attitude is an evaluative judgment about an object, person, or idea, and it can affect how someone approaches or avoids a situation; however, it is not permanent and can be changed. In attitude research, psychologists study how these attitudes affect behavior. In the theory of reasoned action, intention is determined by both a person's attitude and the perceived expectation of behavior, also known as subjective norm.[27] However, this may not be able to determine the behavioral output. Going one step further, the theory of planned behavior adds a third element called perceived behavioral control, which is the person's perception of their ability to do a particular action.[28] If the learner perceives barriers to their ability to make a behavior change, they are less likely to do so, thus making guidance and mentorship by the teacher delivering negative feedback a critical component of the discussion.

Increasing Comfort During Constructive Feedback

It is our job as educators to use strategies to increase comfort when delivering constructive criticism. Feedback should be delivered in a nonthreatening manner that is constructive rather than destructive. It should also be limited to 1 to 3 key points, so that the learner is not overwhelmed; similar to other medical education delivery, a learner's cognitive load, or ability to process new information, should be taken into account.[15] The ultimate goal is performance improvement and helping the learner to be a better clinician. Emphasizing that negative feedback on a particular behavior is not an attack on their personality is necessary to address early in the conversation, or the learner may become self-protective and not be open to suggestions for improvement.[4] Acknowledging emotional reactions and separating the learner from the observed action can be a first step to finding common ground and helping them to be receptive to an action plan to remedy the behavior. Avoiding negative feedback is not a viable solution; the behavior will only continue if unchecked and could lead to poor evaluations and—even worse—suboptimal patient care. Taking a role of "coach" rather than "supervisor" can help the trainee to see that they have support in being a better clinician.[29]

LIMITATIONS

What Can We Really Change?

Despite the promotion of reciprocal conversation between teacher and leaner, feedback is often teacher driven.[5] Teachers should empower their learners to seek and identify feedback. Instilling deliberate metacognition and reflection in action helps to promote the learner's self-monitoring drive.[4,5] Feedback should aim to have the student reflect on their own behaviors, while the teacher should seek to assess the learner's own insight.[3]

A curriculum designed to help learners recognize, receive, and respond to feedback at a metacognitive level, and faculty development on exploration of learner's insight, will help to ensure that feedback is meaningful and encourage personal and professional growth.

RECEIVING FEEDBACK AS A TEACHER

An often-neglected aspect of feedback is the idea that it should be bidirectional. Teachers may not ask for feedback, and learners often will not offer it unsolicited. If educators are not taking time to self-assess and reflect on performance as attending physicians, then they may not realize if there are behaviors that are negatively affecting others.[6] At times, learners may fear giving constructive feedback to their teachers out of a fear of a repercussion in their evaluations. It may end up being vague and generally positive to avoid specific criticism. Therefore, it is important to guide the learner in giving specific information that will help to improve as an educator. Asking probing questions like "What could I have done differently to improve or enhance your learning experience?" may elicit more specific information about actionable improvements.[30]

If the learner is willing to give constructive feedback, be an active listener that does not interrupt, but probes for more information by asking "Tell me more." It may help to take notes, repeat back what was heard to ensure understanding, and ask questions.[31] Paying attention to nonverbal reactions is important to minimize emotional response. Remember that the feedback is about observable behaviors as the supervising physician and not worth.[6] Taking responsibility and verbalizing realistic changes for the future exemplifies the teacher's status as a role model that is striving to be the best physician they can be.

SUMMARY

Although there are many barriers to providing feedback in the inpatient setting, coaching learners to improve their behavior and become better clinicians is one of the most important duties. Ensuring that the feedback is specific, timely, based on first-hand information, given privately, and delivered with empathy helps to make it a more valuable experience for both teacher and learner. Asking for feedback can be difficult to remember, but reminding trainees that medicine is lifelong learning and acting as examples of perpetual improvement helps hospitalists to be the best role models for the team. In the end, it is the teacher's responsibility to give and receive feedback proficiently, because the ultimate beneficiaries are the patients.[17]

REFERENCES

1. Ende J. Feedback in clinical medical education. JAMA 1983;250(6):777–81.
2. van de Ridder JM, Stokking KM, McGaghie WC, et al. What is feedback in clinical education? Med Educ 2008;42(2):189–97.
3. Cantillon P, Sargeant J. Giving feedback in clinical settings. BMJ 2008;337:a1961.
4. Bing-You RG, Trowbridge RL. Why medical educators may be failing at feedback. JAMA 2009;302(12):1330–1.

5. Archer JC. State of the science in health professional education: effective feedback. Med Educ 2010;44(1):101–8.
6. Algiraigri AH. Ten tips for receiving feedback effectively in clinical practice. Med Educ Online 2014;19:25141.
7. Branch WT Jr, Paranjape A. Feedback and reflection: teaching methods for clinical settings. Acad Med 2002;77(12):1185–8.
8. Kogan JR, Conforti LN, Bernabeo EC, et al. Faculty staff perceptions of feedback to residents after direct observation of clinical skills. Med Educ 2012;46(2):201–15.
9. Barton KL, Schofield SJ, McAleer S, et al. Translating evidence-based guidelines to improve feedback practices: the interACT case study. BMC Med Educ 2016;16:53.
10. Nicol DJ, Macfarlane-Dick D. Formative assessment and self-regulated learning: a model and seven principles of good feedback practice. Stud High Educ 2006;31(2):199–218.
11. Dweck CS. Self-theories: their role in motivation, personality, and development. Psychology press; 2013. p. 29–38.
12. Crommelinck M, Anseel F. Understanding and encouraging feedback-seeking behaviour: a literature review. Med Educ 2013;47(3):232–41.
13. Sargeant J, Lockyer J, Mann K, et al. Facilitated reflective performance feedback: developing an evidence- and theory-based model that builds relationship, explores reactions and content, and coaches for performance change (R2C2). Acad Med 2015;90(12):1698–706.
14. Bing-You RG, Paterson J, Levine MA. Feedback falling on deaf ears: residents' receptivity to feedback tempered by sender credibility. Med Teach 1997;19(1):40–4.
15. Kaul P, Gong J, Guiton G. Effective feedback strategies for teaching in pediatric and adolescent gynecology. J Pediatr Adolesc Gynecol 2014;27(4):188–93.
16. Bing-You R, Hayes V, Varaklis K, et al. Feedback for learners in medical education: what is known? A scoping review. Acad Med 2017;92(9):1346–54.
17. Anderson PA. Giving feedback on clinical skills: are we starving our young? J Grad Med Educ 2012;4(2):154–8.
18. Sargeant J, Mann K, Manos S, et al. R2C2 in action: testing an evidence-based model to facilitate feedback and coaching in residency. J Grad Med Educ 2017;9(2):165–70.
19. Milan FB, Parish SJ, Reichgott MJ. A model for educational feedback based on clinical communication skills strategies: beyond the "feedback sandwich". Teach Learn Med 2006;18(1):42–7.
20. Clark W, Hewson M, Fry M, et al. Techniques for the three function model. McLean (VA): American Academy of Physician and Patient; 1998.
21. Barnett PB. Rapport and the hospitalist. Am J Med 2001;111(9):31–5.
22. French JC, Colbert CY, Pien LC, et al. Targeted feedback in the milestones era: utilization of the ask-tell-ask feedback model to promote reflection and self-assessment. J Surg Educ 2015;72(6):e274–9.
23. Ende J, Fosnocht KM. Clinical examination: still a tool for our times? Trans Am Clin Climatol Assoc 2002;113:137–50.
24. Thomas JD, Arnold RM. Giving feedback. J Palliat Med 2011;14(2):233–9.
25. Johnson CE, Keating JL, Boud DJ, et al. Identifying educator behaviours for high quality verbal feedback in health professions education: literature review and expert refinement. BMC Med Educ 2016;16:96.

26. Bing-You R, Ramesh S, Hayes V, et al. Trainees' perceptions of feedback: validity evidence for two FEEDME (Feedback in Medical Education) instruments. Teach Learn Med 2018;30(2):162–72.
27. Maio G, Haddock G. The psychology of attitudes and attitude change. Thousand Oaks (CA): SAGE; 2009.
28. Cameron KA. A practitioner's guide to persuasion: an overview of 15 selected persuasion theories, models and frameworks. Patient Educ Couns 2009;74(3):309–17.
29. Tekian A, Watling CJ, Roberts TE, et al. Qualitative and quantitative feedback in the context of competency-based education. Med Teach 2017;39(12):1245–9.
30. Wilkinson ST, Couldry R, Phillips H, et al. Preceptor development: providing effective feedback. Hosp Pharm 2013;48(1):26–32.
31. van der Leeuw RM, Slootweg IA. Twelve tips for making the best use of feedback. Med Teach 2013;35(5):348–51.

Teaching at the Bedside

Strategies for Optimizing Education on Patient and Family Centered Rounds

Thuy L. Ngo, DO, MEd[a,*], Rebecca Blankenburg, MD, MPH[b], Clifton E. Yu, MD[c]

KEYWORDS

• Bedside teaching • Medical education • Adult learning

KEY POINTS

- Bedside teaching is an educational interplay between teacher, trainee, and patient.
- There are multiple components of bedside teaching including preparation before the patient encounter, teaching, and debriefing afterward.
- There has been a steady decline in bedside teaching because of various constraints, despite known benefits of enhancing clinical education for multiple groups of learners.
- Barriers to bedside teaching include teacher preference or bias, time constraints, perceived patient preferences, and the perception that teaching is not valued at the institution.

DECLINE IN BEDSIDE TEACHING

In 2001, the Institute of Medicine released the report *Crossing the Quality Chasm: A New Health System for the 21st Century*, which focused on improving delivery of patient care through innovation and reinventing the health care system.[1] One of the guiding principles of the report was that "transparency is necessary," that is to say patients and their families should be given information such that they are able to make informed decisions about their care. One of the ways to achieve this is through family-centered rounds (FCR), which shifts the focus from a provider-centered approach to one that more directly involves patients and families in dialogue about their care. For more

Drs R. Blankenburg and C.E. Yu do not have any relevant disclosures. Dr T.L. Ngo serves on the Primary Care Advisory Board for Welch Allyn.

[a] Pediatric Emergency Medicine, Johns Hopkins School of Medicine, 1800 Orleans Street, G-1509, Baltimore, MD 21287, USA; [b] Pediatric Hospital Medicine, Stanford School of Medicine, 725 Welch Road, MC 5906, Palo Alto, CA 94304, USA; [c] Walter Reed National Military Medical Center, Uniformed Services University of the Health Sciences, 8901 Wisconsin Avenue, Bethesda, MD 20889, USA
* Corresponding author.
E-mail address: thuy.ngo@jhmi.edu

Pediatr Clin N Am 66 (2019) 881–889
https://doi.org/10.1016/j.pcl.2019.03.012
pediatric.theclinics.com

information on FCR, See Jennifer L. Everhart and colleagues' article, "Patient- and Family-Centered Care: Leveraging Best Practices to Improve the Care of Hospitalized Children," in this issue: Communication with Patients, and Lauren A. Destino and colleagues' article, "Family Centered Rounds: Past, Present and Future," in this issue: Bedside Rounds.

Although teaching on rounds has been a cornerstone of medical education for over a century, medical providers perceive that patients and families do not regard bedside teaching (BST) favorably,[2] and that it prolongs rounds. As such, teaching at the bedside has steadily declined over the last 50 years. According to Ahmed,[3] time spent at the bedside in the early 1960s comprised 75% of teaching time compared with just 16% by 1978, and is much less now. In addition to patient and family factors, there are multiple issues that have contributed to the decline of BST: rapid patient turnover, prioritization of early patient discharge to improve inpatient throughput, increasing reliance on technological data for diagnosis and management, discomfort with teaching at the bedside, and an increase in duties by senior physicians including research and administrative responsibilities.[2,3] In addition, resident duty hour restrictions have led to a reduction in time spent performing direct patient care by trainees, further contributing to the decline in BST.[4,5] Despite these concerns, BST remains an integral part of teaching on the inpatient unit, with both patients and learners finding it beneficial.[6] In this article, basic tenets for successful implementation of BST, in addition to strategies to alleviate the perceived barriers to its use, are presented and discussed.

PRINCIPLES OF BEDSIDE TEACHING

Despite the use of BST as far back as seventeenth-century Italy, the modern day practice of bedside teaching is widely attributed to Sir William Osler in 1892, who stated that "medicine is learned by the bedside and not in the classroom … the best teaching is taught by the patient himself."[7] BST is the educational interplay between teacher, trainee, and patient (**Fig. 1**).[8] The teacher in this instance can be the attending, senior residents, or even junior residents depending on the structure of the medical team. The trainee can be a resident or student. The patient can include not just the patient but also family members. Successful BST involves preparation before rounds, maintaining a safe learning environment that encourages inquiry, and lastly debriefing and providing feedback from the interaction (**Box 1**).[9]

BST should focus on teaching that will benefit the patient. Through use of a Delphi method comprising physicians, nurses, families, and health literacy experts in July 2014, Khan and colleagues[10] found that BST areas benefitting families include teaching physical examination maneuvers and clinical reasoning, role modeling communication

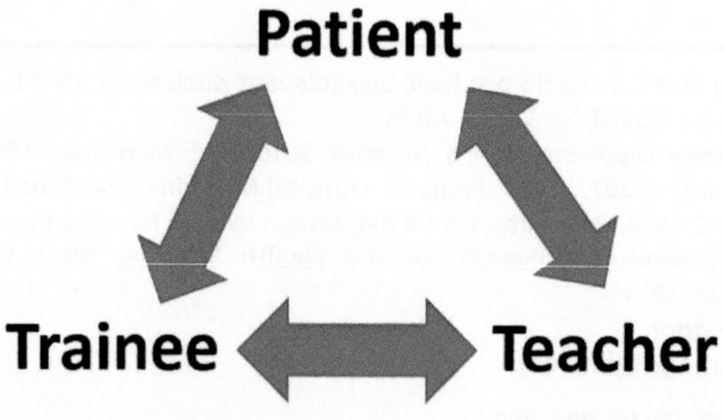

Fig. 1. Bedside teaching team. The bedside teaching team involves engagement and interaction by all members to insure success.

Box 1
Components of bedside teaching

Pre-rounds	Preparation • Faculty development to increase comfort with BST • Be familiar with curriculum, learner skill level Planning • Define goal of BST: What will be taught? What will be emphasized? • Plan on how to keep all learners engaged • Choose appropriate patient(s), obtain assent from patient/family • Determine how much time to spend with each encounter Orientation • Tell learners what objective of BST is • Assign roles to learners • Establish "rules," remind learners of safe learning environment
Rounds	Introduction • Introduce medical team • Orient patient/family to learning goals of BST Interaction • Role model physician-patient interaction, communication • Role model how to integrate family members into the encounter Observation • Observe skills of learner: communication, history taking and physical examination skills, fund of knowledge, professional behaviors, and respect of the family unit Instruction • Challenge learners • Teach professional behaviors • Teach skills that can only be learned at the bedside • Emphasize group learning aspect of BST Summarization • Discuss what was taught to learners and patient • Discuss patient plan of care
Post-rounds	Debriefing • Answer questions as they arise • Allow learners to discuss frustrations from encounter • Allow time to "reset" before next encounter Feedback • Ask learners what went well, ask what can be improved • Commend aspects of encounter that were successful • Discuss strategies for improvement Reflection • Discuss what worked well with BST • Discuss with learners if anything should be modified for next session Preparation • Plan for next patient encounter or next BST session

Adapted from Ramani S. Twelve steps to improve bedside teaching. Med Teach 2003;25:112–5; with permission.

skills and professional behaviors, and assessing learners' clinical reasoning, communication skills, and professionalism (**Fig. 2**). Many of these skills are difficult to simulate outside of the patient's room and even more difficult to teach in a didactic setting. BST also takes advantage of adult learning theory principles, such as situated learning, which posits that learning is more effective when situated within an authentic activity or context such as the bedside setting can provide, while at the same time providing increased transparency to patients and their families. This is also a time when the teacher can model respectful behaviors to the patient: speaking in nontechnical terms to increase the patient's understanding of their illness, understanding privacy issues, and allowing patients to be modest with their bodies, and allowing the patient to participate in their care and provide feedback on the interaction to trainees. For a more in-depth discussion on communication, See Jennifer K. O'Toole and colleagues' article, "Communication with Diverse Patients: Addressing Culture and Language," in this issue: Communication with Patients.

There are additional topics that benefit from discussion outside of the patients' room, between patients, or during team huddles. These include priming trainees before going into the room, debriefing after exiting a room, discussing sensitive psychosocial issues, and teaching about pathophysiology, process improvement, and systems-based practice. In addition, providing feedback about decisions made by the overnight team, issues around the admission process, or other systems issues are appropriate to discuss between patients. Given the time constraints on FCR and hospital administration emphasis on early discharge, there are some topics that should be addressed at other times of day outside the rounding process, including presentation skills and longer teaching sessions covering topics that require more in-depth discussion.

Before Bedside Teaching Rounds

Preparation is imperative for BST success. Factors such as communication of overall curricular and rotation goals, the trainees' own goals for the rotation, trainees' skill levels, and the makeup of the inpatient service will aid in planning and directing BST.

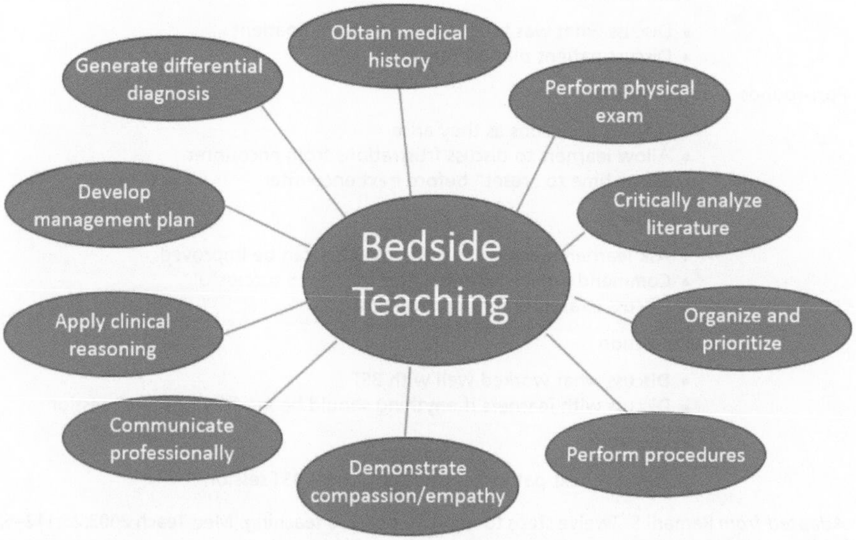

Fig. 2. Knowledge and skills acquired during bedside teaching.

Understanding that many elements can interrupt BST necessitates having a flexible plan and the ability to adjust quickly. The focus of BST can include emphasis on (see **Fig. 2**):

- History taking: emphasizing key features for particular diagnoses
- Physical examination findings: focusing on particular organ systems so that the team can compare and contrast their physical examination findings between patients
- Clinical reasoning: discussing key features and differential diagnosis; devising a plan of care (see **Box 2** for helpful models)
- Contingency planning: identifying key steps to take for each patient given real or hypothetical events that could arise during the day/night
- Communication skills: focusing on specific communication skills, for example, showing empathy, demonstrating shared decision-making, disclosing medical errors
- Ethics: discussing key ethical issues related to the patients on service
- Procedures: emphasizing those that can be performed at bedside, such as arterial puncture, venipuncture, intravenous catheter placement, lumbar puncture, point of care ultrasound, and extremity splinting

Choosing and orienting patients is also crucial before entering the room. This can be performed by anyone on the team but should include reviewing the teaching nature of the encounter and also giving the patient and family the opportunity to decline. The patient and family members should be offered the opportunity to participate in BST and encouraged to ask questions. Lastly, orientation of trainees before BST should always take place, this includes describing expectations for participation and behavior while in the presence of the patient. Roles can be assigned before entering the room to keep all team members engaged.

During Bedside Teaching Rounds

During rounds, a skilled teacher can simultaneously help guide patient care decisions, assess learner abilities, and teach. Allowing the trainee to play a key role (eg,

Box 2
IDEA

IDEA: A helpful model for eliciting clinical reasoning

I: Interpretive summary

D: Differential diagnosis

E: Explanation of reasoning

A: Alternatives

This model can be used to help learners demonstrate their clinical reasoning on rounds, in other teaching sessions, and in notes. In bedside teaching, it is helpful for the patients to hear a prioritized differential and why 1 diagnosis is more likely than another. For example, a patient presents with chest pain, a symptom that has differential diagnoses that range from life threatening to psychosomatic. Allowing the learner to summarize and synthesize the history, physical examination findings, and pertinent laboratory and radiological data will allow the teacher to assess the learner's skills and fund of knowledge. Discussing and prioritizing the differential using clinical reasoning allows the patient to have a clearer understanding of their illness and understand further plans of care.

Data from Baker E, Ledford C, Fogg L, et al. The IDEA assessment tool: assessing the reporting, diagnostic reasoning, and decision-making skills demonstrated in Medical Students' Hospital admission notes. Teach Learn Med 2015;27:163–73.

presenting the patient, teaching a physical examination maneuver) allows two things to occur. First, it establishes the trainee as the primary medical provider for the patient, instilling patient trust in their abilities and knowledge. Second, the teacher is given the opportunity to observe the trainee's interactions with the patient. This includes their ability to problem solve, their communication and negotiation skills, and their attitudes toward the patient, family, and other team members.[10]

When teaching at the bedside, creating a safe learning environment is essential to prevent appearing unsure in front of the patient and other team members, as this may undermine their abilities as the primary medical provider. To create a safe learning environment, one can:

- Provide positive reinforcement by applauding good work
- Avoid asking vague questions
- Ask questions to the entire team
- Be honest with one's lack of knowledge to allow others to be forthcoming with their own limitations
- When errors are made, provide gentle corrections without ridicule
- Focus BST on elements that will benefit the family, for example, physical examination skills, clinical reasoning, and role modeling communication skills and professional behaviors

After Bedside Teaching Rounds

Summarizing what was taught at the patient's bedside can be done in the room; however, synthesizing this learning after leaving the patient's room can be invaluable. At this point, team members can also plan to critically evaluate the literature to further develop the plan of care, allow time for questions and observations from the encounter, and clarify or reinforce key teaching points.

Team members should be encouraged to participate in a debriefing of the encounter and discuss what went well and what can be improved on following the encounter. Trainees may want to reflect on their deficiencies and voice frustrations. This is also a time when feedback can be given to the team or to individuals, as needed, regarding their communication skills, clinical reasoning, physical examination skills, and their integration of the patient and family. The teacher should also solicit feedback from team members to see if adjustments need to be made based on the needs of the team.

BENEFITS

Williams and colleagues[11] conducted focus group discussions with clerkship students and junior residents and found a common belief that BST is a valuable and underused teaching tool. Many junior trainees found BST to be an essential component of their learning. Seeing attendings and senior residents interacting with patients allowed them to model professional behaviors as well as many clinical skills.[9] Focus group participants cited several missed opportunities for BST with variable reasons for its omission; however, they also noted that, when it does occur, it stands out as an exceptional teaching moment.[11]

Heckmann and colleagues[12] performed an educational intervention study to see if there was value added to BST and how it affected students' performance on their clerkship. They looked at sixth year medical students in Germany who were rotating through a 4-month neurology elective. Baseline performance scores were obtained from a written and clinical skills state examination. The average score was 75%. Students were then divided into 2 groups. The control group received the usual curriculum consisting of standard didactic teaching. The study group diverted from the didactic curriculum and focused on history taking, physical examination, and other ways of diagnosing neurologic disease. Their learning was also supplemented with daily BST and case presentations with an attending neurologist. At the end of the rotation, students again took the written and clinical skills state examination. The study group had statistically significant gains in their scores compared with the control group (16.3% gain vs 6.3% gain in scores).

CHALLENGES AND SOLUTIONS

Many challenges and barriers exist to implementing BST, including teacher preference or bias, time constraints, perceived patient preferences, and the perception that teaching is not valued at the institution.

Personal Preferences

Not every attending or senior resident is skilled at BST or even has the desire to perform BST on rounds. Some teachers may also feel uncomfortable discussing a topic they are not an expert in, preferring the classroom where they can limit teaching to subject matter they are comfortable teaching.[13] Expectations can be set for both teacher and trainee in terms of knowledge, skills, and attitudes that should be taught during the rotation, with specific emphasis on those that can be taught and evaluated at the bedside. In addition, faculty development programs should be implemented to increase BST teaching skills and strategies for attendings and residents. Institutional awards for excellence in teaching may also encourage high level teaching on BST.

Trainees may not see the benefits to BST, particularly as it pertains to physical examination skills when laboratory and diagnostic testing are increasingly more available. The onus reverts to the teacher to emphasize the importance of these skills, not only in discussions with the patient but also when generating a differential diagnosis and devising a management plan.

Time Constraints

With high patient volumes, rapid patient turnover, institutional expectations for early discharges, decrease in resident duty hours, and other resident responsibilities, BST can seem extraneous when time is limited.[2,3] In time-motion studies of pediatric residents working on inpatient services, it was found that learners spent only 13% of their time on direct patient care,[4,5] whereas 40% of their time was spent in front of a computer managing patient administrative issues. Faculty can also have competing responsibilities, including outpatient clinic, administrative, and/or research duties. Reducing faculty responsibilities while attending on the inpatient service may help minimize this tension. Efficient teaching techniques such as the One-Minute Preceptor,[14] although originally devised for the outpatient setting, can also be used during BST on the inpatient setting to make teaching more efficient (**Box 3**). With some proactive planning, BST can be limited to a fraction of the patients on the team who are either new to the service and/or have active issues of particular educational benefit. This more deliberate approach allows for preparation by the teacher, orientation of the patient, and work completion without additional time added. Lastly, with the widespread use of the electronic medical record, attending physicians have often reviewed the record before rounds, making extensive and time-consuming patient summaries unnecessary. By emphasizing more focused and concise case presentations, more time can be made available for BST as well.

Box 3
The one-minute preceptor method

1. Get a commitment
2. Probe for supporting evidence
3. Reinforce what was done well
4. Give guidance about errors and omissions
5. Teach a general principle
6. Conclusion

An example on bedside rounds would be:

Teacher: What do you think is going on with this patient? [Get a commitment] Learner: I think the patient has asthma.

Teacher: Why do you think the patient has asthma? [Probe for supporting evidence]

Learner: I think the patient has asthma because he is breathing quickly and hard, and he has a history of asthma.

Teacher: It's great that you are thinking broadly about this patient. Specifically, it is appropriate to think about asthma anytime you have a patient with respiratory distress. [Reinforcing what was done well]

Teacher: I am surprised that he has a fever—anytime I see a fever with respiratory distress, I like to broaden my differential to consider pneumonia and viral illness. [Give guidance about errors or omissions]

Teacher: The most common organisms for pneumonia in this age group are *Mycoplasma pneumoniae* and *Streptococcus pneumoniae*. [Teach a general principle]

Data from Neher J, Gordon K, Meyer B, et al. A five-step "microskills" model of clinical teaching. J Am Board Fam Pract 1992;5:419–24.

Patient Concerns

For patients who are not oriented to BST or who have not experienced it before, the process can be disorienting or intimidating. Trainees may feel like they are being judged on their presentation or may feel embarrassed if they are unable to answer questions, which could potentially undermine their status as the patient's physician. In addition, if there are sensitive issues to discuss, this could create an environment of distrust between patient and medical team or perhaps false information as the patient does not want to disclose sensitive issues in front of a larger audience.

To alleviate these concerns, it is important to request permission and to orient the patient to BST so that they understand that patient care and medical education are not mutually exclusive. Including the patient in BST, whether it be eliciting their opinions or asking for permission to perform or practice physical examination skills, can increase buy-in on the patient's part and can also build trust between the patient and the medical care team. It is equally important to orient trainees to BST and to create a supportive learning environment that allows for knowledge and skills acquisition in a safe space.

SUMMARY

BST is an extremely important form of teaching, allowing learners to consolidate concepts while linking that learning to particular patients, allowing for more immediate future recall and application. In addition, when done well, BST can engage patients and families, create better patient understanding of their medical condition, and inspire greater trust in the medical team.

REFERENCES

1. Institute of Medicine. Crossing the quality Chasm: a new health system for the 21st century. Washington, DC: National Academy Press; 2001.
2. Peters M, ten Cate O. Bedside teaching in medical education: a literature review. Perspect Med Educ 2014;3:76–88.
3. Ahmed Mel-B K. What is happening to bedside teaching? Med Educ 2002; 36(12):1185–8.
4. Destino L, Valentine M, Sheikhi FH, et al. Inpatient hospital factors and resident time with patients and families. Pediatrics 2017;139(5):1–10.
5. Starmer AJ, Destino L, Yoon CS, et al. Intern and resident workflow patterns on pediatric inpatient units: a multicenter time-motion study. JAMA Pediatr 2015; 169(12):1175–7.
6. Gonzalo JD, Chuang CH, Huang G, et al. The return of bedside rounds: an educational intervention. J Gen Intern Med 2010;25:792–8.
7. Stone MJ. The wisdom of Sir William Osler. Am J Cardiol 1995;75:269–76.
8. Garout M, Nuqali A, Alhamzi A, et al. Bedside teaching: an underutilized tool in medical education. Int J Med Educ 2016;7:261–2.
9. Ramani S. Twelve steps to improve bedside teaching. Med Teach 2003;25:112–5.
10. Khan A, for the Patient and Family Centered I-PASS Study Group. Changes in communication and patient safety following implementation of inter-professional Patient and Family Centered I-PASS. Academic Pediatric Association Platform Presentation, Pediatric Academic Societies Conference. San Francisco, CA, May 7, 2017.
11. Williams KN, Ramani S, Fraser B, et al. Improving bedside teaching: findings from a focus group study of learners. Acad Med 2008;83:257–64.
12. Heckmann JG, Bleh C, Dutsch M, et al. Does improved problem-based teaching influence students' knowledge at the end of their neurology elective? An observational study of 40 students. J Neurol 2003;250:1464–8.
13. Linfors EW, Neelon FA. The case for bedside rounds. N Engl J Med 1980;303: 1230–3.
14. Neher J, Gordon K, Meyer B, et al. A five-step "microskills" model of clinical teaching. J Am Board Fam Pract 1992;5:419–24.

Pediatric Hospital Medicine

Where We Are, Where We Are Headed: State of the Specialty, Looking Forward

Matthew W. Ramotar, BA[a,*], Theodore C. Sectish, MD[b]

KEYWORDS

- Pediatric hospital medicine • Health care quality • Inpatient care

KEY POINTS

- Pediatric Hospital Medicine is having an major impact on patient care, quality, safety, and education in academic and community hospital settings.
- Pediatric hospitalists are drivers of change as clinicians who apply evidence-based medicine to standardize practice and promulgate evidence-based guidelines and optimize the function of inter-professional teams.
- Pediatric hospitalists recognize the importance of patient-and family-centeredness of care and the need to incorporate principles of health literacy into all aspects of clinical care and research.
- Pediatric hospitalists assume prominent roles as hospital leaders, educators, and researchers and provide a critical role in promoting improvements in health and health care outcomes.
- Clinical care will undoubtedly remain the major focus of Pediatric Hospital Medicine and with subspecialty status, the field will be expected to accelerate innovations in systems-based practice, advance clinical learning environments, and drive further improvements in quality of care.

BACKGROUND

Hospital medicine as a subspecialty emerged 23 years ago and is the fastest growing subspecialty in all of medicine.[1,2] The number of hospitalists increased because of

Disclosure Statement: Dr T.C. Sectish holds equity in and has consulted with the I-PASS Patient Safety Institute. The I-PASS Patient Safety Institute is a company that seeks to train institutions in best handoff practices and aid in their implementation. Dr T.C. Sectish has additionally received monetary awards, honoraria, and travel reimbursement from multiple academic and professional organizations for teaching and consulting on physician performance and handoffs. Dr M.R. was supported by grant CDR-1306-03556 from the Patient-Centered Outcomes Research Institute (principal investigator: Christopher P. Landrigan).

[a] I-PASS Study Group, Division of General Pediatrics, Department of Medicine, Boston Children's Hospital, 300 Longwood Avenue, Enders, 1st Floor, Boston, MA 02115, USA; [b] Boston Children's Hospital, 300 Longwood Avenue, Hunnewell, 2nd Floor, Boston, MA 02115, USA
* Corresponding author.
E-mail address: matthew.ramotar@childrens.harvard.edu

Pediatr Clin N Am 66 (2019) 891–895
https://doi.org/10.1016/j.pcl.2019.03.013 **pediatric.theclinics.com**

pressures from a changing health care financial landscape as influenced by policy makers, payers, accreditation bodies, and advocacy organizations. Traditionally, inpatients remained under the care of their primary care physicians (PCPs). Health systems, however, began shifting away from this model in the 1990s to one in which care was managed by physicians based in the hospital who were dedicated to providing inpatient care. Thus, the field of hospital medicine grew. In this issue of *Pediatric Clinics of North America*, we describe the role of pediatric hospitalists as clinician educators and how they promote clinical care, education, communication, quality improvement, and patient safety in the inpatient setting. With this context in mind, this article considers the potential future of pediatric hospital medicine (PHM) in its continued evolution.

In December 1999, the Institute of Medicine reported that medical errors cause up to 98,000 deaths in the United States each year. The report, *To Err is Human*, was transformational for the patient safety movement and marked a turning point for the US health care system.[3] *Crossing the Quality Chasm* followed the report in 2001, which documented the failings of the American health care system and described a vision for improvements in 6 dimensions of health care quality: patient safety, care effectiveness, patient-centeredness, timeliness, care efficiency, and equity.[4] The message received widespread attention in the lay press and engaged providers across all levels of care, launching a national movement for health care system redesign. Hospital medicine was positioned perfectly to address these challenges.

In 2003, a group of physicians self-identifying as pediatric hospitalists convened the first annual PHM meeting, marking the formal inception of the field. Like the hospital medicine movement, pediatric hospitalists first emerged within organizations in response to economic pressures and spread across the US health care system out of the need for improved patient safety and provision of high-quality patient care. Contributing factors to the rapid growth of pediatric hospitalists include the economic pressures to contain costs and reduce length of stay, changing population of hospitalized children, PCPs deferring hospital privileges to focus on outpatient practices, reduced resident duty hours, and the demonstration that individuals who focused their practice on inpatient care could provide high-value care.[5]

CURRENT STATE

Pediatric hospitalists have since emerged as a distinct group of practitioners within pediatrics. The number of pediatric hospitalists has expanded largely in the past 10 years.[5] In December 2016, the American Board of Pediatrics voted to recommend that the American Board of Medical Specialties recognize PHM as a distinct subspecialty. Particular consideration was given to the changing population of hospitalized children, the evolution of the pediatric workforce, and health policy and economic trends affecting the future of pediatric inpatient care; evidence of the effect of hospitalists on aspects of safety and quality of pediatric care; and knowledge and skills expected of pediatric hospitalists with respect to the current knowledge and skills learned during pediatric residency training. Deliberations were guided by the overarching question, will children be better served by establishing a distinct PHM subspecialty? PHM fellows will undergo advanced training in areas related to health systems practice and ultimately be expected to address health system issues.

Pediatric hospitalists have been front and center in the patient safety and quality movement, driving change as clinicians, applying evidence-based medicine to standardize practice and promulgate evidence-based guidelines, and playing a central role in optimizing the function of interprofessional teams. Pediatric hospitalists have championed the importance of patient- and family-centeredness of care and the need to incorporate principles of health literacy into aspects of clinical care and research.[6] Moreover, pediatric hospitalists serve as frontline clinicians, hospital leaders, educators, researchers, and mentors for the next generation of pediatricians.

Pediatric hospitalists have roles across all levels of care. Clinical care remains the focus for most pediatric hospitalists, although specific patient duties are varied. Although most pediatric hospitalists serve as general pediatricians for hospitalized children, some provide care on subspecialty services or are actively involved in the care of surgical patients.

Beyond delivering care, pediatric hospitalists have critical roles in education and often are chosen for educator roles, such as residency program directors or clerkship directors, or in leadership roles within the hospital, such as quality and patient safety officers or other operational roles on units or with information technology.

Pediatric hospitalists are also involved in research, particularly health services research. A group of them founded the Pediatric Research in Inpatient Settings, which is supported by the Children's Hospital Association, the Academic Pediatric Association, and the American Academy of Pediatrics.[7] This organization promotes multicenter studies and maintains a database to facilitate meaningful research to answer questions that inform future patient care.

Since inception, pediatric hospitalists have played a critical role in promoting improvements in health and heath care outcomes. Safety targets have included central line-associated bloodstream infections, ventilator-associated pneumonia, catheter-associated urinary tract infection, and medication errors, as well as misidentification of patients, falls, and failures in communication. One area that remains a focus of research is patient safety, most notably in transitions of care (handoffs). Safety gaps from discontinuous care represent a notable example. According to the Joint Commission, communication failures are the leading root cause of hospital sentinel events, the most serious harmful medical errors that can lead to patient injury or death. To address this, Christopher Landrigan and his team[8] developed a bundle of communication interventions known as I-PASS (Illness Severity; Patient Summary; Action List; Situation Awareness and Contingency Planning; Synthesis by Receiver), which focused on improving communication between resident-physicians at changes of shift, or "handoff." The bundle included a training program, changes to verbal and written handoff processes, and a reinforcement and culture change campaign, all organized around the mnemonic I-PASS. Following its implementation in 9 hospitals, injuries due to medical errors (preventable adverse events) decreased by 30% across study sites, and multiple measures of care processes improved.[9] A critical component in improving the handoff process was attaining a shared mental model by the teams giving and receiving critical patient information.

Physician-to-physician handoff failures, however, are but one of many types of miscommunications that occur in hospitals. Another major source of sentinel events is provider-family miscommunication. Pediatric hospitalists have demonstrated the positive impact patient- and family-centered communication and collaboration can have on measures of safety and quality, as well as interprofessional communication processes and experiences with care. An important contribution comes from the Patient- and Family-Centered I-PASS study, in which a team of parents, nurses, and physicians, including health services researchers, medical educators, pediatric hospitalists, communication experts, and health literacy experts, coproduced and tested an intervention to standardize provider-family communication on family-centered rounds organized around the I-PASS mnemonic, Patient- and Family-Centered I-PASS. In Patient- and Family-Centered I-PASS, the study group introduced a structured communication program on rounds that emphasized health literacy, family engagement, and bidirectional communication. Through use of a rigorous, systematic 2-step safety surveillance methodology that incorporated family safety reporting,[10,11] Landrigan and his team found that harmful medical errors dropped by 38% across 7 North American hospitals following implementation of the intervention.[6] In addition, the group found improvements in multiple aspects of family experience and hospital communication processes, without negative impacts on teaching on rounds or the duration of rounds.

LOOKING FORWARD

Looking forward, the future of PHM will evolve in part as a response to the changing health care system, but the field will continue to grow in several key areas—clinical care, education, interprofessional teams and hospital leadership, and quality and patient safety.

Clinical care will undoubtedly be the major focus. As providers on inpatient units to general pediatrics and, increasingly, subspecialty care and the care of children with medical complexity, pediatric hospitalists will remain the key providers of care and will continue to strive for improved outcomes.

Hospitalists have assumed a prominent role as educators in academic medical centers and the ongoing role of the pediatric hospitalist as an educator must not be understated. In the academic environment, where there are trainees, residents, and now, hospital medicine fellows, it is of the utmost importance to understand principles of education to teach communication skills and best practices using workplace-based assessment, simulation-based training, and ongoing feedback to help learners improve and be engaged. The challenge of including hospital medicine fellows in the teaching environment will be finding ways to integrate them into inter-professional teams while maintaining the autonomy and independent clinical decision making of the supervising resident. To mitigate this challenge, programs should include leadership training for their hospital medicine fellows.

The pivotal role of the pediatric hospitalist as a member of interprofessional teams and hospital leaders will continue to evolve as the health care system strives to provide high-quality, high-value care. PHM will succeed if it can function in a way to close the gaps from discontinuities in care and further promote redesign of the health care system.

An ongoing priority for pediatric hospitalists will be spearheading research and quality improvement initiatives aimed at redesigning delivery to optimize patient outcomes. These initiatives would be coproduced with individuals with expertise in implementation science, human factors, and systems engineering, as well as patients, family members, and nurses. Beyond health services research, pediatric hospitalists would ideally engage as collaborators in, or leaders of, comparative effectiveness and bedside-to-community research additionally focused on health conditions commonly seen in hospitalized children.

SUMMARY

Although PHM is in its adolescence, it is already having a major impact on patient care, quality, safety, and education. In the years since *To Err is Human*, *Crossing the Quality Chasm*, and the first 136 members convening the inception of PHM, tremendous strides have been made by the field toward reducing preventable patient harm and improving quality of care. Nevertheless, there remains much room for improvement within the US health care system. As a step toward addressing this gap, the American

Board of Pediatrics recommended recognition of PHM as a distinct new subspecialty in 2015. Fellows of PHM will undergo advanced training in health care systems and systems-based practice, and be expected to accelerate improvements and innovation in quality improvement science and inpatient care. The ongoing major focus for the field will be establishing systems conducive to the training and wellbeing of providers and effective delivery of evidence-based care to hospitalized children.

REFERENCES

1. Wachter RM, Goldman L. The emerging role of "hospitalists" in the American Health Care System. N Engl J Med 1996;335(7):514–7.
2. Wachter RM, Goldman L. Zero to 50,000 — the 20th anniversary of the hospitalist. N Engl J Med 2016;375:1009–11.
3. Institute of Medicine Committee on Quality of Health Care in America. In: Kohn LT, Corrigan JM, Donaldson MS, editors. To err is human: building a safer health system. Washington, DC: National Academies Press (US); 2000.
4. Institute of Medicine (US) Committee on Quality of Health Care in America. Crossing the quality Chasm: a new health system for the 21st century. Washington, DC: National Academies Press (US); 2001. Available at: http://www.ncbi.nlm.nih.gov/books/NBK222274/. Accessed June 27, 2018.
5. Barrett DJ, McGuinness GA, Cunha CA, et al. Pediatric hospital medicine: a proposed new subspecialty. Pediatrics 2017;139(3):e20161823.
6. Khan A, Spector N, Baird J. Patient safety after implementation of a coproduced family centered communication programme: multicenter before and after intervention study. BMJ 2018;363:k4764.
7. Simon TD, Starmer AJ, Conway PH, et al. Quality improvement research in pediatric hospital medicine and the role of the Pediatric Research in Inpatient Settings (PRIS) network. Acad Pediatr 2013;13(6 Suppl):S54–60.
8. Starmer AJ, O'Toole JK, Rosenbluth G, et al. Development, implementation, and dissemination of the I-PASS handoff curriculum: a multisite educational intervention to improve patient handoffs. Acad Med 2014;89:876–84.
9. Starmer AJ, Spector ND, Srivastava R, et al. Changes in medical errors after implementation of a handoff program. N Engl J Med 2014;371(19):1803–12.
10. Khan A, Coffey M, Litterer KP, et al. Families as partners in hospital error and adverse event surveillance. JAMA Pediatr 2017;171(4):372–81.
11. Khan A, Furtak SL, Melvin P, et al. Parent-reported errors and adverse events in hospitalized children. JAMA Pediatr 2016;170(4):e154608.